A Jerry Baker Good Health Book

HEALING REMEDIES

Hiding in Your Kitchen

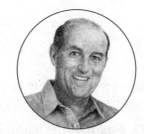

www.jerrybaker.com

Other Jerry Baker Books:

Jerry Baker's Cure Your Lethal Lifestyle!
Jerry Baker's Top 25 Homemade Healers
Healing Fixers Mixers & Elixirs
Grandma Putt's Home Health Remedies
Nature's Best Miracle Medicines
Jerry Baker's Supermarket Super Remedies
Jerry Baker's The New Healing Foods
Jerry Baker's Cut Your Health Care Bills in Half!
Jerry Baker's Amazing Antidotes
Jerry Baker's Anti-Pain Plan
Jerry Baker's Oddball Ointments, Powerful Potions, and Fabulous Folk Remedies
Jerry Baker's Giant Book of Kitchen Counter Cures

Grandma Putt's Green Thumb Magic
Jerry Baker's The New Impatient Gardener
Jerry Baker's Supermarket Super Gardens
Jerry Baker's Dear God...Please Help It Grow!
Secrets from the Jerry Baker Test Gardens
Jerry Baker's All-American Lawns
Jerry Baker's Bug Off!
Jerry Baker's Terrific Garden Tonics!
Jerry Baker's Backyard Problem Solver
Jerry Baker's Green Grass Magic
Jerry Baker's Great Green Book of Garden Secrets
Jerry Baker's Old-Time Gardening Wisdom

Jerry Baker's Backyard Birdscaping Bonanza
Jerry Baker's Backyard Bird Feeding Bonanza
Jerry Baker's Year-Round Bloomers
Jerry Baker's Flower Garden Problem Solver
Jerry Baker's Perfect Perennials!

Jerry Baker's Solve It with Vinegar!
America's Best Practical Problem Solvers
Jerry Baker's Can the Clutter!
Jerry Baker's Cleaning Magic!
Jerry Baker's Homespun Magic
Grandma Putt's Old-Time Vinegar, Garlic, Baking Soda, and 101 More Problem Solvers
Jerry Baker's Supermarket Super Products!
Jerry Baker's It Pays to Be Cheap!

To order any of the above, or for more information on Jerry Baker's
amazing home, health, and garden tips, tricks, and tonics, please write to:

Jerry Baker, P.O. Box 1001, Wixom, MI 48393

Or, visit Jerry Baker online at:

www.jerrybaker.com

A Jerry Baker Good Health Book

HEALING REMEDIES

Hiding in Your Kitchen

1,784 Cupboard Cures, Pantry Perks, Fridge Fixers, and Spice Rack Remedies for a Healthier, Prettier You!

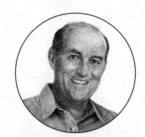

www.jerrybaker.com

Published by American Master Products, Inc.

Executive Editor: Kim Adam Gasior
Editor/Writer: Cheryl Winters-Tetreau
Copy Editor: Nanette Bendyna
Production Editor: Debby Duvall
Interior Design and Layout: Alison McKenna
Indexer: Nan Badgett

Publisher's Cataloging-in-Publication
(Provided by Quality Books, Inc.)

    Baker, Jerry, author.
      Healing remedies hiding in your kitchen : 1,784 cupboard cures, pantry perks, fridge fixers, and spice rack remedies for a healthier, prettier you! / Jerry Baker.
      pages cm
      Includes index.
      ISBN 978-0-922433-26-1

    1. Health. 2. Beauty, Personal.   I. Title.

RA776.B19245 2015   613
    QBI15-600207

Printed in the United States of America
2 4 6 8 10 9 7 5 3 1   hardcover

Contents

Contents

Introduction

It's a great time to be alive! And if you're anything like me—and I'm betting you are—you do everything within your power to stay fit and healthy as the years go by. Lucky for us, medicine has made enormous strides over the last decade. New drugs and treatments have been discovered to help us deal with diabetes, heart disease, bone degeneration, and much, much more. And scientists are exploring all aspects of our DNA and brains with the goal of discovering new ways to tackle inherited diseases, mental illness, and mood disorders. But let's face it, accidents and illnesses still put a hitch in our giddyup from time to time. And when that happens, most of us head straight to the drugstore to pick up the latest, greatest Big Pharma remedy—and empty our wallets to pay for it!

HEALTH

So what if I told you that just about everything you need to live a long, healthy life can be found right in your kitchen? Don't believe me? Well, how about these gems:

■ Sip **COFFEE** to help guard against dementia and Alzheimer's disease! Read all about this amazing remedy on page 3.

■ Stop indigestion in its tracks with the bracing **LEMON** tonic on page 81. It'll ease your discomfort lickety-split!

■ Boost your bone density and help ward off osteoporosis with a sprinkle of **CURRY** powder. See page 159 for a few tasty ideas.

In fact, from the fridge and freezer to the countertops and cupboards, your kitchen holds a wealth of healing ingredients that can help you fight a host of ills, from heart disease and high blood pressure to indigestion and insomnia—even cancer!

In this book, you'll find hearty helpings of *Healthy Hints* that offer some of your kitchen's most surprising healers, like the frozen **PARSLEY** anti-bruise cubes on page 176. They're the perfect pain-relieving help for folks who seem to bruise as easily as a ripe banana.

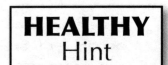

HEALTHY Hint

BEAUTY

As if that weren't enough, you'll be glad to learn that your kitchen also holds an array of products that are perfect for a bevy of homemade beauty concoctions. You don't have to spend your hard-earned money on fancy potions and lotions from the department store or the local beauty aisle—instead, do your hair, skin, and nails a big favor and whip up chemical-, dye-, and preservative-free versions, like these:

■ Get rid of dead skin cells with the super-simple dry-**MILK** scrub on page 240. Your skin will glow!

■ De-stress your tresses with the ultra-luxe **EGG** and **BANANA** hair mask on page 238.

■ Beat back brittle nails with the **VEGETABLE OIL** cure on page 314. You just might fix your dried out nails for good!

BEAUTY
Bonus

Throughout this book, you'll find plenty of *Beauty Bonuses*, like the one on page 230. Did you know that **RED WINE** can help you fight wrinkles?! No, not by drinking it, but by mixing it with egg whites and honey to make a rejuvenating facial mask. Beautiful!

And that's not all! Whether you're looking for feel-great potions or look-lovely lotions, there's something for everyone. In addition to the hundreds of tips, tricks, and tonics within these pages, we added fantastic features like:

Kitchen Counter Cures reveal dozens of recipes for fixing what ails you, as well as handy how-tos for creating your own beauty products. For example, the Gout-Be-Gone Preserves recipe on page 64 is an ultra-simple—and tasty—way to let **APPLES** relieve the pain and swelling gout sufferers are often prone to. Just grab a spoon and dig in!

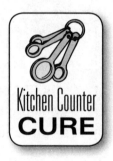

Kitchen Counter
CURE

An apple a day can keep the beautician away, too. Turn to page 247 for a nifty night cream that helps your aging skin retain its youthful elasticity so you can wake up beautiful every morning.

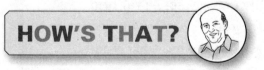

HOW'S THAT?

Find my answers to your most vexing health and beauty questions in *How's That?* boxes. One of my favorites is on page 155, which addresses the preposterous suggestion that **CINNAMON** can make you a better driver. (It's true, because the spicy scent soothes your jangled rush-hour nerves!) And if you think that's crazy, what about the dilemma you'll find on page 303? The answer is yes: Cold **MAYO** straight from the fridge really can take the sting out of sunburn!

Back in the Day... And last, but certainly not least, I share my Grandma Putt's tried-and-true home remedies in ***Back in the Day***. Try the old-time **GRAPE** juice tip on page 78 the next time you need to heal a stubborn cut. And women have been using the farm-fresh facial treatment on page 330 for decades to tone, nourish, and soften their skin. The key ingredient? Believe it or not, it's **ONION** juice!

SPOTLIGHT ON
DIY REMEDIES

Now I know that you know this, but it bears repeating: The homemade healers and beauty solutions in this book are not meant to replace any medical care and/or treatments you are currently using. Especially if you have diabetes, high blood pressure, cancer, or any other long-term condition, be sure to speak with your health-care provider before using any formulas in this book.

For the rest of you, please remember that any home remedy takes a little time to work. But if your symptoms don't improve—or they actually get worse—after one week, seek medical help. And if you have any adverse skin reactions to a beauty treatment, stop using the remedy immediately.

I hope this whets your appetite for all the surprises that await you in your kitchen. So let's head there now and get on the road to good health and good looks!

CHAPTER 1

Cures from Countertops & Cupboards

If you're like many Americans over the age of 50, you start each morning by lining up your pills on the kitchen counter, then gulping them down— one for blood pressure, one for cholesterol, one for gout; the list goes on and on. Well, it's not just those meds that can keep you healthy. Your counters and cupboards contain products that'll promote your well-being. First, talk with your doctor, then give my kitchen-fresh fixes a try.

ON COUNTERTOPS

Yes, Please Have a Banana

Have a **BANANA** today. In fact, have one every day! The potassium in the mellow yellow fruit helps prevent thickening of the artery walls and works with sodium to regulate your body's fluids. The result—a healthier heart!

Peel Away Pounds

Trying to lose weight? Then wake up and smell the **BANANAS**! Studies have shown that dieters who sniffed a banana whenever they felt like munching on food lost an average of 30 pounds in six months.

A Bunch of A-Peeling Healing Solutions

To look at a **BANANA** peel, you'd never take it to be a first-class first-aid worker. In fact, these super skins are world champs at solving a number of common mishaps—and that's no monkey business! In each use below, apply the banana peel inner side down, with the moist side on your skin:

- **Fire ant bites.** Place the peel on the bite, and leave it in place for 20 minutes. Then wash the area, and apply a new peel if needed.

- **Minor cuts and scrapes.** Simply put a piece of peel on the wound, and secure it in place with a bandage or strip of cloth. Change the peel every three to four hours until the pain is gone.

- **Plantar warts.** At bedtime, tape a piece of peel over the wart. Cover the peel with a bandage or a tight sock, and leave it on overnight. Repeat the procedure each night until the wart vanishes, which shouldn't take more than two or three treatments.

- **Poison ivy.** Lay peels all across the rash-covered area, keeping them in place with bandages or pieces of cloth. Before you know it, the rash will dry up, and the itch will be history!

Back in the Day...

Old-timers relied on this DIY first-aid kit in a jar to deal with bruises, sore joints, and insect stings. To mix up a batch, fill a jar with chopped **BANANA** peels, pour in enough rubbing alcohol to cover the peels, and put a lid on it. Stash the jar in your medicine cabinet (without straining out the solids), and let the mixture "brew" for two weeks before you use it. Then, whenever trouble strikes, dip a cotton ball or pad into the solution, and dab it on wherever you're sore, swollen, or stung.

Caffeination Nation

Here's proof that coffee is America's favorite beverage: Almost 83 percent of U.S. adults drink **COFFEE**. Of those, 63 percent drink it every day. That's a whole lotta java going down! While the trend of teens indulging in drinks with a dangerous amount of caffeine is not good news, adults who consume two to four 8-ounce cups per day have a few more reasons to smile. Take a look at what the brew can do for you:

- **Delay dementia.** Moderate coffee consumption (1 to 3 cups per day) may help reduce the risk of developing dementia and Alzheimer's disease. The antioxidants in coffee may also help prevent brain-cell damage.

- **Discourage diabetes.** Frequent coffee consumption (4 or more cups per day) has been linked to a lowered risk of developing type 2 diabetes. Again, it's coffee's antioxidants that may play a role in regulating blood sugar. And even decaf does the trick!

- **Diminish inflammation.** If you take aspirin for painful conditions like sciatica, you'll get quicker relief if you take those tablets with a cup and a half or so of coffee. Why? Because the caffeine in the java helps your body absorb the medication more efficiently. You'll feel the full effects in 30 minutes, and they'll last for up to five hours. *Note: Aspirin and caffeine can worsen reflux, gastritis, and ulcers.*

HEALTHY Hint

WHEN TO CURB THE CAFFEINE

Yes, it's true that studies consistently show drinking a lot of caffeinated or decaffeinated **COFFEE** is associated with a *low* risk of type 2 diabetes. But if you already have type 2 diabetes, are a daily coffee drinker, and are having trouble controlling your blood glucose, try switching to decaf. Start by blending regular coffee with decaf (several national brands offer "half-caff" blends). Gradually increase the amount of decaf until you've weaned yourself from the high-test type altogether.

Why not just go cold turkey and give up coffee completely? Because drinking decaf can help stabilize your body's glucose response—and you still get to enjoy that satisfying coffee taste and aroma.

On Countertops

Make Mine Decaf

Not all the news about **COFFEE** is grande. For some folks, the caffeine in their morning mug can do more harm than good:

- It can increase irritability and anxiety.

- You can get hooked on the caffeine fix and then suffer withdrawal symptoms, such as crushing headaches and intense fatigue, when you try to cut back.

- It can take up to six hours for caffeine to clear your system. So if you're having trouble sleeping, keep an eye on the clock when you're pouring that cup of joe.

- Coffee made with a French press, or by any other method that doesn't use a filter, contains higher levels of a compound called cafestol that can increase your LDL ("bad") cholesterol levels. So stick with the tried-and-true drip method, and always use a paper filter.

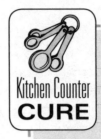

Kitchen Counter CURE

Stop the Stink

Here's a good way to eliminate body odor and cut way back on the cash you spend on deodorant: Kick the **COFFEE**! Drinking coffee increases the activity of your sweat glands, so if you're at all concerned about being a bit, you know, fragrant, consider drastically decreasing the amount of joe you drink, and the foul funk should fade fast.

If the stink is *on* you instead of *in* you, say from chopping onions, scaling fish, or mincing garlic, grab a few coffee beans and roll them between your hands. No beans? No problem. Just grab a handful of leftover grinds and rub them into your skin, then wash your hands to remove the much less offensive coffee aroma.

Get Up and Go!

That morning cup (or two) of **COFFEE** isn't just good for providing a caffeine jolt—it's also an easy way to conquer constipation. If you need to get things moving again, brew your coffee as strong as you can handle, and don't load it up with sugar and cream. A splash of skim milk will suffice if you just can't drink it black. Then sip while it's still nice and hot, and your next stop will be the bathroom. Now that's one fine cup of coffee!

Pungent and Potent

It's not a coincidence that folks in **GARLIC**-loving territory (like the Mediterranean region) tend to live longer and have fewer chronic health problems than those of us who don't regularly partake of the pungent bulb. Studies show that incorporating garlic into your diet can be a magic bullet for health and longevity. In fact, eating as few as one or two cloves a day can help boost your immune system, control blood sugar, and reduce your risk of developing heart disease, cancer, and more.

Banish High Blood Pressure

Here's a folk remedy that can't be beat for reducing blood pressure: Soak 1/2 pound of peeled **GARLIC** cloves in 1 quart of brandy for two weeks, shaking the mixture a few times a day. Then strain it, pour it into bottles with tight-fitting stoppers, and take up to 20 drops daily in a glass of water.

Battle Bad Cholesterol

Scientific studies have shown that eating just one fresh **GARLIC** clove a day can reduce your LDL ("bad") cholesterol levels by 17 percent, thereby lessening your heart attack risk by 25 percent. Not bad for a stinkin' bulb!

HOW'S THAT?

Q *Jerry, my father told me that when he was a kid, folks got rid of toothache pain with* **GARLIC**. *Have you ever heard of this crazy "cure"?*

A Yes, I have. And while this is far from the tastiest way to ease the pain of a toothache, it is one of the quickest. If you want to give it a try, just peel a garlic clove, crush it, and apply it directly to the gum above or below the affected tooth. Then hold it in place until the ache subsides. The relief should last long enough for you to get to a dentist's office—where, no doubt, the receptionist will promptly hand you a free sample of mouthwash and ask you to use it—NOW!

Reliable Asthma Relief

To help ward off your asthma symptoms, try taking a daily dose of this **GARLIC** syrup. Here's your five-step game plan:

Step 1. Separate and peel the cloves of three garlic bulbs.

Step 2. Put them in a non-aluminum pan with 2 cups of water. Simmer until the garlic cloves are soft and there is about 1 cup of water left in the pan.

Step 3. Using a slotted spoon, transfer the garlic to a jar with a tight-fitting lid.

Step 4. Add 1 cup of apple cider vinegar* and ¼ cup of organic raw honey to the water in the pan, and boil the mixture until it's syrupy.

Step 5. Pour the syrup over the garlic in the jar, put the lid on, and let it sit overnight, or for at least eight hours.

Every morning, on an empty stomach, swallow one or two of the garlic cloves along with 1 teaspoon of the syrup. * *For medicinal purposes, always use unfiltered apple cider vinegar (available in health-food stores and in the health-food sections of most supermarkets) rather than the clear, filtered kind that's on the shelves in the main grocery aisle.*

Back in the Day...

When you feel as though you've got a four-alarm fire blazing in your throat, reach for this equally fiery mixture to help extinguish the flames. Crush one **GARLIC** clove, and put it into a glass along with 1 teaspoon of salt and a tiny pinch of cayenne pepper. Fill the glass with warm water and stir. Gargle with the solution, and repeat as needed. (But if your throat doesn't feel better in a day or so, call your firefighter—er, doctor.) *Note: This same garlic-infused potion will also speed the healing of a chest cold or bronchitis. Just massage the fiery solution onto your chest several times a day.*

Aromatic Head Cold Clobberers

When your sinuses are throbbing and you just can't clear your head, reach for one of these time-tested **GARLIC** remedies:

■ Several times a day, crush a garlic clove, put your nose up close to it, and inhale deeply. You might not like what you're smelling—but neither will the cold germs!

■ Keep a whole peeled garlic clove in your mouth, tucked between your teeth and cheek. Don't chew the clove, but gently bite into it every once in a while to release a little garlic juice. Replace the clove with a fresh one every three to four hours.

■ Crush six peeled garlic cloves, and mix them into $1/2$ cup of vegetable shortening. Spread the mixture on the soles of your feet, and cover them with a warm towel or flannel cloth. Then put plastic wrap under your feet to protect your bedding or, if you're sitting up, your carpet or footstool. Repeat the procedure every five hours until your cold is gone. *Note: I know you're wondering, and the answer is "Yes!" You'll still have dragon breath even though you apply the garlic to your feet, so chew some gum during this treatment if you want minty fresh breath!*

HEALTHY
Hint

WHEN TO STEER CLEAR

Even a healthy, potent bulb like **GARLIC** can be quite harmful under certain circumstances. Whether you cook with it, eat it fresh, or take garlic tablets, capsules, or extracts, keep these powerful pointers in mind:

Don't mix with meds. If you're taking any kind of medication, in either prescription or over-the-counter form, be sure to consult your doctor before you dose yourself with a garlic remedy.

Just say "no." Avoid garlic entirely if you have a bleeding ulcer or any bleeding disorder.

Put the brakes on. If you start to experience indigestion or stomach irritation, ease off on your intake until you find your comfort level.

On Countertops

Health

Toss Off Tinnitus

Tinnitus is almost never a serious health condition, but it is one of the most annoying afflictions under the sun. But never fear—here's a bell-blocking cure. Put six large peeled **GARLIC** cloves in a blender with 1 cup of cold-pressed extra virgin olive oil, and blend until the garlic is finely minced. Pour the mixture into a sterile glass jar, put the lid on, and refrigerate it for seven days. Strain out the solids, and pour the liquid into several sterilized eyedropper bottles.

Then each night at bedtime, pour a small amount of the aromatic oil into a bowl, wait a few minutes for the chill to wear off, and put 3 drops into each ear. Plug the openings with cotton balls, leave them in overnight, and remove them in the morning. Within two weeks, your bells should stop ringing. *Note: To sterilize the jar, lid, and eyedropper bottles, simply place them in a large pot of boiling water for a few minutes, and let them air-dry before you add the oil. Also, always keep the prepared garlic oil in the refrigerator, where it will last up to a month.*

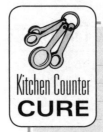

Kitchen Counter CURE

Lovely Liniment

If you suffer from rheumatism—or you just want to be prepared for treating muscle aches and sprains—this healing potion belongs in your medicine chest. Put 1 cup of high-quality extra virgin olive oil into a glass jar with a tight-fitting lid. Peel and crush four **GARLIC** cloves, and add them to the oil. Cover the jar, and leave it in a warm place for a full week. Strain the oil into a clean bottle with a lid, and store it in a cool, dark spot. Then once or twice a day, massage a teaspoon or two of the oil onto your achy breaky body parts.

Undo Ulcers

Although **GARLIC** is a big no-no for anyone with a bleeding ulcer, it is a highly effective way to help relieve mild ulcers and prevent new ones from forming. That's because garlic's antibacterial properties fight the *H. pylori* bacterium that causes these annoying (and painful) stomach sores. The recommended dose is two small crushed cloves a day, in whatever form you care to take them.

SPOTLIGHT ON
ACHES & PAINS

Are you suffering from sciatica or arthritis? Have you been a bit too ambitious out in the garden or indoors at the gym? No matter what the cause of your aching muscles and joints, relief is at hand—from your kitchen cupboards and drawers!

◆ Ease the pain of sciatica with **GARLIC** milk. Mince two cloves of peeled garlic, put them in about 1/2 cup of milk, and drink it down without chewing the garlic (to avoid having the odor on your breath). Take a dose each morning and evening, and within a week, you should feel much better.

◆ Give gout the heave-ho: Twice a day, drink a glass of 100 percent cherry juice with two cloves of minced **GARLIC** in it. Be sure not to chew the garlic, so it won't wind up on your breath.

◆ Subdue shin splints and other muscle injuries by applying **CASTOR OIL** to the affected area. Cover it with plastic wrap, and top it off with a heating pad set on low. The heat will help the oil penetrate your skin and act directly on your muscles to ease the pain and stiffness. Leave the pad on for 20 to 30 minutes, then wash the oil off with soap and water. Repeat the treatment several times a day as needed.

◆ When you've been working or playing too hard in the hot sun, give your aching muscles a nice cool treat. Mix 2 cups of **WITCH HAZEL**, 2 teaspoons of light corn syrup, 1/2 teaspoon of castor oil, and 3 or 4 drops of essential oil (eucalyptus, peppermint, rosemary, and wintergreen are good choices) in a jar with a tight-fitting lid. Shake well, and massage the potion into your sore body parts for almost-instant relief.

◆ Before you start a chore that you have to do on your knees—like weeding the garden or painting the porch—put on your work pants, and fasten a soft rectangular sponge to each knee with **DUCT TAPE**. It'll help cushion your joints, and the whole shebang is easy to pull off when you're done!

On Countertops

A Tea-sy Way to Ease—*Urp!*—Indigestion

Don't let indigestion spoil your evening. Instead, brew up a batch of **ANGELICA TEA** to alleviate your after-dinner distress. Here's the R_X: Put 1 teaspoon of the dried herb (or 3 teaspoons of crushed fresh leaves) in 1 cup of boiling water. Let it steep for about 10 minutes, strain out the herb, and enjoy a cup after every meal. By the way, sipping angelica tea also works wonders for relieving monthly woes and easing cold and flu symptoms. *Note: Angelica is available in health-food stores and herbal-supply stores.*

Halt Hot Flashes

Ladies, if you've entered that phase of life in which hot flashes, mood swings, and flat-out crankiness are intruding, make the transition into menopause a bit smoother with **ANGELICA**. Women in China have been sipping angelica tea since long before hormone replacement therapy (HRT) came on the scene. If you'd like to give it a try, use the brewing instructions above (see "A Tea-sy Way to Ease—*Urp!*—Indigestion"), and sip the hot tea three times a day.

Angelica Conquers Constipation

When your internal "plumbing" goes haywire, don't reach for an over-the-counter laxative. Instead, hightail it down to your local health-food or herbal-supply store and pick up a bottle of **ANGELICA** tincture (or order it for overnight delivery from a reputable herbal website). Drink 20 to 30 drops mixed in 1 cup of water three times a day until things are moving along normally again.

HEALTHY Hint

ACQUIRE ANGEL BREATH

Looking for an easy way to sweeten up your breath without using a commercial mouthwash filled with alcohol and chemicals? Look no further! Just put 3 tablespoons of **ANGELICA** seeds in a teapot or other heat-proof container, and pour 2 cups of boiling water on top. Cover, and steep until the brew cools to room temperature. Strain it into a glass bottle with a tight-fitting lid, and use the solution as you would any other mouthwash.

Black Tea Staves Off Strokes

A number of studies have found that drinking **BLACK TEA** regularly can reduce the risk of heart disease and stroke. Scientists believe it works because the tea's antioxidants maintain the health of your circulatory system and reduce the risk of clogging up your arteries and/or developing blood clots. And here's more good news—even if you prefer decaffeinated tea, you'll still get the same healthy benefits.

Boost Your Bones

Ladies, drinking even a single cup of **BLACK TEA** per day may preserve your bone density—especially if you sip it every day for 10 years! The natural phytoestrogens in tea may help your bones remain thicker by boosting calcium absorption even as your natural estrogen decreases during menopause. So raise a cup to your skeletal health—cheers!

Wake Up to Tea

If you have chronic sinusitis, you wake up most mornings stuffed up and hacking as your sinuses try to drain. Get rid of the gunk by drinking hot **BLACK TEA** first thing. It will warm your body and activate the cilia, the tiny nasal hairs that whisk irritants and bacteria from your nose.

HOW'S THAT?

Q *I know the classic remedy for a black eye is to slap a steak over it, but we're vegetarians! Is there anything else besides beef that'll get the job done?*

A Where's the beef? Nobody should waste a steak on a bruise: Simply soothe your shiner with tea. After brewing a cup of **BLACK TEA**, let the tea bag cool for a few minutes, then squeeze out the excess moisture. Lie back, close your eyes, and hold the damp tea bag against the puffy peeper for 10 minutes or so.

SPOTLIGHT ON
HEART DISEASE

You've heard this before: To keep your heart healthy, you should eat right, get daily exercise, and keep your weight under control. Yes, it takes work, but there are also some less strenuous ways to tend to your ticker. Start with these heart-friendly choices:

◆ Drink **COFFEE**. Enjoying one to three cups of java per day may keep your blood vessels clear, which lowers blood pressure. Plus, coffee drinkers have fewer strokes than non-drinkers. But don't go overboard—more than five cups a day may increase your risk of developing heart disease.

◆ Tipple some **BLACK TEA**. One study found that people who drank one or more cups of black tea daily were half as likely to have a heart attack as those folks who were not tea drinkers. Scientists speculate that tea's powerful antioxidant package may help keep cholesterol in your blood from mucking up your arteries.

◆ Sip **CHAMOMILE TEA**. Almost everyone experiences heart palpitations (a.k.a. arrhythmia) at one time or another. If you've received a clean bill of health from your doctor and still your heart starts thumping, or seems to skip a beat or two, make 2 cups of strong chamomile tea, and while it's brewing, shred three or four cabbage leaves and steam them. Combine the tea and the leaves in a bowl, and sip the soup. It won't be the tastiest dish you've ever had, but it should tune up your ticker in a hurry. *Note: If your palpitations persist, or if they're accompanied by chest pain, dizziness, or fainting spells, seek immediate medical help!*

◆ Have a handful of **NUTS**. All nuts are packed with unsaturated fat that helps keep your heart in good working order. Studies show that people who snacked on nuts (especially almonds, walnuts, and pecans) five or more times a week cut their heart attack risk in half compared with folks who said "No thanks."

3 Cheers for Catnip!

Catnip isn't just a kitty's delight, and though it turns your lazy feline into a rowdy cat, it has the opposite effect on us folks. **CATNIP TEA** saves the day in so many ways, and it's a snap to make: Place 1 teaspoon of dried catnip leaves or 1 tablespoon of fresh catnip in a mug. Pour 6 ounces of boiling water over the leaves, and let it steep for 10 minutes. Strain out the solids, and enjoy. To enhance the flavor, you can add a lemon slice and/or a spoonful of honey.

Then, the next time you find yourself tossing and turning, get up and brew some catnip tea. Its mild sedative properties will have you in dreamland in no time, and you won't feel groggy when the alarm goes off in the morning. *Note: Catnip is available in health-food stores and herbal-supply stores.*

HEALTHY Hint

CATNIP CAVEAT

CATNIP should not ever be used in any form by women who are pregnant or nursing, or by women who have heavy menstrual bleeding. In addition, do not take catnip if you are on lithium or any sedative medications.

Some people experience headaches, vomiting, and a general feeling of illness when taking catnip. If you develop any of these side effects, stop using catnip immediately and see your health-care professional.

On Countertops

Nip Coughs in the Bud

When your hacking just won't quit, brew a cup of **CATNIP TEA**. Steep 2 teaspoons of dried catnip leaves in 1 cup of boiling water for 15 minutes. Strain out the leaves, then add honey to taste. You can drink up to 3 cups a day until your cough subsides.

Catty Cure for Cuts

For years, people have used **CATNIP TEA** as an external antiseptic. Simply brew the version in "Nip Coughs in the Bud" (above), and let the tea cool to room temperature. Then pour some on a cotton ball to clean out your cut and speed up the healing process.

One Weird Weight-Loss Trick

If you need to drop a few pounds (and who doesn't?), this recipe is just the ticket. It's a concoction of herbs that tone the digestive system and can help stop mindless munching between meals and prevent overeating. Sip this warm tea before breakfast, lunch, and dinner: Mix equal parts of centaury, **CHAMOMILE**, dandelion root, and fennel. Steep 2 teaspoons in 1 cup of hot water for 20 minutes, then strain. Drink 1/4 to 1/3 cup and pour the remaining brewed tea down the drain. Store the leftover dry blend in an airtight container away from sunlight, and use within a week. *Note: If you take diuretics or potassium supplements, don't use dandelion; if you have ragweed allergies, steer clear of chamomile.*

Take a Break from Back Pain

Back pain is so crippling that it can interfere with your happy life and make you just plain miserable. So don't wait—relieve the agony with this terrific tea. Mix 1 part dried **CHAMOMILE** flowers (available in health-food stores and herbal-supply stores) with 1 part dried peppermint leaves, 1 part grated fresh ginger, and 1 cup of water. Add 1 teaspoon of the mixture to 1 cup of just-boiled water. Cover, and steep for 10 minutes. Store any remaining herbal blend in a container with a tight-fitting lid. Drink 1 cup of the tea three or four times a day to ease your pain and put a smile on your face!

Back in the Day...

Long before the medical community started diagnosing seasonal affective disorder (SAD), folks often felt gloomy and tired during the long winter months. And along with the blues and blahs came intense cravings for carbohydrates. One effective old-time antidote: Whenever a carb craving strikes, drink a cup of **CHAMOMILE** tea. It'll divert your attention from food and give you a much-needed energy boost at the same time.

Tame Tummy Troubles

Here's just what the doctor ordered for curing a cranky gut and other intestinal woes—**CHAMOMILE** tea. The dose is 3 or 4 cups a day until you feel chipper again. This versatile beverage can also:

- **Alleviate menstrual cramps.** At the first twinge of monthly discomfort, start sipping cups of chamomile tea. Continue throughout the day until your cramps are gone.

- **Relieve indigestion.** Drink 1 cup of chamomile tea after each meal until you're feeling better. Or if you have a chronically sensitive digestive system—and no serious underlying medical condition—make a post-meal cup part of your regular routine.

Fabulous Flu Bath

In addition to clearing stuffed-up nasal passages and soothing aches and pains, a nice long soak in an herbal bath will help you get a good night's sleep. And that's exactly what you need when your body is racked with the flu or fighting any kind of virus!

Start with a clean jar that has a tight-fitting lid. Put 1 teaspoon each of dried **CHAMOMILE**, dried lavender, dried rosemary, ground cinnamon, and ground ginger in the jar and shake it to thoroughly blend. To use: Add 1 teaspoon to a panty hose toe or a coffee filter, and close it tightly with a twist tie. Toss the pouch into a tub of hot water, and let it steep for 10 minutes. Then sink into the fragrant brew, and chase away the flu!

HEALTHY Hint

CHAMOMILE CAUTION

CHAMOMILE is one of the most effective, healthful herbs you can use, but there are a couple of things you need to be aware of. First, chamomile contains coumarin, which reacts with blood-thinning drugs. So if you are taking any of those meds, consult with your doctor before you consume it in any oral form. Second, because chamomile is a member of the ragweed family, you should use this herb with caution if you suffer from pollen allergies. It won't cause you any long-term harm, but it may trigger some sneezing or wheezing, or even contact dermatitis if you use it topically.

Towel Off a Sore Throat

It seems that everybody and his uncle has a favorite sore-throat cure. Well, my Grandma Putt taught me one of the best: Make a quart of a strong **CHAMOMILE** infusion (just quadruple the recipe for "Tea Times Two," below), and strain it into another pan. Let the brew cool just enough so that you can handle it, then soak a clean towel in the solution. Wring it out, and wrap it snugly around your neck. As soon as the towel cools off, warm up the tea, remoisten the towel, and reapply it to your throat. The chamomile will help draw out the pain, and the heat will ease the tension that's built up in your throat muscles. Repeat the procedure as needed until you feel better. (It shouldn't take more than one or two additional dips.)

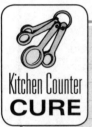

Kitchen Counter CURE

Tea Times Two

An herbal infusion is simply an extra-strong tea that's ideal for topical use—although you can also drink it, as long as the herbs are edible and you like your tea strong. This **CHAMOMILE** recipe makes 1 cup of brew, but you can double, triple, or even quadruple the recipe if you need more for a particular use (like soaking your feet), or if you simply want to keep a supply on hand.

2 heaping tbsp. of dried chamomile
8 oz. of just-boiled fresh spring water

Put the chamomile in a ceramic or glass mug, jar, or pitcher, and pour the water over it. Cover, and let the mixture steep for 10 to 15 minutes. Strain, and pour it into a clean container. Cool the brew before you use it on your skin, but drink it at whatever temperature suits your fancy. Either use the infusion right away, or store it in the refrigerator, tightly covered, where it will keep for about five days. Let the tea come to room temperature before you use it, or feel free to heat it up if you want to drink it or use it as a soak.

Soothe Sore Eyes

Do seasonal allergies make your eyes irritated, weepy, and swollen? Reach for the herb with potent anti-inflammatory powers that make it a perfect choice for reducing redness, puffiness, and irritation. It's **CHAMOMILE**, and it couldn't be easier to use. Simply steep two chamomile tea bags in 1 cup of just-boiled water for three minutes. Remove them from the water, and tuck them into the fridge to cool for about five minutes. Then lie down, and put a bag over each eye. Relax for 15 minutes or so, and jeepers creepers—your peepers should be back to normal.

Choose Your Poison

Rather, when your poison has chosen you—and it came from poison ivy, poison oak, or poison sumac—**CHAMOMILE** can clear up the itchy, burning rash. Just steep 2 tablespoons of dried chamomile in 2 cups of boiling water for about 10 minutes. Let the tea cool to a comfortable temperature, then soak a clean washcloth in it. Lay the cloth gently on your afflicted skin, and leave it on for 15 minutes or so. Repeat as often as needed until your rash has healed.

HOW'S THAT?

Q *A friend told me that* **CHAMOMILE** *can help with my rosacea flare-ups. Is this advice true?*

A As you know, there is no cure for this chronic acne-like condition. But with regular treatment from a dermatologist and your Johnny-on-the-spot response to facial flushing—the trigger mechanism for a full-fledged attack—your rosacea flare-ups can be controlled. To make a fast-acting weapon, toss a handful of dried chamomile into 3 cups of boiling water, remove it from the heat, and steep for 10 minutes. Strain the brew into a container with a tight-fitting lid, and stash it in the fridge. Then whenever the need arises, dip a soft cotton cloth in the cold solution, and apply it to the affected area until you feel relief.

Cures from Countertops & Cupboards

SPOTLIGHT ON
COLDS & FLU

You cough, you sneeze, your head is pounding, and you ache all over. When a bad cold or the flu comes a-calling, it's no fun to be down for the count. Try some of these homemade kitchen healers to ease your woes and get you back on your feet fast.

◆ When congestion is backing up into your ears, try this potent treatment. Spread ½ teaspoon of prepared horseradish or mustard on three or four slices of **GARLIC** and eat them. Wash the concoction down with a cup of hot peppermint tea. You should feel a flow of relief almost immediately.

◆ Once a head cold sets in, your poor noggin really takes a beating. As soon as that familiar throbbing starts, mix ½ teaspoon of **ANGELICA** tincture in ¾ cup of hot water, and drink it down. Not only will it ease the pain in your noggin, but it will also lift your spirits—and just maybe boost your flagging energy!

◆ One super sore-throat soother you should reach for is **GREEN TEA**. It's among the best sore-throat remedies because it's loaded with bioflavonoids. And don't forget to stir in a drizzle of honey to coat your throat and help numb the pain.

◆ When you've got a cough that's keeping you awake at night, sip this simple sleeping aid. Heat 1 cup of **RED WINE** (don't let it boil!), and stir in lemon juice, cinnamon, and sugar to taste. Drink it slowly while it's hot, and you'll not only quiet your cough, but also sleep like a baby—guaranteed!

◆ Once you're on the road to recovery, you'll want **EUCALYPTUS OIL** in your arsenal. It calms you down, lifts your mood, and boosts your energy. Simply mix 15 to 20 drops of the oil per ounce of distilled water in a spray bottle, and spritz yourself every day until the recuperation period is over.

A Cuppa to Curb Cancer

Scientists who study health risks have found that in countries where people drink lots of **GREEN TEA**, folks rarely get certain cancers. In the lab, mice given green tea were protected against cancers of the skin, lungs, esophagus, stomach, colon, bladder, liver, mammary glands, and more. While full-scale human studies have yet to take place, it sure can't hurt to drink more green tea and keep your cells in tip-top shape. *Note: If you have clotting disorders or take heart medications, check with your health-care professional before drinking green tea.*

Tea Targets Cancer Meds

Polyphenols are special cancer-battling compounds, and **GREEN-TEA** leaves are loaded with them. These compounds help cancer drugs attack bad cells and spare healthy ones. In addition, green tea protects the liver, so it's able to function optimally as your body's detox center. Try to drink 3 to 5 cups daily.

Aid for Arthritis Pain

HEALTHY
Hint

LESSEN CATARACT CONCERNS

No nutrient can cure cataracts, but studies show that quercetin, a powerful antioxidant, may help delay their formation or slow their development. And dried **GREEN-TEA** leaves (as well as black-tea leaves) contain more quercetin than any other food. There's just one catch: *Brewed* tea contains almost no quercetin. But you can still enjoy its benefits in two ways:

Sip the leaves. Brew your tea using loose leaves, and don't strain it before sipping. Just drink it down, leaves and all.

Stir the leaves. Add a teaspoon or two of tea leaves to a delicious smoothie recipe, or stir them into your favorite flavor of yogurt.

You can fend off the agonizing pain of arthritis by drinking plenty of **GREEN TEA**. Medical studies show that it contains the strongest known form of antioxidants and that consuming 4 to 6 cups a day seems to reduce the incidence of rheumatoid arthritis.

Put a Headache on Ice

Take a throb-stopping tip from the German Tea Association and freeze brewed **GREEN TEA** in ice cube trays. Then whenever a headache hits, wrap one of the cubes in a paper towel, and press it alternately against your neck, temples, and forehead. Hold it in place for at least 15 seconds in each spot, and your ache should ease off. *Note: This same remedy can also relieve stress, whether it's accompanied by a headache or not.*

Give Dental Health the Green Light

Stop tooth decay dead in its tracks by tippling tea. **GREEN TEA** contains tannins that kill decay-causing bacteria and stops them from producing a sticky substance that helps acid-generating bacteria adhere to your teeth. Drink a cup, hot or cold, after every meal to keep your choppers chomping.

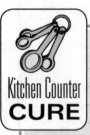

Kitchen Counter CURE

Green-Tea Toothpaste

Besides preventing plaque-forming microbes from attaching to the teeth (see "Give Dental Health the Green Light," above), **GREEN TEA** is an excellent toothpaste base. So make your mouth even fresher and cleaner than it is by brushing with this potent paste.

> 3–3 1/4 oz. of loose green tea
> 1 cup of boiling water
> 1 tsp. of baking soda
> Peppermint extract (optional)

Put the tea in a small heat-proof bowl, pour the water over it, and steep for at least 30 minutes. Drain out the solids, and stir the baking soda into the liquid tea to make a paste. Add the extract if you want a minty flavor. Then twice a day, dip your toothbrush into the paste, and brusha, brusha, brusha the germs away!

Mint May Mitigate Cancer

Mint contains limonene, a powerful anti-cancer agent that may help block the development of breast tumors and possibly even shrink them. Limonene hinders cancer cells from using a protein they need to survive. In addition, **PEPPERMINT** packs another breast cancer fighter, luteolin, which may inhibit the production of inflammatory compounds linked with the development of cancer. Scientists are still testing these compounds, but you can put the power of mint to work today by sipping peppermint tea and mixing fresh mint leaves into salads, smoothies, and sauces.

Mighty Mint Back-Pain Tamer

When your back is out of whack, reach for this minty tea toddy. Pour 1 cup of boiling water over 1 teaspoon of **PEPPERMINT** leaves, cover, and steep for 10 minutes. Drink 1 cup three or four times a day to relieve your pain.

Curb Cramps and Queasiness

The next time you're feeling queasy or have stomach cramps, sip **PEPPERMINT** tea. Use leaves or prepackaged tea bags to make a strong cuppa. Take it straight, because sugar can dampen your immune system and increase your risk of infection. Peppermint contains menthol, which helps ease spasms in your digestive tract.

Back in the Day...

Grandma Putt knew a thing or two about mint. In fact, she grew a variety of mints in her herb garden and regularly brewed refreshing teas from them. Her favorite was **PEPPERMINT**, because she knew that simply sniffing the mint leaves, whether fresh or dried, can:

Increase your energy level. The aroma of peppermint boosts alertness and get-up-and-go power by working directly on your sensory nerves.

Help you lose weight. In one study, 3,193 volunteers who regularly sniffed the scent of peppermint lost an average of 30 pounds in six months.

HEALTHY Hint

TEATIME WITH HERBS

Hundreds of herbs can be brewed into healthful, regenerative teas. Here's a handful to get you started. (For more about herbs and their uses, see Chapter 4: Spice Rack Relievers, on page 152, and Chapter 5: Healing Plants, on page 172.) The following ingredients are available in most health-food stores and herbal-supply stores.

Keep digestion on track. Mix 1 teaspoon of **SLIPPERY ELM** powder in a glass of warm water or juice, and drink it one to three times a day to thwart constipation and soothe intestinal tissues.

Take the edge off arthritis and bursitis pain. Grate about an inch of fresh **GINGER** and steep it in hot water for 10 minutes, then strain. Drink it once or twice a day, hot or cold, to get the full effects of ginger's anti-inflammatory power.

Put the kibosh on back pain. Make a **WILLOW BARK** tea by steeping 2 teaspoons of willow bark in 1 cup of boiling water for 10 minutes, then strain and sip. It's a natural source of aspirin-like salicylates, which ease pain. But unlike aspirin or ibuprofen, willow bark won't irritate your stomach while it's working on your back. *Note: Don't use willow bark if you take aspirin.*

Heal wounds. **PLANTAIN**, an antibacterial plant containing allantoin, is often referred to as "nature's Bactine®" because it's good for healing all kinds of wounds. Brew a beverage (made from packaged plantain tea), let it cool, and apply it to your injured skin.

Put pinkeye to pasture. Combine equal parts of **CALENDULA**, **CLEAVERS**, **ECHINACEA**, and **EYEBRIGHT**. Steep 1 teaspoon of the mixture in 1 cup of hot water for 10 minutes. Strain, and drink 2 to 3 cups daily until your pinkeye is history.

Chase the blues away. Make a tea with one or a combination of these herbs: **BORAGE, LAVENDER, PASSIONFLOWER, ROSEMARY, SKULLCAP, VERVAIN**. Steep 1 teaspoon of herbs in 1 cup of boiling water for 10 minutes, then strain. Drink 2 to 3 cups per day.

Halt a Heart Attack

Most folks have heard that if they ever suspect they're having a heart attack, they should call 911 and then pop an **ASPIRIN**. But not everyone knows just *how* to take that pill. According to *The American Journal of Cardiology*, you should chew the pill, not swallow it whole. Chewing releases aspirin's active ingredients and has a more immediate anti-clotting effect. It may not taste great, but it just might save your life!

A Bedtime Boon for Blood Pressure

In a recent study, participants who took **ASPIRIN** each night for three months registered a 5.4-point drop in their systolic blood pressure. But those folks who took the same dosage every morning saw no change at all. Don't start dosing yourself, but if your doctor has already prescribed aspirin to lower your blood pressure, ask whether you would be better served by taking it at night.

A Potent Paste for Pain

The agonizing pain of shingles can have you all but climbing the walls. Fortunately, this healing mix can help you stay grounded. Simply crush two **ASPIRIN** tablets into a powder and combine with 2 tablespoons of rubbing alcohol to make a paste. Apply the mixture to the affected areas three times daily and you'll soon heave a sigh of relief. *Note: Do not apply to any broken skin.*

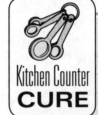

Kitchen Counter
CURE

Pump Up the Pain Relief

When your head is pounding to beat the band, try pairing **ASPIRIN** with caffeine. The combination of two aspirins with two cups of coffee can relieve a headache 40 percent better than the pain reliever does on its own. In addition to revving up your motor in the morning, caffeine helps your body absorb medications. The full effects kick in about 30 minutes after you finish your second cup, and can last from three to five hours.

A Sensational Sciatica Solution

Your sciatic nerve is your body's biggest nerve, and it can also produce one of its biggest pains. But—as unlikely as it may seem when that "fire" is shooting down your leg—you *can* relieve the discomfort. Just mix equal parts of **CASTOR OIL**, arnica oil, and St. John's wort oil, and gently massage the mixture onto the nerve track. Begin at your buttocks, and go down the back of your leg. If you have a disk problem, massage the oil into that area, too. Repeat as needed for soothing relief. *Note: You can buy arnica oil and St. John's wort oil in health-food stores and herbal-supply stores, as well as from numerous websites.*

Calm Carpal Tunnel Syndrome

Has too much time spent tapping away at your computer keyboard or doing other repetitive tasks left you with the pain and discomfort of carpal tunnel syndrome? If so, here's good news: A **CASTOR OIL** compress can deliver relief directly to the site of your pain, and it's an easy fix. Start by soaking a soft cloth in the oil, and heat it in the microwave until it's warm, but not hot. Wrap the oil-soaked cloth around your wrist, cover it with plastic wrap, and leave it in place for several hours—then alter your routines as much as you possibly can!

HEALTHY Hint

CASTOR OIL CAUTION

If you will be swallowing **CASTOR OIL** or using it in or around your eyes, ears, or mouth, make sure you use only 100 percent pure castor oil. If you're using it as a muscle rub or anywhere on your skin, look for cold-pressed or cold-processed oil (which is also safe to ingest), available in health-food stores and online. Avoid "refined" castor oil— more than 95 percent of the compounds that give the oil its healing power are removed during the refining process. And whatever you do, steer clear of the industrial-grade castor oil found in hardware and home-improvement stores. It is unsafe for both oral and topical use.

Get Some Shut-Eye

Have trouble falling asleep at night? Just rub a little **CASTOR OIL** over your eyelids at bedtime. It'll help you relax deeply so that you can get a restful night's slumber without using any drugs.

Conquer Canker Sores

Medical gurus tell us that canker sores are probably brought on by stress. Well, there's no "probably" about one thing: You can get rid of the annoying eruptions by dabbing them with **CASTOR OIL** frequently throughout the day until they're gone.

Silence the Ringing

Church bells and sleigh bells are one thing. But bells that ring…and ring …and ring in your ears are something else again—namely, tinnitus, and it can be the very dickens to get rid of. One remedy that has proven effective for many folks is **CASTOR OIL**. Just before bedtime each day, put 3 or 4 drops of the oil into each ear. Plug the openings with cotton, and keep it in place overnight. After a month or so, the ringing should have lessened considerably.

HOW'S THAT?

Q *Every once in a while, I get an earache that's not quite bad enough to send me to my doctor, but still bugs the heck out of me. Do you have a good homemade healer?*

A When a mild ear infection strikes, reach for this gentle, but powerful, remedy. Heat (but don't boil!) 1 tablespoon of **CASTOR OIL** and 1 tablespoon of milk in a non-aluminum pan. Let the mixture cool to a comfortable temperature. Put 4 drops into your inflamed ear every hour, and plug the opening with cotton. *Note: If your ear pain is severe and persistent, get medical attention pronto.*

A Royal Flush

CASTOR OIL was once considered the King of Laxatives—because for decades folks took it regularly to keep things moving right along. The problem is that your internal plumbing can become dependent on it if you use it for an extended period of time. If you would like to try this classic remedy, proceed with caution and take just 1 teaspoon of the oil in the morning (mixed in fruit juice to disguise the bitter taste). You should have a bowel movement within four hours or so. If not, you can continue the treatment once a day for two more days, but no longer! If you're not back to your usual elimination routine by then, call your doctor. *Note: If you are pregnant, don't take castor oil before speaking with your doctor; it is a strong stimulant that can bring on labor.*

Cast Off Corns

The mighty moisturizing power of **CASTOR OIL** makes it a perfect choice for softening up tough, painful corns. Your action plan: Cover the offending bump with a commercial, non-medicated corn pad (the kind with a hole in the center to corral the oil). Then use a cotton swab to reach inside the hole and coat the corn with a thin layer of castor oil. Cover the pad with adhesive tape to keep the fluid in continuous close contact with the corn. Follow this routine, with a fresh dressing and application of oil, every day until the corn has flown the coop.

Back in the Day...

Unlike warts on your hands or face, which are merely unsightly, plantar warts can make every step you take a painful experience. The nasty things start as little black dots on the soles of your feet—usually in clusters. Don't be tempted to scrape them off with a fingernail—you'll only make the infection spread. Instead, try this old-as-the-hills vanishing trick: Simply rub **CASTOR OIL** on the spots several times a day. Before you know it, they'll be gone with the wind!

Pack Away Your Problems

A **CASTOR OIL** pack is just what the doctor ordered for relieving inflammation and promoting internal healing anywhere on—or in— your body. Follow my four-step procedure:

Step 1. Pour castor oil into a bowl, and add a soft, clean cloth that's big enough to cover the problem area.

Step 2. Lay the oil-soaked fabric on your bare skin, and add a sheet of plastic wrap over it. Make sure you've got complete coverage—you don't want oil stains on your clothes or sheets!

Step 3. Top the plastic wrap with a heating pad set on low. Make sure it isn't set on high. You want it to be just comfortably warm.

Step 4. Leave the pack in place for 20 to 60 minutes. Repeat as needed once or twice a day until you feel relief.

PICK A PACK OF POWER

Physicians and naturopathic professionals routinely prescribe **CASTOR OIL** packs to treat a passel of problems (see "Pack Away Your Problems," above, for the how-to). Once you've made the pack, here are the most common uses for this powerful remedy.

ANNOYING HEALTH PROBLEM	THE R$_x$
Arthritis and bursitis pain	Cover the affected area, and leave the pack in place for 45 to 60 minutes, once a day.
Chest cold	Lay the pack on your chest, and lie down for about 60 minutes.
Constipation	Keep a tummy-sized pack on your abdomen for 20 minutes or so. That should be plenty of time to get the show on the road.
Tender breasts (caused by fluctuating hormones before menopause)	Lay a pack across your breasts, and leave it on for 60 minutes or so.

In Cupboards

Good Health Over Easy

When it comes to overall good health, an **EPSOM SALTS** bath is the closest thing you'll ever find to a magic bullet. That's because the magnesium in the salts is absorbed through your skin to benefit every part of your body. The pleasant R_x for maximum benefit: Three times a week, pour 2 cups of Epsom salts into a tub of warm water, and soak for 20 minutes. If you like, add 1/2 cup of your favorite bath oil. But don't use soap of any kind—it will interfere with the action of the salts. Besides improving your blood circulation, lowering your stress level, and relieving general aches and pains, this powerful soak can help alleviate a lot of other health conditions, including these:

- Arthritis

- Bruises

- Gout

- Hives

- Kidney stones

- Sciatica

HEALTHY Hint

EASY ON THE EPSOM

While magnesium is essential for good health, it is possible to give yourself an accidental overdose, especially if you are taking any medications that also contain the chemical. So if you're under medical care for a chronic health condition—especially high blood pressure, heart disease, or diabetes— consult with your doctor before you use **EPSOM SALTS** in any form. (Same goes for any woman who is or might be pregnant, or who is nursing.)

Stop Back Spasms

If there's anything worse than a plain old backache, it's being stabbed in the back by muscle spasms. Give that "knife" the heave-ho with this simple routine: Pour 2 cups of **EPSOM SALTS** in a tub full of hot water, ease yourself in, and have a good soak. You'll start to feel relief almost instantly. Afterward, lie down for 30 minutes or so with an ice pack on your back.

Fight Fibromyalgia

Fibromyalgia makes you so tired and achy that you can barely move. Inactivity leads to poor sleep, which in turn makes your muscles ache even more. Here's one way to break the cycle: Before bedtime, soak for 15 minutes in a tub laced with ½ cup of **EPSOM SALTS**. Stick with this routine until you're regularly sleeping through the night.

Ease Trigeminal Neuralgia Pain

This agonizing condition occurs when a vein or artery compresses the trigeminal nerve on the side of the face. **EPSOM SALTS** can help reduce the pain. Mix equal parts of Epsom salts and water that's as hot as you can stand. Dip a clean towel in the solution, wring out the water, and lay the towel at the base of your neck, where the nerve originates. Keep the compress in place until it cools down, then repeat as needed.

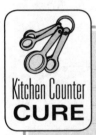

Kitchen Counter CURE

Rheumatism-Reduction Soak

Can you tell that a weather change is on the way because your toes, or maybe your knees or elbows, ache? You don't want to be a famous weather prognosticator at the price of painful, swollen joints! One of the most effective ways to relieve the swelling and discomfort of occasional bouts of rheumatism is to relax in this simple **EPSOM SALTS** soak.

> **2 cups of Epsom salts**
> **1 cup of baking soda**
> **1 cup of sea salt**

Mix all of the ingredients in a bathtub under warm running water. Then settle in and soak for 20 minutes or so. To treat just your foot or elbow in a basin, or to make enough solution for a compress, use the same dry ingredients in the same proportions, but use only 1 or 2 tablespoons of the mixture per gallon of water. Store the leftovers in an airtight container, and leave the weather forecasting to Al Roker.

Shove Off Shingles

If you had chicken pox as a kid, your body is still harboring the virus that caused it—and it could come back to haunt you in the form of painful, blistery shingles. For those of you who get a case of the shingles, help lessen the pain by making a paste of **EPSOM SALTS** and water, and smooth it directly on your affected skin. Repeat the process as often as possible until your flare-up fades away.

Soften Psoriasis Scales

Those scaly areas of skin on your hands and feet that are caused by psoriasis are as good as gone. Just sprinkle 1 cup of **EPSOM SALTS** in your bathwater and soak. After patting the itchy areas dry, rub them with some warm peanut oil, and top off the oil with a paste made from baking soda and castor oil. Put on white cotton gloves and socks and say "nighty-night." After a few days, your scales should disappear. *Note: Don't use this treatment on raw, irritated, or broken skin.*

Back in the Day...

When I was growing up, I was the unlucky kid who got bronchitis, complete with that deep, window-rattling cough that sounds like a barking seal and brings up gobs of mucus. You know the drill: Your muscles ache head to toe from nonstop hacking; you have a slight fever—and your voice sounds as raspy as Marlon Brando's. The next time you're battling bronchitis, do what Grandma Putt always prescribed for me. Climb into a steaming tub laced with 1 cup or so of **EPSOM SALTS**, plus 2 drops each of eucalyptus, thyme, and rosemary oils. The steam will increase the flow of nasal mucus; the molecules from the oils will dilate your internal airways, thereby easing your breathing; and the megadose of magnesium in the Epsom salts (absorbed through your skin) will relax your stressed-out bronchi. Of course, if your bronchitis lasts more than a week with no letup, see your doctor right away to rule out (or head off) pneumonia.

SPOTLIGHT ON
CORNS & CALLUSES

While corns and calluses aren't a major health issue, they sure can be painful—not to mention unsightly. Your goal is to soften them up so you can put on your shoes and walk around without irritation. With that in mind, treat your feet with my neat, from-the-kitchen remedies:

◆ Mash five uncoated **ASPIRIN** tablets with equal parts of water and lemon juice (just enough to make a thick paste), and apply it to the annoying spot. Wrap the area in a warm towel, put a plastic bag over your foot, and leave it on for 10 minutes or so. Take off the wrappings, and gently scrub the bump away with a pumice stone.

◆ Fill a basin with 32 ounces of just-boiled spring water and 8 heaping tablespoons of dried **CHAMOMILE**. Let the herb steep for 10 to 15 minutes, or until the water has cooled enough for you to put your feet in. Then sit back in a comfortable chair and soak your dogs.

◆ Pour 1/2 cup of **EPSOM SALTS** into a basin of warm water, and soak your feet for 20 minutes or so. Then use a pumice stone to gently rub away the softened layers of skin. Dry your feet, and add 2 drops of peppermint oil to a handful of shea butter or cocoa butter, then rub it into your feet thoroughly to lock in the much-needed moisture.

◆ Slice off a sliver of peeled **GARLIC** that's the same size as the corn, put it on top of the blasted bump, and secure it with a bandage. Replace the mini-poultice every day until the corn gives up and drops off.

◆ Once each day, tape a moist **TEA** bag on the spot and leave it on for 30 minutes or so. Within about two weeks, the bothersome corn should be gone. You can use either a freshly soaked tea bag or a cooled one that's left over from your morning cuppa.

Buddies Banish Back Pain...

With a little help from **EUCALYPTUS OIL**. Put 20 drops of the oil in a cup, add 4 tablespoons of olive oil, and heat it in the microwave for a few seconds. (It should feel warm—not hot.) Then have a friend or your spouse gently massage the oil onto the painful area of your back. After the hands-on healing session, you should feel a whole lot better! *Note: Do not apply eucalyptus oil directly to your skin; always "dilute" it with another oil, such as olive, almond, or coconut, to prevent skin irritation.*

Eucalyptus Conquers Coughs

Got a cough that just won't quit? Then rub the outside of your throat with a mixture of 5 drops of **EUCALYPTUS OIL** and 1 tablespoon of olive oil. Besides getting rid of the built-up mucus, it'll help you relax enough to get some much-needed rest.

If your sinuses are making you miserable, use this same rub on your face at bedtime, keeping it well away from your eyes. Apply it over the sinus area with a light touch (don't rub), and keep it well away from your eyes.

HOW'S THAT?

Q *Jerry, I really don't like using commercial insect repellents when I venture out into the wild. Is there a natural alternative that will work just as well?*

A Of course there is! Just mix up a batch of this all-natural spray and you'll be pest-free. Start with a glass spray bottle (the oils in this recipe will eat away at plastic over time). Then add 3/4 teaspoon of **EUCALYPTUS OIL**, and 1 1/2 teaspoons each of citronella, jojoba, and lavender essential oils. Shake well, then pour 8 ounces of distilled witch hazel into the bottle and shake again. You can spray this repellent on your clothing and your skin—just be sure to keep it away from your eyes, nose, and mouth. Reapply as needed, shaking the mixture well before each use.

Bust Up Bronchitis

If the diagnosis is bronchitis, help break up your chest congestion with a **EUCALYPTUS OIL** rub. Mix 10 drops of the aromatic oil with 1 tablespoon of olive oil and rub it on your chest, over your lungs. The expectorant effect will have you coughing the mucus up and out, making your coughs more productive and reducing the amount of nonproductive coughing spasms.

Come to Your Senses

When a head cold has your air passages so congested that your senses of taste and smell have all but vanished, try this trick: Sprinkle a few drops of **EUCALYPTUS OIL** on a cotton ball, and tuck it into a clean, empty pill bottle. Carry it around with you, and whenever you feel the need, remove the cap and take a few quick whiffs. You'll be tasting the wine and smelling the roses quick as a wink!

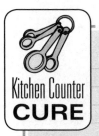

Kitchen Counter
CURE

Sinus-Clearing Bath Oil

Whether the sinus-clogging culprit is a nasty head cold or annoying seasonal allergies, a nice long soak in this soothing solution will help clear your airways—and relax your mind and body to boot!

> **8 drops of EUCALYPTUS OIL**
> **8 drops of peppermint oil**
> **8 drops of tea tree oil**

Put the three essential oils in a small bottle, screw the lid on tightly, and shake the bottle until the mixture is thoroughly blended. Then head to your bathroom and start filling the bathtub with water that's as hot as you can handle, pouring the oil under the spigot. Settle into the tub, and soak for at least 20 minutes, breathing deeply to inhale the wonderful (and wonderfully clearing) aroma.

Cures from Countertops & Cupboards

Feel Better with Fish

If you're battling the blues, here's uplifting news: Cold-water fish, such as salmon and tuna, are loaded with essential fatty acids that help your brain receive serotonin, the feel-good brain chemical. But there is a downside—you'd have to eat a boatload of fish to get the antidepressant effects. Instead, eat fish as often as you can, and take 1 gram (1,000 milligrams) of **FISH OIL** capsules or liquid every day. Look on the label for a concentration that contains half EPA and half DHA omega-3 fatty acids. *Note: Fish oil can thin your blood, so avoid it if you take aspirin or prescription blood thinners.*

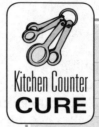

Kitchen Counter CURE

Give Bruises the Brush-Off

As soon as you bang your shin—or any other part of your body—fetch some **FISH OIL.** It's a first-rate way to reduce inflammation in and under your skin. Take 1 to 2 tablespoons of pure fish oil a day until the bruise is gone. (You can mix the oil with fruit juice to minimize the fishy taste.)

Go Fishing for Psoriasis Relief

Recent studies have shown **FISH OIL** to be effective in healing psoriasis, and a combination of fish oil liquid and avocado oil seems to be especially successful. Put the dynamic duo to work for you with this three-step procedure:

Step 1. Pour fish oil into one bowl and an equal amount of cold-pressed avocado oil into another bowl. Set the two containers close together, so you can reach them both quickly.

Step 2. Using your very clean fingers, apply the avocado oil to the psoriasis lesions in gentle circular motions. Immediately follow up with the fish oil, using the same circular pattern. Work on one small area of skin at a time.

Step 3. Wait until the oils have dried thoroughly—at least 10 minutes—before you let clothing or other fabric touch your skin. Or, if you really need to scurry in a hurry, wait three to five minutes, then lightly pat the treated area with a damp cloth to remove any excess oil.

A Gel of a Healer

Accidents do happen. So next time you get a minor skin wound or burn, turn to **PETROLEUM JELLY**. It keeps the moisture level of your injured skin close to that of normal skin, which speeds healing. It also reduces inflammation, seals out infection-causing germs, and helps prevent scarring. Use it as follows:

■ **Wounds.** Clean the wound thoroughly, and apply an antibiotic ointment. Then cover it with a generous layer of petroleum jelly, and top that with a bandage. Change the dressing several times a day, or whenever it's gotten wet.

■ **Minor burns.** This treatment is only intended for minor first-degree burns—the kind you get from a brief encounter with a steam iron, hot pan, or barbecue grill. Run cold water on the burn site for at least five minutes. When it's cooled down completely, very gently rub petroleum jelly over the affected area. Then wrap the burn loosely in a single layer of light gauze, and tape it in place. *Note: For anything more serious, get medical help ASAP (see "Pitfalls of Petroleum Jelly," at right).*

Send Psoriasis Plaques Packin'...

And fast! Twice a day, bathe the affected areas, pat them dry, and immediately rub on several layers of **PETROLEUM JELLY**. Within a week, the plaques should vanish.

HEALTHY
Hint

PITFALLS OF PETROLEUM JELLY

While **PETROLEUM JELLY** is tops for helping burns heal faster, you should never use it on a fresh burn unless it is very minor, and only after cooling it completely, as described in "A Gel of a Healer" (at left). That's because heat remains in your skin for some time after the initial impact and continues to damage the area. If you apply petroleum jelly (or any other kind of fat, including butter or oil) to a burn too soon, it will hold in the heat and cause more damage to the underlying tissue.

Dry Up the Drip

Here's a formula to halt postnasal drip. Melt ¼ cup of **PETROLEUM JELLY** in a small saucepan over medium-low heat, stirring frequently. Remove it from the stove and stir in 10 drops each of eucalyptus, peppermint, and thyme essential oils. Let cool to room temperature and pour it into a clean glass jar with a tight-fitting lid. Apply a small dab to the inside of each nostril up to three times a day. The petroleum jelly keeps the oils from being absorbed into your skin, thereby allowing you to inhale their drip-stopping essence over a prolonged period of time.

Bar the Door against Blisters

To fight the friction that causes blisters, smooth a nice light layer of **PETROLEUM JELLY** over each foot before you put on your socks and shoes. And be sure to lace up your shoes tightly.

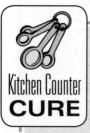

Kitchen Counter CURE

Achy-Muscle Massage Gel

Whether you got your muscle pain from hiking up a mountain trail, working in your yard, or standing on your feet for hours cooking a Thanksgiving feast, this ointment is your ticket to fast relief.

    1 tbsp. of glycerin
    1 tbsp. of PETROLEUM JELLY
    1 tbsp. of water
    ½ tsp. of almond extract
    ⅛ tsp. of wintergreen oil

Mix the glycerin, petroleum jelly, and water in a microwave-safe container. Nuke the mixture on high for 30 seconds, then add the extract and essential oil, and stir until smooth. While it's still warm, massage the gel onto your sore body parts. If you have any leftover gel, store it in a jar with a tight-fitting lid, and warm it up before using it again. But it's best to make fresh batches throughout the day and apply the gel until you're ache-free.

Mind Your Mouth

The antiseptic, anti-inflammatory, and astringent powers of **WITCH HAZEL** make it a first-class healer for gingivitis and other gum problems. Mix 1/2 to 1 teaspoon of food-grade witch hazel and 2 or 3 drops of clove oil in 1 cup of lukewarm water. Use the mixture three or four times a day, as you would mouthwash, until your gums are back to normal. *Note: If you're being treated for gingivitis, consult your dentist before using this remedy.*

A Witchy Trick for Laryngitis

Cat got your tongue? Or is it a case of laryngitis? Get your voice back pronto with the same **WITCH HAZEL**–clove oil solution described in "Mind Your Mouth" (above). But instead of swishing the potion around in your mouth, gargle with it three or four times a day (but don't swallow it!). Before you know it, you'll be whistlin' Dixie again.

Relieve External Hemorrhoids

Don't let this annoying affliction get you down. **WITCH HAZEL** can greatly reduce the pain and itch and help dry up any bleeding. Combine equal parts of witch hazel with either aloe gel, glycerin, or petroleum jelly, and gently rub the mixture onto the trouble spots.

Back in the Day...

For generations, folks have suffered from varicose veins. If you're one of them, you know this circulation problem can be pure agony. Fortunately, old-timers like my Grandma Putt knew a thing or two about the healing properties of **WITCH HAZEL**. The simple routine: Chill a bowl of witch hazel in the refrigerator for an hour or two, then soak washcloths in it. Sit back in a comfortable chair, put your legs up, and lay the cold compresses on the affected areas. Keep them in place for 15 minutes or so, and the pain should be gone, or at least greatly diminished. Repeat the procedure as often as necessary.

Cures from Countertops & Cupboards

Hazel to the Rescue!

Straight from the bottle, **WITCH HAZEL** can perform heaps of health-care feats. Here's a handful of everyday problem solvers:

- **Black eye.** Soak a washcloth in witch hazel, and hold it over your eye. The pain and swelling will vamoose. Just make sure you don't get any in your eye, though, because it will sting like crazy!

- **Bruises.** Dab witch hazel on the mark three times a day, and it'll be gone in no time at all.

- **Cuts and scrapes.** Pour a generous amount of witch hazel on the wound, let it air-dry, and then cover it with a bandage.

- **Sore, strained eyes.** Soak two small cotton pads in witch hazel, and put one over each closed eye. Lie back and relax for 10 minutes or so, and you're good to go!

Sack Psoriasis Plaques

Mix equal parts of alcohol-free **WITCH HAZEL** and glycerin USP (available in pharmacies) in a wide-mouthed container. After your shower or bath, pat your skin dry, and rub the mixture thoroughly into the affected areas—avoiding any open lesions. (The potion should disappear entirely; if your skin is greasy, you've used too much.) Repeat daily. Within three weeks, redness and scaling should be reduced by 80 to 90 percent. After that, use the treatment once a week or as needed to help prevent flare-ups.

HEALTHY Hint

FAST FIX FOR SUNBURN PAIN

Feeling a bit crispy-fried after spending a day at the beach? Then it's time to grab some gauze and **WITCH HAZEL**. Dip the gauze (or cheesecloth) in the witch hazel, and gently wrap it around the affected area. As the cloth dries, repeat the procedure until you feel relief—which will be a lot sooner than you think. Follow up with a rich moisturizing lotion. If the sun has done its number on a part of your body that cannot be easily wrapped, pour some witch hazel into a spray bottle, and spritz your sore skin.

Cool Aid for Hot Muscles

When you've been working or playing hard in the hot sun, give your aching muscles a nice cooling treat. Here's how: Mix 2 cups of **WITCH HAZEL**, 2 teaspoons of light corn syrup, 1/2 teaspoon of castor oil, and 3 or 4 drops of essential oil (eucalyptus, peppermint, rosemary, and wintergreen are good choices) in a jar with a tight-fitting lid. Shake well, and massage the potion into your sore body parts for almost-instant relief.

Colonoscopy Prep Made Easy

Believe you me, prepping for a colonoscopy is far more unpleasant than the procedure itself. It entails a 24-hour process of cleaning out your colon by drinking only clear fluids and a foul-tasting "beverage," and the routine can make your rear end as sore as the dickens. You can buy commercial hemorrhoid pads to relieve the discomfort, but here's a better (and cheaper) idea: The evening before you start prepping, mix together a few drops of lavender oil per ounce of **WITCH HAZEL**. Dip a dozen or so large cotton pads in the solution, put them into a ziplock freezer bag, and then stash them in the freezer. The next day, use chilled pads right out of the bag as often as needed to bring powerful relief to your sitting area. *Note: If you have any pads left over, save them in the freezer for soothing future cuts, scratches, or insect bites, and as handy wipes for hemorrhoid relief.*

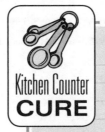

Kitchen Counter CURE

Nix the Nosebleeds

Almost everyone gets a nosebleed from time to time. So make like a Boy Scout and be prepared with this classic remedy: Mix 6 drops of cypress oil (available in health-food stores and herbal-supply stores) per 2 tablespoons of **WITCH HAZEL** in a bottle, and stash it in the medicine chest. Then whenever the need arises, shake the bottle well, moisten a cotton ball with the potion, and gently insert it into the bleeding nostril. Sit up straight, with your head tilted just slightly forward. Within two or three minutes, the blood should stop flowing. *Note: To speed up the process, squeeze the soft tissue of your nose firmly, but gently, between your thumb and forefinger.*

Cures from Countertops & Cupboards

Tape Away Warts

Yes, there are plenty of over-the-counter wart-removal potions, but why spend the money? Instead, pull out a roll of **DUCT TAPE** to get the job done. Put a piece of the tape right over the wart and leave it on for six days. (If the tape falls off, replace it with a fresh piece.) At the end of the sixth day, remove the tape, soak the wart in water, and gently rub the spot with an emery board or pumice stone. Leave the area bare overnight, and apply more duct tape in the morning. Repeat this routine for two months—unless the wart disappears sooner.

Sticky Help for Injured Fingers

Whether you caught your finger in a door, or jammed it playing ball, you can easily make a splint for your sore digit with the help of **DUCT TAPE**. Here are two options:

1. Place a wooden craft stick on each side of the injured finger, then wrap duct tape around your finger and over the sticks until they are well secured.

2. No craft sticks? No worries! Just wrap duct tape firmly around your hurt digit and the one next to it. Then continue what you were doing or hightail it to the emergency room.

HEALTHY Hint

DIY FIRST AID

If you keep a roll of **DUCT TAPE** in your glove box, you'll be prepared to offer aid for someone (or yourself!) when minor mishaps occur. Besides using the tape to fashion finger splints (see "Sticky Help for Injured Fingers," at left), you can apply this handy helper as an impromptu bandage. Just cover the cut with whatever clean, absorbent material you have on hand, such as facial tissue, a folded paper towel or napkin, or a scrap of fabric, then use the tape to hold it securely in place.

If the wound is large and gaping, don't worry about the absorbent material. Just take a page from countless EMT training manuals—use duct tape to "suture" the skin closed, then get to the emergency room pronto!

Tacky Tick Removal

Whenever you spend a day in the great outdoors, you should always do a complete and thorough tick check from head to toe. If one or more of the tiny terrors has landed on you, don't panic. Instead, just reach for the nearest roll of **DUCT TAPE**. Tear off a piece of tape that's about 5 inches long and wrap it around your index and middle fingers, sticky side out. Then press the tape firmly against your sleeve, pant leg, or bare skin, and quickly pull off the tick(s). Repeat with fresh tape until you're tick-free. By the way, this technique is also great for getting ticks off your dog before they have the chance to burrow under Fido's coat and into your pet's skin.

Back in the Day...

When it was invented during World War II, the original name for **DUCT TAPE** was "Duck" tape because it repels water, like a duck. After the war, the tape was used extensively in civilian industries and became known as "duct" tape because of its use on, of course, ductwork. Its water-shedding reputation still comes in handy, and not just for ductwork! For instance, use this terrific tape as a:

Bandage saver. When you need to keep a bandaged area from getting wet, cover it with plastic wrap, and seal it securely with duct tape. Now you can hop in the shower or even go for a swim, and you'll keep your wound nice and dry.

Cast repairer. More than one doctor has passed this tip along to patients who end up with a broken cast—use duct tape to repair it. It's tough enough to hold it together until the cast is ready to come off, and it's easy to keep clean because dirt wipes right off. Simply wrap the tape around and around until the cracked area is covered.

Cast protector. Duct tape also does the job when you need to keep your cast dry in the shower. Just stick your casted arm or leg into a large plastic garbage bag, gather the open top tightly around your exposed skin, and securely tape it shut.

Foil Frostbite

Take a tip from Alaskan snowmobilers, and be sure to carry a roll of **DUCT TAPE** on your next cold-weather hike. It's a real skin saver when the temperatures drop and you run the risk of frostbite. Simply use the tape to cover your nose, cheeks, and any other exposed skin. Tear a piece small enough to cover the tip of your nose and apply, then use another piece or pieces to cross over the bridge of your nose. Use multiple pieces to form squares over your cheeks, and longer strips if you need to cover your forehead. You may look a bit silly, but this is one heck of a skin protector—no fooling!

Save a Life

If you ever find yourself in a situation where you need to give someone CPR and you don't have a mask handy, a strip of **DUCT TAPE** could help save a life. Fold a foot-long length of the tape over on itself so that the sticky sides meet. Quickly cut a horizontal slit in the middle of the tape, through both layers, place the tape over the victim's mouth, and administer breaths through the slit.

HOW'S THAT?

Q *Hey, Jerry, I've heard about doing arm exercises with cans of soup, but with* **DUCT TAPE?** *Can a roll of tape really give me a good workout?*

A I wouldn't exactly call it a *workout*—but for folks who haven't been doing *any* kind of exercise, this is one super-simple way to ease into arm strengthening. Best of all, you can do it right in your kitchen! Grip a jumbo roll of duct tape and fully extend your arm out to the side, keeping it in line with your shoulder. Hold the position until your arm begins to tremble. Then repeat with the other arm. Do this every other day for a few weeks, and you should be able to keep your arms steady for longer periods. You'll also begin to see a little more muscle definition.

Get Steamed

When you're battling a ferocious head cold, inhaling steam is one of the best ways to open up your congested airways and soothe irritated tissues. Just heat a pot of water on the stove until it's simmering, then carefully move it to a table or counter (with a protective towel or mat underneath). Drop 1 or 2 tablespoons of **MENTHOLATED RUB** into the water and stir. Lean over the pot with a towel draped over your head and shoulders, and breathe in the fragrant steam. Keep your eyes closed so the menthol doesn't make them sting. If the heat is too much for your skin, move the towel to release trapped steam.

Rub Out a Head Cold

Sure, inhaling steam breaks up head congestion (see "Get Steamed," above), but if you need to be out and about, you can make yourself a portable "vaporizer." Just dip a cotton ball into a jar of **MENTHOLATED RUB** so that it picks up a good dollop of the stuff. Put the coated ball into a clean pill bottle, cap it tightly, and tuck it in your pocket or purse. Then anytime you start to feel congested, remove the cap and take a few deep breaths. Bingo—your airways will be free and clear!

Forget Fungus

When foul fungi have infected the nails on your fingers or your toes, **MENTHOLATED RUB** can charge to the rescue. Twice a day, coat the afflicted nail(s) and surrounding skin with mentholated rub. It should solve the problem in no time flat. *Note: If the infection does not clear up after a few weeks, call your doctor.*

HEALTHY
Hint

REBUFF BUGS

The **MENTHOLATED RUB** that's been easing chest colds for decades is also a terrific insect repellent. Just smooth the stuff onto your skin (but not on your face) to fend off mosquitoes, ticks, and equally nasty bloodsucking bad-guy bugs. Be sure to wash your hands thoroughly if you're going to be handling any food while you're in the great outdoors.

Make Drug Labels Long-Lasting

If you take prescription drugs of any kind, you certainly don't want to have the label smeared by wet hands, or defaced by the liquid medicine itself as it dribbles over the side of the bottle. So stop trouble in its tracks with **TRANSPARENT TAPE**. The minute you get your meds home from the drugstore, cover the label with a generous piece of tape.

Tape Trick to Kick the Habit

Trying to quit smoking? Congratulations! And here's a tip to help you on the road to success: As a first step, keep your package of cancer sticks closed with **TRANSPARENT TAPE**—and use lots of it. That may not stop you from taking a cigarette, but it'll slow you down, and will at least force you to think about the consequences each time you do!

Coax Out a Splinter

If you're not a fan of digging into your skin with a needle to get at a sliver, take the easy way out with **TRANSPARENT TAPE**. Cover the splinter with a piece of tape, making it long enough so that you can grasp one end to remove it. Press down on the tape to ensure it's making contact with your skin. Keep it on overnight. Come morning, grab one end of the tape and quickly pull it off; the splinter should glide right out.

Back in the Day...

As Grandma Putt was getting on in years, she found that the directions on medicine bottles (prescription and otherwise) seemed to grow smaller and smaller. But she didn't take that shrinkage lying down! Instead, she wrote the information she needed on a piece of paper, in letters and numbers that were big enough to read—even without her spectacles on—and fastened the paper to the bottle with **TRANSPARENT TAPE**. These days, the print on most drug packaging has shrunk even more, so give Grandma's easy-reading trick a try.

Calming Brewski Bath

The next time you're feeling so tense and stressed out you could scream, relax with a **BEER**. Rather, make that beers, plural. Now I'm not talking about heading downtown to the nearest pub! This is a more calming cure: Pour three bottles of brew into a bathtub of warm water, lean back, and think lovely thoughts.

Bid Bunions Adieu

About to open an ice-cold can of **BEER**? Before you pull the tab, give your sore tootsies a treat: Lay the can sideways on the floor, slip off your shoes and socks, and put your aching foot on the can. Then roll it back and forth for several minutes. The cold will help reduce inflammation, and the motion will give your foot a good massage. Just be sure to let the can rest upright for a few minutes before you open it, or you'll get a fizzy shower! (And then open it over the sink to be safe.)

Roll Away Aches and Strains

Besides bunions (see "Bid Bunions Adieu," above), good ol' **BEER** can ease the pain of sore muscles just about anywhere on your body. For back and shoulder pain, put a can in the crook of your back or between your shoulder blades and lean back against a wall, rolling it around as you do so. Or roll a can along the back of your neck, along your calves, or wherever you need to loosen up tight muscles and encourage healing blood flow.

Kitchen Counter CURE

Upset-Tummy Tamer

You probably know that sipping on a carbonated beverage like soda can help ease indigestion and settle your stomach. What you may not realize is that **BEER** works just as well as soda does. In fact, beer packs an extra punch because the alcohol can help buffer your stomach pain. *Note: Do not drink beer if you have an ulcer or gastritis, which can worsen with the use of alcohol.*

Warm Up for a Cold

Coughing? Sneezing? Longing to crawl into bed? Well, before you call it a night, head to the liquor cabinet and pull out a bottle of **BOURBON**. Pour a generous shot into a mug, add boiling water, a squeeze of fresh lemon juice, and honey to taste. Then slowly sip the steaming toddy, turn out the lights, and sleep like a baby. Your cold symptoms should be tamed by morning. Repeat this R_X nightly until you're feeling chipper.

Emergency Anesthetic

If the knife slips while you're slicing and dicing during meal prep, make like a chef and grab a bottle of **BOURBON**. Pour a drop or two of the alcohol directly on your cut to help clean it out and numb the pain. Then wrap the wound to keep it sterile while you finish KP duty.

Clean Your Mouth

You can kill the germs that cause gingivitis with this tasty tip: After your regular toothbrushing, swish a shot of **BOURBON** around in your mouth for at least 30 seconds, then spit it out.

Back in the Day...

During Prohibition, doctors across America lobbied strongly for the right to prescribe alcohol for health purposes. In fact, a survey taken in 1921 showed that 51 percent of physicians advocated prescribing **BOURBON** or whiskey, and 26 percent believed that beer was "a necessary therapeutic agent."

All forms of alcohol were also used as stimulants in hypothermia cases because they cause vasodilation (widening of the blood vessels) and the feeling of warmth. We now know that vasodilation speeds heat loss and actually worsens hypothermia. Yet, even today, outdoorsmen often carry hip flasks of spirits to warm themselves on cold winter days. Don't be one of them! Instead, bring along a thermos of hot coffee, tea, or cocoa.

Drink Up, Ladies!

Drinking 100 percent **CRANBERRY JUICE** (*not* a juice cocktail or blend) can help cure and/or prevent urinary tract infections and water retention. A 10-ounce glass a day should prevent bacteria from building up in your urethra, and it will also help fluids flow out of your body. Keep this healthy habit going during happy hour by using cranberry juice as a mixer.

Wage War on Wounds

In olden days, Native Americans used cranberry poultices to pull toxins from arrow wounds. Chances are you won't get too many arrow injuries as you go about your day, but the antibacterial properties of **CRANBERRY JUICE** work just as well to disinfect modern-day cuts, scrapes, and puncture wounds. Simply soak a gauze pad with 100 percent cranberry juice, place it over the cut, and secure it with adhesive tape. Change the dressing every few hours until the wound has healed.

CRANBERRY JUICE TO THE RESCUE!

Pure, unsweetened **CRANBERRY JUICE** is just what the doctor ordered for relieving a number of nagging health conditions. Just remember to use 100 percent cranberry juice (not juice combos), with no sugar or preservatives added. And, as always, consult with your health-care provider before using any of these treatments.

CONDITION	DOSAGE
Asthma	2 tbsp. 30 minutes before each meal and at the onset of an asthma attack
Canker sores	One 8-oz. glass between meals
Kidney and bladder infections	6 oz., three times a day
Nausea and vomiting	Frequently throughout the day to replace lost fluids and nutrients

From the Liquor Cabinet

Health

I Heard It Through the Grapevine...

That good health can be mine—and yours!—by simply sipping on purple **GRAPE JUICE** every day. This delicious drink, like red wine (see page 51), is bursting with flavonoids, those plant compounds that help prevent your blood from clotting and gunking up your arteries. That means less chance of having a heart attack down the road. Here are two other ways the purple juice can keep you in the pink of health:

- Drinking grape juice makes your arteries more flexible, which can improve blood flow and reduce angina pain.

- Both purple and red grape juices have been found to make LDL ("bad") cholesterol less likely to stick to artery walls.

Your daily dose: just 5 ounces of 100 percent purple (or red) grape juice each and every day. And don't forget to include the purple juice when you're tending bar. Search online for tasty grape juice cocktails.

HEALTHY Hint

GRAPE NEWS FOR CUTS

To heal a cut or stubborn sore, saturate a gauze pad in purple **GRAPE JUICE**, apply it to the wound, and fasten it in place with adhesive tape. Replace the dressing every day, but don't wash the affected area. Before you know it, the nasty "owie" will be gone and forgotten.

Relief for Slow Healers

Once, I had a cut on my heel that just wouldn't close up—until a retired doctor who lived down the street suggested a remedy that worked like a miracle. Here's all there is to it: Every night before bedtime, soak your foot for half an hour in a porcelain bowl (not metal) filled with enough purple **GRAPE JUICE** to cover the sore. Gently pat the spot dry with a soft cotton cloth (use something old—it will get stained by the juice). Don't rinse off the juice, and don't get the area wet when bathing. Healing time varies with the depth of the cut, but it should be gone after two to three weeks of nightly treatments. If the cut is still not healed after this regimen, have your doctor take a look at it.

Fight the Flu

Before cold and flu season starts, arm yourself with this immunity-boosting tonic: Mix $3/4$ cup of **VODKA**, $1 1/2$ tablespoons of dried echinacea root (available in health-food stores and herbal-supply stores), and $3/4$ cup of distilled water in a glass jar with a tight-fitting lid. Store it in a cool, dark place for two weeks, and strain the tincture into glass bottles. Then, at the first sign of cold or flu symptoms, mix 2 or 3 drops in a glass of water, and drink to your health!

Raise a Glass to Vodka!

This potent libation acts as both a local anesthetic and disinfectant, so it's just the ticket for treating blisters and minor wounds. So raise a glass of **VODKA** to these two quick fixes:

- **Blister buster.** To dry up a fresh blister fast, dab it with some vodka and let the alcohol air-dry on your skin. Repeat throughout the day.

- **Wound healer.** Pour vodka onto a gauze pad, and press the pad against the injured area. Hold it in place with adhesive tape. Change the dressing two or three times a day, until the wound heals.

HOW'S THAT?

Q *I love the convenience of those little bottles of hand sanitizer, but have you read their labels? I wonder if those impossible-to-pronounce ingredients are doing more harm than the bacteria I'm trying to kill. Is there a more natural solution that I can take on the road?*

A Heaven knows, there *are* plenty of commercial hand sanitizers out there. And I also wonder about all of those unpronounceable ingredients! That's why I use this simple—and safe—DIY spray: Mix $1/4$ cup of **VODKA** and $1/2$ cup of water, and stir in 20 drops each of lavender oil and tea tree oil. Pour the potion into a 4-ounce spray bottle or two 2-ounce bottles. Use as you would any other hand sanitizer.

HEALTHY Hint

BAR BUDDIES

Whether you have a well-stocked display or just a few bottles of liquor and mixers collecting dust on a pantry shelf, you still have the makings for a handful of first-aid friends, like these:

Quiet a queasy stomach. If a stomach bug has got its grip on you, go for **APPLE JUICE**. Pour a big glass and sip it slowly. In no time flat, your tummy should be feeling better. Why? Because apples contain compounds that work wonders when it comes to fighting stomach flu and other viruses. So drink up!

Stop flu in its tracks. Put 1/2 pound of peeled, chopped garlic and 1 quart of 90-proof **COGNAC** in a dark brown bottle. Put on the cap, and seal it with heavy tape to make sure it's airtight. During the day, keep the bottle in a light, warm spot (preferably in the sun). Then move it to a cool, dark place for the night. After 14 days and nights of this routine, open the bottle and strain out the garlic. Pour the infused cognac back into the bottle, and label it with the date (it should retain full potency for a year). To use, take 10 to 15 drops, mixed in a glass of water, three times a day (one hour before each meal) for the duration of flu season. If you already have the flu, take 20 drops an hour before each meal for five days. Then switch to taking 10 to 15 drops three times a day, as described above.

Help a hangover. On "the morning after the night before," some folks will settle for nothing less than the "hair of the dog." If you're part of that crowd, give this old-time remedy a try: Combine 1 ounce of Pernod®, 1 ounce of white **CRÈME DE CACAO**, and 3 ounces of milk in a blender. Add three ice cubes, and blend on high speed. Then pour the potion into a glass, toss it back—and cross your fingers!

Lessen leg cramps. If a painful leg cramp jolts you wide awake, don't just lie there squirming. Instead, hobble into the kitchen, pour an 8-ounce glass of **TONIC WATER**, and drink it down. The quinine in the fizzy mixer should be enough to uncramp your muscles. If you don't care for the taste of plain tonic, jazz it up with a squirt of orange juice, a wedge of lime—or a shot of gin!

Ease Chemo Aftereffects

Hopefully, you're not among the more than 1 million Americans diagnosed with cancer each year. But if you are, you know that chemotherapy and/or radiation treatments can really do a number on you. While your doctor may prescribe anti-nausea and other medications, there are natural remedies you can also try, and one of the best is **WINE**.

To improve your appetite and corral a host of cancer-fighting nutrients from your meal, enjoy some red wine before dinner. Not only can it help stimulate your appetite, but the pigments that give red wine its color may help to correct the imbalance of B vitamins that often occurs after cancer treatments, and that may contribute to mouth irritation, anemia, and nerve problems. In addition, red wine contains an antifungal compound that's converted by the body into a powerful cancer-fighting agent. *Note: If you have breast cancer, you should avoid alcohol because it may boost estrogen levels and fuel cancer.*

Hammer High Cholesterol

According to a study at the University of California, Davis, drinking three to six glasses of red **WINE** a week lowers LDL ("bad") cholesterol, most likely because of its high concentration of plant compounds that bind to and prevent the absorption of cholesterol. And here's the best part for all you wine lovers: While eating grapes is fine, the alcoholic version appears to work better at releasing these compounds and raising HDL ("good") cholesterol levels.

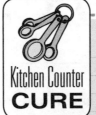

Kitchen Counter CURE

Soak Your Cares Away

You don't have to drink **WINE** to reap its healthful benefits. Just pour 4 cups of red wine and 1 cup of raw honey into your bathtub as you fill it with very warm water. Settle in and relax for 30 minutes. The warm, steamy air will open your airways and pores so they can absorb the wine's beautifying antioxidants and complex amino acids. The honey will help your skin retain moisture. When you're done soaking, rinse off with clear water, and pat yourself dry.

From the Liquor Cabinet

CHAPTER 2

Fridge & Freezer Fixers

Most of us reach into the fridge several times a day, or stand at the open door thinking, "What am I in the mood for?" Maybe we should all be asking this instead: "What healthy healer will make me feel terrific today?" Believe it or not, your fridge holds unbeatable cures for colds and hay fever, high blood pressure, psoriasis pain, and more.

DAIRY PRODUCTS

Build Better Bones

Like all dairy products, **BUTTERMILK** contains a healthy dose of calcium. In fact, 1 cup of low-fat buttermilk contains 28 percent of the Daily Value of calcium. Getting enough calcium in your diet helps slow bone loss as you age, helps support new bone growth, and lessens your chance of developing osteoporosis.

Douse Stomach Distress

When your stomach feels like it's on fire after a spicy meal, reach for **BUTTERMILK**. Sipping a cold glass of this rich, tangy milk will calm your irritated stomach, plus give you a much-needed calcium boost.

Dismiss Psoriasis

More than seven million Americans have psoriasis. If you're one of them, you know the rashes and plaques caused by this disease are unsightly and uncomfortable—and sometimes downright painful, too. Well, you can find major psoriasis relief in your fridge—from good old **BUTTERMILK**. Here's your trio of options:

1. Pour 2 to 4 cups of buttermilk into a tub of warm water, and soak for 20 minutes. Gently pat your skin dry, and smooth on a rich, natural moisturizing lotion.

2. If you prefer showers to baths, fill a clean plastic squirt bottle with buttermilk, and use it as a body wash. Again, follow up with an intensive-care moisturizer.

3. To treat psoriasis on your scalp or a small area of your body, saturate a soft all-cotton cloth with buttermilk, apply it directly to the site, and hold it there until the pain and itch subside.

In each case, repeat the process as needed. Also, start adding buttermilk to your daily drink menu. There is no specific dose (at least not yet), but studies show that it seems to relieve psoriasis pain. *Note: If what you think is a psoriasis patch suddenly appears, and you have not been diagnosed with the disease, see your doctor immediately. It could be a more serious, look-alike condition.*

HEALTHY
Hint

BUTTERMILK BASICS

For all the good it can do you, **BUTTERMILK** also has two drawbacks—fat, which increases your cholesterol levels, and sodium, which can make your blood pressure spike. Even low-fat buttermilk contains 2.2 grams of total fat per serving, with 60 percent of that made up of harmful saturated fat. In addition, buttermilk contains a whopping 466 milligrams, or 20 percent, of your daily sodium limit. That's much higher than the sodium count for regular low-fat milk, which contains just 107 milligrams per cup. Both saturated fat and sodium can be bad for your heart, so as a remedy, buttermilk comes with a caution: Use buttermilk in moderation and stick with the low-fat version.

An Eggs-tra Brain Boost

If you can't remember where you left your car keys, or struggle to remember a neighbor's name or your sister's phone number, it's time to get crackin' and cook up some **EGGS**. Their yolks contain high levels of choline, a nutrient that aids brain development. Research shows that rats fed choline-rich diets had better memories, even in old age. Do our human brains work in the same way? We don't know for sure just yet, but we do know that eating eggs several times a week won't raise your cholesterol, and may actually boost your brainpower.

Vitamin D Over Easy

EGGS are one of the few natural food sources of vitamin D, which is essential for calcium absorption and for maintaining optimum bone health. Vitamin D also improves memory. Our bodies produce vitamin D when we expose our bare skin to sunlight. But if you're like the majority of folks who spend most of their time indoors, you're missing out on vital sunlight exposure, and increasing your risk of developing osteoporosis. So help your bones—eat more eggs!

Save Your Sight

Age-related macular degeneration (AMD) is the leading cause of blindness in American adults aged 60 and older. Lutein and zeaxanthin are two carotenoids critical for preventing AMD, and **EGGS** contain both, which are absorbed more easily from eggs than they are from green vegetables.

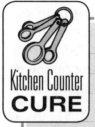

Kitchen Counter CURE

Scramble Up Some Skin Savers

In addition to boosting brains, bones, and vision, **EGGS** are equally good for your skin. Here are two ways to use them:

• Apply a thin layer of whisked egg whites to a minor cut. The egg whites will dry, creating a film that protects your cut, and they provide nutrients that will help the skin heal quickly.

• Place an eggshell into a glass of apple cider vinegar and leave it to soak for a day or two. Remove the eggshell, and use a cotton ball to dab the vinegar on minor skin irritations or itchy skin several times a day.

Soothe a Stye

To treat a stye, doctors often prescribe a hot compress, applied three or four times a day. And you'll find just what the doctor ordered in your refrigerator: an **EGG**. Pull one out, and hard-boil it. Wrap the hot egg (still in its shell) in a washcloth, and lay it against your sore eye for 10 minutes. When it's time for your next egg-laying session, put the piece of "hen fruit" back in a pot of water, and reheat it.

Eggy Sunburn Relief

Make up a supply of these comforting sticks once summer rolls around, and keep them on hand to supply instant relief whenever sunburn strikes (they work well on minor kitchen burns, too):

Step 1. In a small bowl, beat an **EGG** until it's frothy. Then slowly whisk in 1/2 cup of warm (but not hot) coconut oil and 1 tablespoon of raw honey until the mixture is the consistency of mayonnaise

Step 2. Set an empty toilet paper roll on end in another bowl, spoon the blend into the tube, and set it (still in the bowl) in the freezer until it's frozen solid.

Step 3. When it's skin-soothing time, peel away the top 1/4 inch of the cardboard, and gently rub the top of the frozen stick over the burned area. Wait 5 to 10 minutes, and rinse with cool water. Repeat as needed until you've banished the burn.

Between uses, cover the cream stick with plastic wrap, and keep it frozen. It will last indefinitely.

Back in the Day...

Got a boil that's driving you nuts? Try this old-time remedy: Remove the shell from a hard-boiled **EGG**, and then gently peel off the delicate skin that's left on the egg. Wet it, and lay it over the boil. It should draw out the pus and reduce the inflammation pronto. *Note: If the pain gets steadily worse, or you see a red streak in the boil, get medical help immediately!*

Bone Up Better with Milk

When you consider the health benefits of **MILK**, the first thing that probably comes to mind is calcium, which is beneficial in the fight against osteoporosis. And you're right—milk and products made from milk, such as cheese and yogurt, supply about one-third of the Daily Value of calcium for folks under 50 and about one-fourth of what you need if you're older. But only milk fortified with vitamin D will help prevent bone loss; without the D, your body can't absorb the calcium. The good news is that the milk you buy in the grocery store—from skim to whole and everything in between—is fortified with vitamin D. So drink up!

DASH from High Blood Pressure

Which do you think works better for lowering blood pressure—taking calcium supplements or drinking milk? **MILK**! All sorts of dietary supplements, including calcium and magnesium, have been tested for their ability to lower blood pressure, but what works best is real food.

In a study called Dietary Approaches to Stop Hypertension (DASH), researchers found that when people with high blood pressure switched their diets from ones high in fat to low-fat diets rich in fruits and vegetables, their blood pressure went down. When they added three servings of dairy foods daily, their blood pressure dropped as much as if they were taking blood pressure medications.

HEALTHY Hint

THINK YOU CAN'T DRINK MILK?

Many adults think they can't digest lactose, the naturally occurring sugar in **MILK**. But the calcium in milk is easier to absorb than the calcium in vegetables, and there's a lot more of it in milk, to boot. That's why a recent study found that adults who avoid milk and other dairy foods have an increased risk of osteoporosis. If you've been avoiding milk, try these tips:

Drink small portions. Many can tolerate ½ cup of milk a day with no problems.

Take the test. Once you can drink ½ cup of milk, gradually increase quantities to test your tolerance.

Mix with meals. Drink your milk with meals. Food will diminish the lactose effect.

Milky Burn Treatment

If you're like me, you've had your share of kitchen mishaps, including minor burns. The next time you singe your fingers on the stove, make a beeline for your fridge and grab the **MILK**. Pour milk into a bowl, dip a clean dish towel in it, and lay the wet compress on your burned skin. Hold it in place for about 20 minutes, then rinse the milk off with cool water. Repeat every two to four hours, until the pain and redness subside. *Note: This treatment is for minor burns only; and if you try this trick, be sure to use whole milk or (better yet) half-and-half—it's the fat content that soothes the burn and helps it heal faster. By the way, this same treatment works like magic on sunburn, too. If you don't believe me, just give it a try the next time you spend too much time sizzling in Ol' Sol's company.*

Mooove Over, Eczema!

When a flare-up strikes, help is as close as your refrigerator. Just mix cold whole **MILK** in a bowl with an equal amount of water, and saturate a gauze pad or soft cotton cloth with the solution. Hold it on the affected area for about three minutes. Perform this procedure two to four more times in quick succession. Then repeat as needed throughout the day. Just be sure to rinse your skin with cool water after each treatment—otherwise, before you know it, you'll smell just like sour milk!

HOW'S THAT?

Q *Jerry, I often have irritated eyelids by the end of the day. Do you have any suggestions on how I can get relief?*

A If the question on your mind is how to cure sore, swollen eyelids, my answer is "Moo"—moo juice, that is. Just soak a couple of cotton pads in ice-cold, whole **MILK**, lie down, put one over each eye, and rest for 5 to 10 minutes. Then, jeepers creepers, those peepers will be back to their old selves again!

Say "Yes" to Yogurt

Besides tasting delicious and providing a good dose of calcium, **YOGURT** is one heck of a healer because of its bugs. Yes, bugs—not the kind that crawl and fly, though. These bugs are microscopic forms of friendly bacteria that help destroy the bad guys that give us diarrhea, yeast infections, and possibly even cancer. Here's the rundown:

- In a study, eating 8 ounces of yogurt containing the bacterial culture *Lactobacillus acidophilus* reduced the risk of yeast infections threefold.

- The active cultures in yogurt may decrease the risk of breast, colon, and liver tumors that are triggered by carcinogens. Further studies are under way.

The key here is to be sure you are buying yogurt with live cultures. How do you know? It's simple. Make sure the carton sports the Live & Active Cultures seal bestowed by the National Yogurt Association (NYA). It guarantees that the product contains a full load of these beneficial bugs.

Bolster Immunity

Beyond bacteria, other compounds (including lipids, peptides, and acids) in **YOGURT** may possess anti-cancer benefits. In fact, yogurt might just rev up the entire immune system. Research is ongoing, but studies suggest that people with compromised immune systems, especially older folks, may be able to increase their resistance to some cancers and other diseases by eating yogurt.

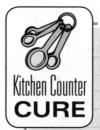

Kitchen Counter CURE

Quick Fix for Canker Sores

If you're constantly coming down with canker sores, eat plain **YOGURT** more often (at least 8 ounces of plain yogurt daily). The helpful bacteria it contains help to fight off the bad bugs that cause these painful sores. For extra healing power, swirl the dairy dynamo around in your mouth before swallowing it. This way, it'll coat your gums, tongue, throat, and the roof of your mouth with beneficial bacteria. *Note: If you don't care for the taste of plain yogurt, mix it with a teaspoon or so of raw honey or a drizzle of pure maple (not pancake) syrup.*

Keep Colds at Bay...

And hay fever, too. Studies have shown that folks who eat as little as 6 ounces of **YOGURT** a day sail right through the cold and allergy seasons. For best results, though, begin your prevention plan before the viruses start circulating and the pollen flies, and keep at it all the way through the peak season.

Rescue the Good Guys

Anyone who's ever taken antibiotics knows that these meds can deliver side effects in the form of diarrhea, an upset stomach, or a yeast infection. The simple solution: Eat $1/2$ to 1 cup of **YOGURT** two hours before or after taking each dose of your medication. Then, after you finish your prescription, eat 1 cup of yogurt each day for two to four weeks. This way, you'll restock your body with a full load of the bacteria that are essential for good health.

> # HEALTHY
> ## Hint
>
> ### THE SCOOP ON FROZEN YOGURT
>
> If you prefer your **YOGURT** in frozen form, keep in mind that the sweeteners and fruit added to frozen yogurt inhibit some of the beneficial cultures. Even so, most frozen yogurts are still a healthier choice than ice cream. They usually offer more calcium, less fat, and at least some active cultures. Choose a brand that mentions "active cultures" on the label. The government requires manufacturers to supply enough of the good guys to meet a minimum standard.

Fight the Fungus

The active cultures in **YOGURT** make a terrific topical treatment for these two common fungal infections:

■ **Athlete's foot.** Rub plain yogurt directly onto the affected skin. For good measure, eat a cup or two of yogurt each day until the pain and itch are gone.

■ **Nail fungus.** Coat the infected nail with a generous layer of plain yogurt, cover it with a piece of gauze or a bandage, and let it soak in overnight. Come morning, rinse off any residue. Repeat the procedure each night until your fungus has flown the coop.

Dairy Products

SPOTLIGHT ON
SKIN PROBLEMS

Looking to relieve skin woes ranging from sunburn to dry, itchy skin? I say "Cowabunga!" Or maybe *cow bonanza* would be a better term. That's because while Bessie and her gal pals provide the milk, Farmer Jones does the job of turning it into dairy products that can hold their own against the pricey stuff you'll find in the skin-care aisle. Take these dairy delights, for instance:

◆ Treat dry, cracked hands and feet to this nourishing routine: Mix ¼ cup of **BUTTERMILK** and ½ cup of dry milk to form a smooth paste. Using a small, soft paintbrush or pastry brush, spread an even layer onto each hand or your feet. Leave it on for 15 minutes, or until it's dried completely. Rinse with cool water, and pat dry.

◆ Make a **SOUR CREAM** mask that exfoliates, brightens, and moisturizes your skin, and also refines your pores, heals any irritation, prevents breakouts, and fades acne scars. The simple formula: Mix 2 tablespoons of sour cream, 2 tablespoons of raw honey, and 1 tablespoon of either unfiltered apple cider vinegar or fresh-squeezed lemon juice. Spread the mixture onto your just-washed face, and leave it on for 20 minutes. Rinse with tepid water, then cool water. Repeat no more than twice a week.

◆ Soothe sunburn with **YOGURT**. Grab a cold container of plain yogurt—preferably the whole-milk kind. Stir in 1 to 2 teaspoons of aloe vera gel, and slather the mixture generously onto the burned area(s). Leave it on for 15 to 20 minutes, or until it dries. Then gently wipe it off with a soft, damp cloth. Repeat the procedure as many times as necessary. Then step into the shower and rinse any residue off with tepid water.

◆ Hydrate dry winter skin and keep it itch-free. In a blender, mix 8 ounces of plain **YOGURT**, ¼ cup of raw honey, 2 teaspoons of bee pollen powder (available online), 2 teaspoons of lemon juice, and 1 teaspoon of hot-pepper sauce. Pour the mixture into a container with a tight-fitting lid, and store it in the refrigerator, where it will keep until the expiration date on the yogurt container. To use, gently rub it onto any dry, itchy patches as needed.

An Apple a Day Keeps Stroke at Bay

Yep, it's true—men and women who eat an **APPLE** every day have a lower risk of embolic stroke (the kind caused by blood clots blocking an artery in the brain) than those who don't bother biting into this fruit. Exactly why apples work this way isn't clear, but while you're waiting for science to figure it all out, eat another apple!

Back in the Day...

It's no surprise that old-timers coined the saying "An **APPLE** a day keeps the doctor away." While folks back then didn't know all the science behind it, they sure knew a good fruit when they found it! Apples contain a truckload of nutrients, enzymes, and biochemical compounds essential to good health. Studies have found that eating apples on a regular basis can help folks by relieving or preventing a lot of common health problems—for instance:

- Asthma
- Cardiovascular disease
- Colds
- Coronary heart disease
- Seasonal allergies
- Stroke

The Appeal of Peels

The best way to eat an **APPLE** is with the skin on. Why? Because apple skins are brimming with quercetin, a plant chemical that fights heart disease by preventing cholesterol from turning into the muck that plasters itself to your artery walls, setting you up for a heart attack. And quercetin helps fight cancer, too.

Boot Out Bad Cholesterol

If you have high levels of LDL ("bad") cholesterol, an increase in **APPLE** intake is just what the doctor ordered. Studies show that eating two large apples a day can reduce LDL cholesterol levels by as much as 23 percent. If you want to eat more, go for it! After all, you'd have to be chomping on apples day and night to eat too many.

Fiber on the Double

Dietary fiber comes in two types: soluble and insoluble, and **APPLES** deliver a sizable supply of both kinds. So what's the difference between the two? Just this:

■ **Soluble fiber** dissolves in water and combines readily with other substances to form a gel-like material that prevents fats and sugars from being absorbed into your body, which can help control diabetes and lower LDL ("bad") cholesterol.

■ **Insoluble fiber** does not dissolve in water. Rather, it absorbs bile and cholesterol in your intestines and carries them out of your body. Insoluble fiber can also help prevent constipation.

Send Artery Plaque Packin'

Arteriosclerosis, a.k.a. clogging of the arteries, is caused by plaque, a combination of LDL ("bad") cholesterol, calcium, fatty food substances, and other matter. It builds up over many years as a result of smoking, lack of exercise, and poor diet. If that description fits your lifestyle (but you haven't been diagnosed with the condition), keep clogs at bay with this old Slavic folk remedy: Once a day, drink a glass of **APPLE** cider boiled with a garlic clove.

Pick a Peck of Pectin

Every time you eat an **APPLE**, you consume the richest source of pectin—a natural fiber that not only controls diarrhea, but also decreases the likelihood of getting colon cancer, reduces high blood pressure, and helps prevent or even dissolve gallstones. What's more, it slows the absorption of nutrients into the bloodstream, thereby helping to keep blood sugar under control. (Diabetics, take note!)

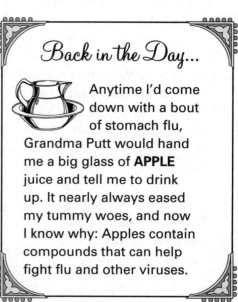

Back in the Day...

Anytime I'd come down with a bout of stomach flu, Grandma Putt would hand me a big glass of **APPLE** juice and tell me to drink up. It nearly always eased my tummy woes, and now I know why: Apples contain compounds that can help fight flu and other viruses.

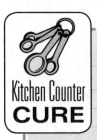

Kitchen Counter CURE

Juicy Flu Stopper

Before flu vaccines came along, folks relied on home remedies like this one to keep trouble at bay. It still works to fend off viruses that cause colds and flu. So even if you get your yearly flu shot, reach for this recipe at the first sign of symptoms.

1 large, tart, juicy APPLE
1 qt. of water
2 shots of whiskey
$\frac{1}{2}$ tsp. of lemon juice
Honey (optional)

Cut the apple into quarters and boil it in the water until it falls apart in pieces. Strain out the solids, and add the whiskey and lemon juice to the remaining apple liquid. Sweeten to taste with honey, if you like. Then get in bed and drink the toddy. If you've acted in time, by morning those germs should be history!

Clear Up Conjunctivitis

A lot of things can cause red, watery, or itchy eyes. But if your orbs are really irritated, it could indicate that you're coming down with conjunctivitis, a.k.a. pinkeye. If you act fast, an **APPLE** poultice just may stop the infection in its tracks. To make it, first dampen a piece of soft, all-cotton fabric that's about 12 inches square. Next, grate a large, peeled apple. Spread the pulp in the center of the cloth, and fold the sides over to form a rectangular mask. Then lie down, lay the poultice over your closed eyes, and relax for half an hour. Within a day or two, your eye problem should clear up. If it doesn't, then get medical help.

Gimme a Q!

Q is for quercetin, the plant chemical in **APPLES** that can relieve runny noses and watery eyes. The big Q also enhances physical endurance by making oxygen more available to the lungs. So if you eat an apple before you hop on the treadmill at the gym, take off on your bike, or hit the hiking trail, you may find that you have a lot more staying power, and that's something to cheer about!

Fresh Fruits

Apples against Alzheimer's

I think it's safe to say that for most folks, there is no more dreaded disease than Alzheimer's. Well, here's some good news: Eating at least two **APPLES** a day may cut your risk of getting this most common form of dementia. Research shows that the quercetin in the fruit helps protect brain cells from oxidation damage caused by free radicals that can lead to the onset of Alzheimer's. If that doesn't give you the incentive to up your apple intake, I don't know what will!

Boost Your Brainpower

Diseases aside (see "Apples against Alzheimer's," above), no matter what your age, you'll do the old gray cells a big favor if you add more **APPLES** to your diet. That's because these fruits contain plenty of boron, a potent mineral that stimulates brain cells, thereby helping you stay active, alert, and in tip-top mental condition.

Ease Your Achin' Joints

The next time your knees, elbows, or other joints start hurting—or, better yet, before the pain starts— eat a few **APPLES**. Their boron, the same trace element that kicks brain cells into high gear, can relieve joint pain and stiffness and actually seems to protect against arthritis.

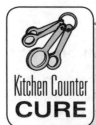

Kitchen Counter CURE

Gout-Be-Gone Preserves

Gout is a form of arthritis that results from the buildup of uric acid in the blood. As you know, if you're prone to this nasty disease, the symptoms can strike with the speed of lightning. This ultra-simple recipe can help relieve the pain and swelling by neutralizing the acid.

**4 APPLES
(any kind will do)
Water**

Peel, core, and slice the apples, put them in a pan, and add just enough water to cover the slices. Simmer them for three hours or more, until they turn thick, brown, and sweet, adding more water as necessary. Store the mixture in the refrigerator. Spread it on toast or bagels, use it as a condiment with chicken or ham—or simply put it in a bowl and dig in with a spoon!

SPOTLIGHT ON
WEIGHT LOSS

At one time or another, just about every American adult has been on a diet to lose weight. And many of us may succeed in dropping some pounds, only to find them creeping back up a few months (or years) later. In this never-ending battle of the bulge, it's time to enlist these fridge-friendly fruits:

◆ Believe it or not, eating **APPLES** actually subtracts calories from your diet. That's because the calories your body uses to break down the fiber in the apple exceed those contained in the fruit. Bottom line: The more apples you eat, the more weight you lose. Just don't get carried away—after all, man (or woman) cannot live by apples alone.

◆ Shed excess pounds painlessly with this tasty—and healthy— **APPLE** cocktail: Mix 64 ounces of 100 percent organic apple juice, 1/2 cup of unfiltered apple cider vinegar, and 1/2 teaspoon of liquid stevia (either plain or your favorite flavor) in a pitcher that has a tight-fitting lid. Store it in the refrigerator, and drink an 8-ounce glass of the tangy-sweet beverage before each and every meal.

◆ Mash an **AVOCADO** and mix it with lemon or lime juice and your choice of herbs. Then use it to replace higher-calorie spreads and toppings like mayo and cream cheese.

◆ Drinking a glass of lemonade (homemade from fresh-squeezed **LEMONS** and sugar is best) between meals can cleanse your system of toxins and impurities, conquer cravings for junk food, and speed weight loss.

◆ Studies show that smelling **STRAWBERRIES** before you exercise causes you to burn more calories. So before you head off on your next power walk, or hit the treadmill at the gym, pull some berries out of the fridge, and take a good long whiff!

Fresh Fruits

Apricots Attack Cancer

Yes, you read that right. **APRICOTS** are loaded with beta-carotene and other carotenoids, which help fight cancer. Here's how:

- **Beta-carotene** gobbles up free radicals, substances that cause cell damage, from fluids located inside and outside the body's fats.
- **Lycopene** may arrest the growth of tumor cells.
- **Other carotenoids** found in apricots may stimulate an enzyme in the immune system that breaks down carcinogens.
- **Diets rich in beta-carotene** may reduce the risk of breast cancer recurrence by one-third, and can also cut the risk of most cancers—including bladder, cervical, lung, and stomach—by about one-half.

Have a Happy Heart

Eating just three fresh **APRICOTS** a day can have heart-healthy benefits. The fruit's beta-carotene and lycopene fight a process that makes LDL ("bad") cholesterol even worse. One study has shown that a diet rich in these reduced the risk of heart disease by more than 20 percent.

Stave Off Stroke

Dried **APRICOTS** provide a heaping dose of potassium, a nutrient that helps lower blood pressure and reduce the risk of stroke. In fact, a 3 ½-ounce serving of these dried fruits has close to 1,400 milligrams of potassium—three times the amount found in a banana!

Back in the Day...

Here's a women's health tip that's been passed down over the years: To avoid getting a yeast infection, snack on **APRICOTS**. The beta-carotene may bolster your immune system enough to ward off infection (see "Apricots Attack Cancer," above, for more about this carotenoid). Studies have found that the vaginal cells of women with yeast infections had significantly lower levels of beta-carotene than did cells taken from women with no infections.

Avocado ABCs

Not so long ago, when folks were avoiding fatty foods like the plague, **AVOCADOS** wound up on dietary no-no lists nationwide. But now we know that while avocados are high in fat, 80 percent of it offers health benefits galore. What's more, these creamy green treats exceed every other fruit in certain plant compounds that may help prevent cancer and heart disease. So how can a food that's high in fat be good for you? Well, most of the fat in avocados is the unsaturated kind, which helps lower levels of LDL ("bad") cholesterol, while maintaining supplies of HDL ("good") cholesterol. It's as simple as that.

Deliver a Dynamic Duo

In addition to their beneficial fat, **AVOCADOS** contain healthy amounts of many essential vitamins and minerals. But the fruit's true superstar status lies in the fact that it contains much larger supplies of two powerful plant compounds:

HEALTHY Hint

LOSE THE BLUES

Whether the problem is caused by your monthly bout with PMS, a wintertime attack of seasonal affective disorder, or a simple case of the blahs, **AVOCADOS** can cheer you up fast. They contain potent supplies of serotonin and tryptophan, two compounds that help boost your brain's natural mood-lifting chemicals. So the next time you're feeling down in the dumps, slice an avocado, drizzle it with some lemon or lime juice, and dig in. *Note: If you're battling prolonged depression, rather than just a short period of the gloomy-doomies, don't fuss with dietary remedies—get professional help pronto!*

- **Beta-sitosterol** inhibits the absorption of cholesterol from your intestines into your bloodstream, thereby reducing your risk of heart disease. Research has also shown that beta-sitosterol can reduce inflammation, boost the immune system, and may hinder the growth of cancerous tumors.

- **Glutathione** is a powerful antioxidant that, among other feats, boosts the immune system, encourages a healthy nervous system, slows the aging process, and may help prevent heart disease, as well as cancers of the mouth and pharynx.

Fruity First Aid

You're cutting into an **AVOCADO**, the knife slips, and you slice into your finger. What do you do? Count your lucky stars, that's what—because you've got first aid at your fingertips. Just break off a little piece of the avocado flesh, and apply it to the cut. The fruit has antibiotic properties that will start working right away to heal the wound. Plus, the soft, mellow pulp will help ease the pain.

Foil Fat with Fat

Trying to drop a few pounds? **AVOCADOS** can help you reduce your calorie intake painlessly if you put them to work in two ways:

- **Spread it on.** Replace high-calorie spreads and toppings with mashed avocado. Simply mix it with lemon juice and Italian seasonings, or your favorite herbs and spices.

- **Bake with it.** Puree an avocado in a blender (or mash it thoroughly with a fork). Then replace either all or half the amount of butter called for in your recipe with the mashed avocado. Although you should notice little if any difference in flavor, the finished product will have a lighter texture and may have a slight greenish tinge.

HOW'S THAT?

Q *Jerry, my pal out in California told me they often make a pack out of AVOCADO leaves to help sore muscles after a workout. Have you heard of this?*

A As a matter of fact, I have. But you don't need to live in California—the leaves from a potted avocado plant will do the trick, too. This poultice will ease the pain of muscle strains and sprains, and headaches: Heat six or eight avocado leaves in water until they're warm, but not hot, and lay them in the middle of a piece of soft, all-cotton cloth that's about 12 inches square. Fold the sides in to form a rectangular pouch, and lay it on your achin' body part. Leave the poultice in place until it cools down. Repeat several times a day as needed. That's all there is to it!

Eat a Sports "Drink"

Amazing **AVOCADOS** contain approximately 60 percent more potassium than bananas, which makes them the heavyweight champion when it comes to relieving muscle cramps. So when your next marathon—or cutthroat badminton match—leaves you with a charley horse, don't down a Gatorade®; grab an avocado instead. (My favorite fast fix is to simply chop a small avocado or half of a large one, and toss the pieces with a half-and-half mixture of olive oil and balsamic vinegar.) Your muscles will say "Thanks!"

More Power from Potassium

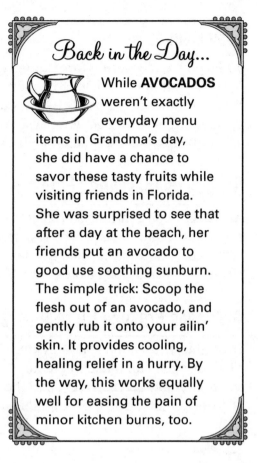

Back in the Day...

While **AVOCADOS** weren't exactly everyday menu items in Grandma's day, she did have a chance to savor these tasty fruits while visiting friends in Florida. She was surprised to see that after a day at the beach, her friends put an avocado to good use soothing sunburn. The simple trick: Scoop the flesh out of an avocado, and gently rub it onto your ailin' skin. It provides cooling, healing relief in a hurry. By the way, this works equally well for easing the pain of minor kitchen burns, too.

You don't have to be a weekend warrior to benefit from the potassium **AVOCADOS** offer up. Eating plenty of these creamy green fruits can help solve some of your most nagging health problems. Like these, for instance:

- **Fluid retention.** The potassium will counterbalance the sodium in your body and help reduce the excess fluids.

- **High blood pressure.** Potassium prevents the thickening of artery walls and also helps regulate your body's fluid levels, which are crucial to regulating blood pressure.

- **Insomnia.** Having trouble sleeping through the night? Eat avocados (and other potassium-rich foods) on a regular basis. This mighty mineral encourages deep, restful sleep.

Easy Does It

When you're recovering from surgery, or suffering from an illness that reduces your appetite level to near zero, pureed **AVOCADO** is just what the doctor ordered. It packs a boatload of the nutrients you need to build up your strength and get your system working smoothly again, yet its flavor and texture are mild enough to sit easy in sensitive stomachs.

Relieve Psoriasis and Eczema

AVOCADO oil contains sterolins that moisturize the skin, keeping it soft and hydrated. That's why it's a prime choice for treating the pain and itching of skin disorders like psoriasis and eczema. *Note: Avocado oil is available in health-food stores, herbal-supply stores, and online.*

Avocados Produce More Amore

Over time, the vagina's natural lubrication tends to diminish, and even slight dryness can make intercourse unpleasant or painful. The simple solution: Apply **AVOCADO** oil to the affected area. It'll solve the problem at a fraction of the cost of commercial products.

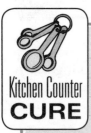

Kitchen Counter CURE

Avocado Healing Cream

Folks who use this powerful concoction claim it fights athlete's foot, eczema, and other skin irritations as well as or better than any commercial product they've found.

> 4 oz. of shea butter
> 2 tbsp. of AVOCADO oil*
> 2 tbsp. of olive oil
> 15 drops of tea tree oil

Combine the shea butter, avocado oil, and olive oil in a double boiler or heat-proof bowl, and heat until the shea butter melts. Remove from the heat, and stir in the tea tree oil. Pour the mixture into a lidded container, such as a small clamp-top canning jar or a 6-ounce herb-storage tin. Refrigerate to cool. Once the cream is firm, take it out of the fridge, and store it at room temperature. *Available in health-food stores, herbal-supply stores, and online.* Yield: About 1/4 cup.

To Your Berry Good Health!

The same compounds that give **BERRIES** their beautiful colors—namely anthocyanins—also earn them their standing in the superfoods category. All berries pack mega-supplies of anthocyanins, which have been shown to reduce the risk of chronic diseases by protecting the body's cells from damage. What's more, they can improve your eyesight and help ward off cancer and coronary heart disease.

Blackberries Battle Cancer

While all berries are great-tasting, healthy treats, **BLACKBERRIES** stand out from the crowd. Why? Because they contain compounds that can help fight cancer. Research shows they neutralize free radicals, the substances that damage cells and provoke cancer-causing mutations in our DNA.

Be Berry Kind to Your Heart

The catechins found in **BLACKBERRIES** help lower cholesterol levels, especially LDL cholesterol (the "bad" version). And when you reduce your cholesterol levels, you lower your risk of heart disease, so bulk up on blackberries!

THE BERRY BOWL

See how your favorite **BERRIES** stack up in vitamins and minerals. Nutritional values are based on a 3 1/2–ounce serving. The equivalent in cups is listed with each berry type.

BERRY	CALORIES	FIBER (g)	FOLIC ACID (mcg)	POTASSIUM (mg)	VITAMIN C (mg)
Blackberries (2/3 cup)	52	4	34	196	21
Blueberries (2/3 cup)	56	3	6	89	13
Raspberries (3/4 cup)	49	4	26	152	25
Strawberries (2/3 cup)	30	2	18	168	57

Fiber with Flavor

Now we all know how important fiber is in our daily diet. But you may not realize that you can get a hefty dose of it from **BLACKBERRIES**. In fact, these super berries pack a whopping 7 grams of fiber in a single cup, which equals one-third of what you need for the entire day— and they taste a lot better than bran! More good news: Fiber fills you up, so you feel satisfied on fewer calories. It also prevents constipation, helps reduce the risk of heart disease, and may even lower your chance of developing colon cancer. Not too bad for a berry!

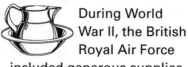

Back in the Day...

During World War II, the British Royal Air Force included generous supplies of **BILBERRY** jam in its pilots' ration kits. Why? Because these blueberry relatives are especially renowned for their power to sharpen your vision and help your eyes adjust quickly from light to darkness. Fresh bilberries are hard to come by in supermarkets, but they are widely available via the Internet in both dried and frozen forms—and they're well worth seeking out if you have eye problems of any kind.

Berries Ease Bursitis Pain

The flavonoids found in all dark-colored berries, including varieties like **BLACKBERRIES**, blueberries, boysenberries, and black raspberries, reduce inflammation and can ease the pain of bursitis—as well as arthritis and muscle strains. As for the amount, the more the better! With berries (or any other kind of fruit), there's no such thing as an overdose. Just make sure you regularly include them in your recommended minimum of five fruit and veggie servings per day.

Stop Hay Fever Right Now

When allergy season rolls around, that's the time to go berry picking. And nothing beats **BLACKBERRIES** for fighting hay fever. These plump purple berries contain ample amounts of quercetin (more than any other berry, in fact), and the big Q is what halts the production of histamine, the substance that makes allergy sufferers sneeze, wheeze, and generally feel miserable.

A Berry Brainy Idea

Studies suggest that eating **BLUEBERRIES** and strawberries regularly may improve your memory, enhance general brain function, and possibly reduce your risk of developing Parkinson's disease. But that's not all! Researchers have also found that eating two or more servings of these berries a week may delay cognitive aging by as much as 2 1/2 years.

Give Bruises the Blues

BLUEBERRIES are rich in bioflavonoids, which are essential for repairing blood vessels. Eating just 1/2 cup of the tasty blue fruits each day will not only speed the healing of your current bruises, but also strengthen your blood vessels so they're better able to fend off future damage. An added bonus: A serving of blueberries can also help reduce swollen varicose veins.

Squelch a Stomachache

The next time your tummy is all a-rumble, reach for a few tablespoons of dried **BLUEBERRIES**. Research has shown the berries can inhibit the ability of bacteria to stick around, helping to reduce the chance of a nasty infection in the lining of your stomach. Pass up fresh or frozen berries, though, because they can aggravate tummy troubles.

HOW'S THAT?

Q *I've heard something about* **BLUEBERRIES** *helping to cure a sore throat. What's the scoop? Do I have to eat a couple of bowls of berries a day?*

A No, this cure is the drinking kind. While plenty of beverages can ease the pain of a sore throat, one of the most effective comfort givers is blueberry juice. If you can't find 100 percent juice at your local supermarket or health-food store, liquefy a handful of fresh or frozen berries in a juicer, blender, or food processor, and drink up. (Add a little water to taste if the flavor is too intense.)

Pick Raspberries for Health

If you're looking for the one berry that can do you the most good, **RASPBERRIES** fit the bill. These small red gems are chock-full of a compound called ellagic acid that destroys cancer-causing chemicals in your body. Research is ongoing to determine if eating raspberries can:

- Reduce the number of colon polyps in people who are at risk for developing colon cancer

- Stave off cervical cancer in women at increased risk

- Fight cell division that causes breast, prostate, and skin cancer

Fruitful Fiber

Just 1 cup of **RASPBERRIES** packs about 6 grams of fiber—20 to 25 percent of what you need for the entire day. That's more than most other fruits provide, except for blackberries (see "Fiber with Flavor" on page 72), and raspberries have a mix of both soluble and insoluble fiber. The soluble type lowers cholesterol, while the insoluble fiber wards off constipation.

Send Allergies Away

RASPBERRIES are rich in quercetin, an antioxidant that helps block the production of histamine. That's the substance that causes the runny nose, itchy eyes, and sneezing during allergy attacks.

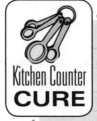

Kitchen Counter CURE

Raspberry-Leaf Tea

This is one of the most versatile—and effective—remedies for treating health woes.

4 cups of water
6 tbsp. of dried RASPBERRY leaves*

Bring the water to a boil, remove from the heat, and add the leaves. Steep for 40 minutes, then strain. Drink the tea hot, put it in the fridge to chill (it will keep overnight), or pour it into ice-pop molds and freeze. Use it to treat the following conditions:

- **For diarrhea,** drink the tea hot or cool, or eat ice pops throughout the day.

- **For high blood pressure,** drink 1 cup per day—hot or cold—for one week, then check your numbers.

- **For leg cramps,** drink 1 cup in the morning and 1 cup at night until cramps are gone.

- **For motion sickness,** drink 1 cup of cool tea twice a day.

* Available in health-food stores, herbal-supply stores, and online.

A Strawberry Boost

Besides being a yummy treat, **STRAWBERRIES** offer up a heap of vitamin C and other antioxidants. And how does that help you stay healthy? Here's the rundown:

- Vitamin C boosts immunity, making wounds heal faster and fending off heart disease and cancer.
- The antioxidants in strawberries may inhibit cancer of the esophagus.
- A Harvard study found that strawberry lovers were 70 percent less likely to develop cancer than those who rarely ate the fruit.
- Studies have shown that eating strawberries may help slow down memory loss as we age.

Berry Good Eye Protection

STRAWBERRIES can help prevent cataracts, the leading cause of blindness in the world. By age 80, more than half of all people in the United States will either have cataracts or undergo cataract surgery. You can do your best to beat those odds by indulging in strawberries every day. Their phytochemicals help strengthen the cornea and retina.

Fight Inflammation

Inflammation in your body can cause arthritis and lead to heart disease. One tasty way to reduce inflammation is to eat **STRAWBERRIES**. A recent study found that women who eat 16 or more strawberries a week are 14 percent less likely to have elevated levels of C-reactive protein, a major indicator of inflammation in the body.

Back in the Day...

Grandma Putt loved her **STRAWBERRIES**, but not just for her delicious pies! She knew that juice from freshly sieved strawberry pulp has a cooling and purifying effect that would bring down a fever. Her recipe: Chop a handful of berries, and whirl them in a blender with a little water. Then strain out the solids, and drink up. Repeat frequently until the thermometer registers a healthy 98.6°F.

Fight Athlete's Foot

When this irritating, burning fungus attacks your toes, fight back by gobbling up plenty of **STRAWBERRIES**. They're packed with vitamin C, which boosts your immune system and helps rout the nasty fungal infection.

Say "Ta-Ta" to Tartar

STRAWBERRIES contain chemicals that help prevent the buildup of tartar on your teeth, thereby fending off tooth decay and gum disease. You can put this healthy power to work in two ways:

1. Simply rub your teeth every few days with the cut face of a strawberry.

2. For a more thorough dental hygiene experience, mash a strawberry, dip your toothbrush in the pulp, and brush as you would with your regular toothpaste. In either case, wait at least half an hour before you rinse—or longer if possible—because the longer the berry juice remains on your teeth, the more effective it will be at removing tartar.

   One word of caution: Commercial strawberries are treated with high levels of pesticides; if you don't grow your own, be sure to purchase organic berries.

HEALTHY Hint

YOUR STRAWBERRY PREPAREDNESS PLAN

Attention, home **STRAWBERRY** growers—or you folks who buy your berries at a berry farm! For those times when you're fresh out of fresh strawberries, keep a supply of strawberry-leaf mouthwash on hand. The leaves contain many of the same plaque- and germ-fighting chemicals that make the fruits so good for your teeth and gums (see "Say 'Ta-Ta' to Tartar," at left.)

To make the brew, put 1 cup of fresh strawberry leaves into a heat-proof glass or ceramic bowl, and cover them with 1 cup of boiling water. Let it steep until the water has reached room temperature, strain it into another bowl, and mix in 2 teaspoons of either vodka or lemon juice (not both). Store the mixture in the fridge, and use it as you would any other mouthwash.

3 Cheers for Cherries!

Fresh, sweet **CHERRIES** are so much more than just a summertime snack. These superfruits should be in everyone's health-care arsenal. Here's why:

- **They fight dementia.** The flavonoids in cherries have antioxidant properties, which help protect brain cells and battle memory loss.
- **They're good for your heart.** Sweet cherries contain 270 mg of potassium, more than strawberries and apples. Potassium helps to prevent thickening of the artery walls and to regulate your body's fluids, thus reducing your risk of hypertension and stroke.

Chomp on Cherries

Need even more reasons to enjoy these delicious, sweet, juicy fruits? **CHERRIES** are chock-full of quercetin, a flavonoid that fights cancer and heart disease. They're also loaded with perillyl alcohol, which may help prevent the development of breast cancer and pancreatic cancer. And cherries are a good source of boron, which is important for bone health.

Sweet Arthritis Relief

You can spend a lot of time, money, and energy trying different ways to relieve arthritis pain and stiffness. But you may be able to solve the problem quickly and deliciously: Eat about 20 sweet bing **CHERRIES** every day. Before you know it, you could be moving smoothly again.

HOW'S THAT?

Q *A friend of mine swears that he sleeps better whenever he eats a bowl of CHERRIES after dinner. Is it all in his head?*

A As a matter of fact, no. Your friend really is sleeping better. Why? Because scientists have discovered that tart cherries contain significant amounts of melatonin, the brain hormone that fights insomnia. Lots of folks take melatonin pills, but I'd rather eat a bowl of cherries, wouldn't you?

Beat Blood Clots

Purple **GRAPE** juice, like red wine, is bursting with flavonoids. These plant compounds help prevent blood clots from clogging your arteries and causing a heart attack. One study showed that drinking just 5 ounces of 100 percent purple grape juice every day for a week reduced blood clotting by 60 percent—better than the reduction brought about by taking aspirin.

A Grape Way to Ease Arthritis Pain

GRAPE skins contain resveratrol, a natural compound that helps reduce inflammation caused by an injury or disease. A study published in *The Journal of Biological Chemistry* confirmed that eating 1 cup of either green or red grapes each day would increase your comfort level considerably. Drinking 100 percent purple grape juice (the recommended dose is one 8-ounce glass per day) does the trick, too.

More Great Grape News

Whether you eat them by the handful or drink 100 percent juice, **GRAPES** have these additional health benefits:

■ They improve blood flow by making arteries more flexible.

■ They decrease LDL ("bad") cholesterol by making it less likely to stick to artery walls.

Back in the Day...

Old-timers used this trick for healing stubborn cuts that just don't want to close up—but aren't infected. Their secret weapon: 100 percent **GRAPE** juice. Here's how to put it to work:

On your heel. Every night before bedtime, soak your foot for half an hour in a porcelain (not metal) bowl filled with enough grape juice to cover the wound. Pat dry with a soft cotton cloth, but don't rinse off the grape juice, and don't get the area wet when bathing.

Elsewhere on your body. Saturate a gauze pad in grape juice, apply it to the wound, and fasten it in place with adhesive tape. Replace the dressing every day, but don't wash the affected area.

Go for the Green

What fruit contains a boatload of vitamin C? Here's a clue: It's not orange. It's green. One medium **KIWI** delivers a whopping 250 percent of your daily requirement for vitamin C—more than twice of what an orange provides. An added bonus: This fruit offers three times the amount of vitamin E that an orange does. And both vitamins C and E act as powerful antioxidants in your body, gobbling up free radicals that can cause cancer, heart attack, stroke, and diabetes.

I Can See Kiwi

In addition to its powerful anti-oxidant vitamins (see "Go for the Green," above), **KIWI** holds another disease-fighting weapon: lutein, which is a powerful carotenoid that's also found in your eyes. Research suggests that lutein may protect your eye tissues from damage that leads to age-related macular degeneration (AMD), the leading cause of blindness in Americans over age 60.

Good Things in a Small Package

In addition to vitamins C and E, the **KIWI** also offers these nutrients:

- **Copper.** It's essential for a strong immune system.
- **Folate.** This B vitamin is important for preventing birth defects.
- **Magnesium.** For bone formation and the regulation of heart rhythm.
- **Potassium.** It's critical for blood pressure control.

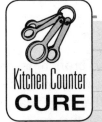

Kitchen Counter **CURE**

A Quick Kiwi Course

If you're not familiar with **KIWI**, here are some tips for buying and preparing:

- When buying kiwi, pick up the fruit and gently press it. It should be slightly soft. Avoid fruit that is very soft; it's overripe and will spoil quickly.

- It's okay to buy kiwi that is still firm. To ripen, put it in a brown paper bag and leave it on your kitchen counter away from direct sunlight and heat. You can add an apple, pear, or banana to the bag to speed ripening. Once the fruit has softened, store it in the refrigerator and use it within a few days.

- To enjoy kiwi, simply cut the fruit in half and scoop out the green flesh with a spoon. Or peel the fruit and cut it into slices.

Bash Bronchitis

When a cold turns into bronchitis, and the tubes in your windpipe become so inflamed and swollen that breathing is a chore, reach for a **LEMON**. Scrub it well, grate 1 teaspoon of the rind, and add it to 1 cup of just-boiled water. Let it steep for five minutes, and sip it down. It will help clear the mucus and bacteria out of your respiratory system. Repeat as needed throughout the day until you're breathing freely again. *Note: Anytime you use citrus peels in an oral or topical remedy, opt for organic produce if at all possible. And, organic or not, always scrub the skins thoroughly.*

Nix the Nausea

The next time you feel as though you're going to vomit, mix a few drops of **LEMON** juice, $1/2$ teaspoon of sugar, and a pinch of baking soda in an 8-ounce glass of water. Drink it down, and heave a sigh of relief because the contents of your tummy will now stay right where they are.

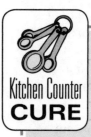

Kitchen Counter CURE

Classic Lemonade

Whether you're making **LEMONADE** to address a medicinal purpose or simply to sip it on your front porch as you watch the world go by, this is the ultimate, old-time recipe.

1 cup of water (for the simple syrup)
1 cup of sugar (or less to taste)
1 cup of fresh-squeezed lemon juice (4–6 lemons)
3–4 cups of cold water (to dilute)

Make a simple syrup by heating 1 cup of water in a pan, and then stirring in the sugar until it's dissolved. Mix the syrup and lemon juice in a pitcher, and add enough cold water to reach the desired strength. Refrigerate, covered, for 30 to 40 minutes. Then take a sip. If the lemonade is too sweet for your liking, add more lemon juice, and use less sugar next time. Serve it up in ice-filled glasses, garnished with lemon slices. *Note: Feel free to multiply the ingredients if you're serving a crowd, but stick to the same proportions.* Yield: 6 servings

Battle a Bladder Infection

If you've ever suffered from a bladder infection—or have one now—you know how important it is to drink plenty of water so that you can flush the impurities from your system. Well, here's a hot tip: You'll speed up that outflow and get back into the pink of health faster if you add a couple teaspoons of **LEMON** juice to each glass of water. You say you don't like the taste of lemons? Cut the dose to 1 teaspoon per 12 ounces of water. Any lemon juice is better than none.

Purge Your Gallbladder

Your gallbladder's mission in life is to store the bile produced by your liver, largely to aid in the digestion of fats. But it doesn't always function smoothly, especially if you eat a lot of fatty foods. So if you wake up feeling tired and nauseated, there's a good chance that your gallbladder has gotten clogged with stale bile and other pollutants. The simple remedy: Take 3 tablespoons of **LEMON** juice 15 to 30 minutes before breakfast each day for a week.

Stop Indigestion in Its Tracks

Spicy foods aren't the only kinds that cause acid indigestion. An overdose of sweet goodies can bring on that burning pain, too. Fortunately, there's a simple way to ease the discomfort. Just mix the juice of half a **LEMON** in 1 cup of warm water, add ½ teaspoon of salt, and drink the potion slowly. To treat chronic indigestion, drink the juice of one fresh-squeezed lemon in a glass of lukewarm water after each meal. The lemon will stimulate the production of gastric juices and the activity of your stomach muscles. By the way, this bracing tonic will also help cleanse your system of toxins and impurities

Cut Your Risk of Skin Cancer

A study at the Arizona Cancer Center found that regularly drinking black tea with **LEMON** slices added to it may reduce your lifetime risk of developing squamous cell skin cancer by (are you ready for this?) as much as 70 percent. Scientists speculate that the secret lies in d-limonene, an antioxidant in lemon peels that has been proven to kill cancer cells. So do as our English cousins do, and always take time for tea. Just remember, this is not intended as a substitute for sunscreen!

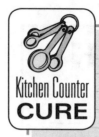

Kitchen Counter CURE

Conquer Cuts

When you cut yourself in the kitchen, help is close at hand. Slice a **LEMON** in two, squeeze some juice onto the wound to disinfect it, then run cool water over the area to stop the sting. Finally, sprinkle powdered cloves over the spot to reduce the pain and help the cut close up more quickly. *Note: This treatment also works like a charm on paper cuts.*

Give Headaches the Squeeze

How? Simply drink a cup of coffee with a few drops of fresh-squeezed **LEMON** juice mixed into it. Sip it slowly, and before you know it, your headache will be history. *Note: Do not use this remedy if you have a sensitive stomach.*

Citrusy Cold Stopper

If you enjoy a spot of rum now and then, you'll love this cold cure: At the first sign of symptoms, mix the juice of 1 **LEMON** with 4 teaspoons of rum (either dark or light) and 3 teaspoons of raw honey. Pour the mixture into a glass of hot water, drink it down, and hop into bed. When you wake up, you should feel as fit as a fiddle.

Calm a Sore Throat

Don't suffer needlessly when it hurts to swallow. Instead, mix the juice of half a **LEMON** and 1 teaspoon of pure maple syrup in 1 cup of warm water, and drink it down. It'll relieve the pain pronto. This same remedy loosens any mucus in your throat and nasal passages to boot!

Real Lemon-Aid

When you're wielding a weapon as powerful as a **LEMON**, it doesn't take much to make a big difference in your health. Just look at some of the pesky problems a lemon wedge or a few drops of fresh-squeezed lemon juice can help you solve—fast.

- **Bee stings.** First, get the stinger out, and then squeeze a few drops of lemon juice onto the sting site. If you've responded quickly enough, you'll head off any pain and swelling.

- **Cold sores.** Dab a little lemon juice on them. Yes, it will burn at first, but your discomfort will last only a few seconds, and the sores will soon be gone.

- **Hiccups.** Tuck a thin slice of lemon under your tongue. Suck it once, hold the juice for 10 seconds, and then swallow it (the juice, not the lemon). Your hiccups will be history!

- **Motion sickness.** Whenever you head off on a car or boat trip, take along a supply of lemon wedges. Then, at the first sign of queasiness, pull out a wedge and suck on it for a minute or two. That should chase the butterflies away.

- **Nosebleed.** Saturate a cotton ball with lemon juice, and gently insert it into the bleeding nostril. The flow should stop instantly.

- **Tired, strained, or burning eyes.** Mix a drop of lemon juice and 4 tablespoons of distilled water (not tap water!) in an eyecup. Wash your eyes with the solution, and you'll be back in business again.

HEALTHY Hint

WHOA, CHARLEY

There are few more annoying, out-of-the-blue ailments than the shooting pain and stiffness of a charley horse. The next time you suffer an equine muscle attack, try this highly recommended healer: Chop three small **LEMONS**, two small oranges, and a small grapefruit, and toss them (peels and all) into a blender or food processor. Pulverize the fruits into a pulp, and mix in 1 teaspoon of cream of tartar. Pour the mixture into a jar with a tight-fitting lid, and store it in the refrigerator. Then take 2 tablespoons of the concoction mixed with 2 tablespoons of water twice a day, first thing in the morning and just before bedtime.

Heal Hemorrhoids

There are scads of folk remedies for hemorrhoids, but legions of folks swear by this old-time favorite: Mix the juice of half a **LEMON** in 1 cup of warm water, and add 1/4 teaspoon of ground nutmeg. Drink the potion twice daily. It works its magic by shrinking the swollen blood vessels that cause the pain and itching, so you'll soon be sitting pretty.

Boost Iron Intake

We all know that it's important for women of childbearing age to have a steady supply of iron in their diets. But teenage girls are at ultra-high risk for iron-deficiency anemia—especially those who have gone vegetarian or decided that they absolutely must lose a few pounds to fit into their size 1 jeans. If you have a daughter or granddaughter who falls into this category, here's one way to help her meet her iron quota: Serve plenty of iron-rich, leafy greens, and douse them generously with **LEMON** juice. Besides perking up the flavor, the lemon will help liberate the minerals, thereby enabling her body to absorb the iron more efficiently.

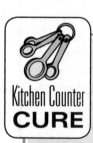

Kitchen Counter
CURE

Electrolyte-Replacement Tonic

Even a mild attack of vomiting or diarrhea whisks crucial fluids and electrolytes right out of a child's body. But this **LEMON** potion will put them back where they belong. Plus, it's healthier and a whole lot cheaper than commercial versions. By the way, adults will benefit from this tonic, too.

> 1 cup of warm water
> 2 tsp. of sugar
> 1 tsp. of sea salt
> 4 cups of lemon juice*

Pour the water into a jar or pitcher, add the sugar and salt, and stir until they're dissolved. Then mix in the lemon juice. Store the tonic, covered, in the refrigerator. After each occurrence of vomiting or diarrhea, pour 2 to 3 ounces of the tonic into a glass, and have the child sip it down. *Preferably fresh squeezed, but in a pinch, frozen lemon juice will do.* Yield: About 5 cups

Time for Lime

When your throat hurts so badly you can hardly swallow, then it's time to try this tasty sore-throat remedy: Mix the juice of 1 fresh-squeezed **LIME** with 1 tablespoon of pineapple juice and 1 teaspoon of raw honey in a glass of water, and drink it down. Repeat as necessary throughout the day and you'll soon be whistling "Dixie."

Stop a Throbbing Headache ...

And I mean instantly! Now this may sound a bit odd, but trust me, it works. Slice a **LIME** in two, and rub one of the cut surfaces across your aching forehead. Zap—end of pain! *Note: If this doesn't do the trick and your head continues to pound for two days or more, call your doctor.*

Dry Up Diarrhea

Next time you're rammed with a case of the runs, give this tangy but effective recipe a try: Squeeze two or three **LIMES**, and pour the juice into an 8-ounce glass. Add enough water to fill it, and stir in 3 teaspoons or so of cornstarch (more if your "plumbing" is especially energetic). Add sugar to taste if you like, and drink up. Repeat once or twice if you need to (but you probably won't).

Keep Your Gums Healthy

LIME peel contains compounds that fight gum disease and whiten your choppers at the same time. The simple routine: Cut a wedge of the fruit, remove the skin, and wipe the inside of the peel over your teeth and gums. *Note: Lemons and oranges perform the same dandy dental work—just be sure to use organic citrus fruits.*

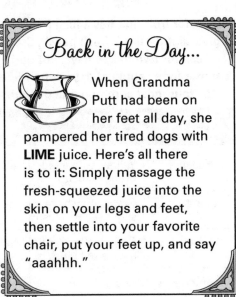

Back in the Day...

When Grandma Putt had been on her feet all day, she pampered her tired dogs with **LIME** juice. Here's all there is to it: Simply massage the fresh-squeezed juice into the skin on your legs and feet, then settle into your favorite chair, put your feet up, and say "aaahhh."

Much Ado about Mangoes

One of the most commonly eaten fruits in the world, **MANGOES** originated in Southeast Asia more than 4,000 years ago, and have been used in folk remedies ever since. If you're wondering why they've had such staying power, the answer is simple: They're loaded with vitamins A and C, nutrients that help fend off cancer and heart disease.

Thwart a Troubled Tummy

Have an upset stomach? Nibble on some fresh **MANGO** slices. The fruit contains an enzyme that can act as a digestive aid. Mangoes are also relatively rich in fiber, which improves digestion by helping food move quickly through the digestive tract.

Aid for Eyesight

Much like their kiwi cousins (see "I Can See Kiwi" on page 79), **MANGOES** contain the antioxidant lutein, along with zeaxanthin, both of which help protect vision. They work by warding off age-related macular degeneration (AMD), the leading cause of blindness in older folks in the United States.

THE MANY FACES OF MANGO

Look for fruit that has a lush fragrance. Press the flesh; a ripe **MANGO** will give slightly, like a fresh peach. Store ripe fruits in the fridge, where they'll keep for two to five days. Put unripe fruit in a paper bag on the kitchen counter for a couple of days; when ripe, transfer to the fridge. Here's a look at the four most common mango varieties available in most grocery stores.

MANGO VARIETY	COLOR WHEN RIPE	FLAVOR	FIBER CONTENT	AVAILABILITY
Haden	Yellow, with a red-orange blush	Mild	Medium	February–June
Keitt	Green; may have a slight yellow blush	Rich	Low	July–September
Kent	Green-yellow; may have a red blush	Very sweet	Low	June–August
Tommy Atkins	Red	Mild	High	April–July

Heart-Happy Oranges

Here's good news for all of you OJ lovers. One study found that women who drank **ORANGE** juice daily got a heart-happy surprise: Their levels of HDL ("good") cholesterol rose by 21 percent. Red wine and dark chocolate are the only other foods known to raise HDL. Orange you glad you know?

Oranges and the Big C

We're all aware that **ORANGES** are high in vitamin C. In fact, just one large orange or a 6-ounce glass of fresh-squeezed orange juice contains your entire daily requirement for the Big C. And while the jury's still out on whether or not vitamin C fights the common cold, we do know that it can:

■ Create collagen, which holds calcium in your bones and teeth

■ Delay the appearance of wrinkles

■ Improve the absorption of iron

Orange Aid for Troubled Tummies

When a bout of nausea or stomach flu strikes, mix $1/2$ cup of fresh-squeezed **ORANGE** juice, 2 tablespoons of clear corn syrup, and a pinch of salt in $1/2$ cup of water. Store the potion in a covered jar in the refrigerator, and take 1 tablespoon every half hour or so until your queasiness is gone.

HOW'S THAT?

Q *Hey, Jerry, do you have any tips for making it through the morning after a night on the town? And please don't tell me I have to swallow a raw egg in a glass of booze.*

A I sure do—and don't worry, I'm not suggesting that you try the old "hair of the dog" cure for a hangover! Instead, prop yourself up at the kitchen counter, and squeeze a glass of fresh **ORANGE** juice. Then mix in 1 teaspoon of fresh-squeezed lime juice and a pinch of cumin, and drink up. Cheers!

Tropical Treasure

PAPAYA is a tropical treat that's available all year long. And if minimizing heart disease and reducing high blood pressure are high on your to-do list, then have a papaya today. It's packed with these nutrients:

- **Folate.** This is the B vitamin that tames homocysteine, which, at high levels, can trigger a heart attack.

- **Potassium.** This mineral is important for lowering blood pressure—and there's more of it in a papaya than in a banana!

- **Vitamin C.** It may help prevent LDL ("bad") cholesterol from clogging your artery walls, and may help your wounds heal faster after surgery. And a papaya has more C than a glass of OJ.

Boost Your Immune System

Fruits, especially **PAPAYA**, top the list of foods that release beta-carotene. And those carotenoids can boost your immune system and protect you from just about anything that can kill you, including cancer. Plus, papaya can help beat vitamin A deficiency, a threat to your vision and skin.

Halt Hiccups

The next time you get a case of the hiccups, eat **PAPAYA**. Its digestive enzymes will quickly relieve your distress. By the way, these same enzymes can help quell belching and bloating, too.

HEALTHY
Hint

COLOR COUNTS

When it comes to choosing **PAPAYAS**, color is key. Look for fruits that are about half yellow. As they ripen, they'll begin to glow a beautiful yellow-orange color. Skip fruit that is all green—that color is a dead giveaway that they've been picked too soon, and your papayas may never ripen. At home, place your fruit in a paper bag with a banana to speed ripening. When the papayas are about three-quarters golden, they'll give slightly when you press near the stem. If they feel soft and mushy, you've waited too long. Cut into the papaya lengthwise, scoop out the black seeds, and the yellow-pink flesh is ready to eat.

Dodge Indigestion

PAPAYAS break down the food compounds in your stomach that cause indigestion. So if you have a chronically slow digestive system, give it a jump-start each morning by eating half a papaya or drinking a glass of 100 percent papaya juice. Or, if you feel discomfort only after you've eaten rich food, down a glass of the juice half an hour or so before you indulge.

Papaya the "Plumber" to the Rescue

The same **PAPAYA** enzymes that ease your digestive discomfort (see "Dodge Indigestion," above) can also stimulate bowel movements. The next time you need to loosen things up, eat some papaya fruit or drink a glass of 100 percent juice to get things moving.

Tropical Booty for Black Eyes

Got a shiner? Eat fresh **PAPAYA** and/or pineapple for two or three days. Aim for at least 2 to 3 cups of diced fruit every 24 hours. The enzymes in these tropical fruits will help you lose the bruise.

If You Need the C…

Your best bet is to eat fresh **PAPAYA** to get the most vitamin C. Otherwise, feel free to enjoy the convenience of the frozen, canned, or dried-fruit options, as well as 100 percent papaya juice. All deliver beta-carotene and beta-cryptoxanthin, and the benefits they offer.

Back in the Day…

Grandma Putt certainly never ate a **PAPAYA**! In fact, most tropical fruits were foreign to her generation. Today, we have access to the world's produce and if Grandma did back then, she would have approved of papayas. And Grandma certainly would have eaten them as often as she could because the vitamin C in papayas is just what the doctor ordered to keep arthritis at bay. In fact, studies show that folks who don't eat vitamin C-rich foods are three times more likely to have arthritis than those who do. Bonus for older folks: Papaya is rich in vitamin A, too, which means it can help protect your aging eyes from failing.

Peachy-Keen Health Heroes

PEACHES are packed with vitamins A and C. Vitamin A helps your eyes see normally in the dark, and protects you from infection by keeping your skin and mucous membranes healthy. It also battles bad guys called free radicals, which cause cell damage that can lead to cancer and heart disease. Vitamin C also has an equally impressive list of accomplishments. It boosts your immune system, helps form and repair red blood cells, and protects you from bruising, cuts, and wounds. In short, this fuzzy fruit is a true health hero, so eat a peach!

Stop Sinusitis

If you've come down with sinusitis, pick up a **PEACH**. A study found that sinusitis sufferers might not be getting enough glutathione, an antioxidant compound found in peaches. So if your sinuses frequently flare up, add peaches to your daily diet.

Block Bronchitis

Tea made from **PEACH** leaves has expectorant properties and has been used for centuries in China to treat chest colds and bronchitis. To make the tea, steep 1 ounce of dried peach leaves (available online) in 2 cups of boiling water for 15 minutes. Strain out the leaves. Sip the tea while it's still hot to help break up congestion. *Note: Tea made from peach leaves can have a strong laxative effect and should not be taken during pregnancy.*

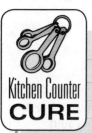

Kitchen Counter CURE

Whip Windburn with Peaches

To ease the pain of nasty windburn, slice a **PEACH** in half, and rub the juicy surface over your skin.

If you're constantly battling dry, flaky skin, make a more potent potion: Peel two peaches, remove the stones, and mash them in a bowl with a teaspoon of heavy cream. Add enough olive oil to make a smooth paste. Smear the mixture onto your face, wait 10 minutes, and rinse with lukewarm water. Follow this routine nightly throughout the winter months and you'll have smooth, clear skin!

Pear Away IBS

Irritable bowel syndrome (IBS) ranks right along with the common cold as a major reason why people miss work or school. Fortunately, IBS is not an actual disease, it does not lead to other, more serious intestinal conditions—and there are plenty of gentle, natural remedies that can relieve its painful spasms. One of the best is **PEARS**. Eating the fresh, ripe fruit can go a long way toward easing your discomfort.

Fabulous Fiber Filler-Upper

One of the healthiest things about **PEARS** is their high fiber content. In fact, they pack a 50-50 blend of the two main types of fiber—soluble and insoluble. The soluble fiber, called pectin, may help lower cholesterol levels, which is a critical way to reduce your risk of heart disease. Soluble fiber also helps bind together bile acids, enabling the pectin to draw cholesterol out of your blood.

Pears for Prostate Protection

Men, listen up. Eating one or two **PEARS** a day can do your prostate good. That insoluble fiber we mentioned earlier (see "Fabulous Fiber Filler-Upper," above) is called lignin. It helps bind up the male hormone testosterone, making it pass more quickly out of the body, and thus possibly lowering your chance of developing prostate cancer.

HEALTHY
Hint

DON'T GET SAD

No one is quite sure why some folks are troubled by seasonal affective disorder (SAD) while others are not, but we do know what triggers it: The absence of light during winter's gray days and long nights causes the pineal gland to turn the hormone serotonin into melatonin. The absence of serotonin disrupts normal sleep patterns and causes depression and a craving for sweets and starches. One of the best ways to alleviate those debilitating symptoms is to eat plenty of **PEARS**, apricots, plums, and apples. All of these tree fruits gradually raise serotonin levels and help keep them there—so you'll lose your desire to crawl into bed and hibernate.

Pineapple Paradise

Depending on the variety, one 4-ounce serving of **PINEAPPLE** has 25 to 150 percent of the vitamin C you need for the day. And, as you know from reading about the other fruits we've featured in this chapter, vitamin C is an antioxidant that gobbles up free radicals, the bad guys that cause cell damage that can lead to heart disease and cancer. It also revs up your immune system, so you can ward off colds, flu, and other infections.

Help Tackle Tumors

PINEAPPLE is also packed with bromelain, an enzyme that may help halt the spread of tumors. Studies suggest that bromelain especially holds promise in fighting lung cancer and leukemia, and testing is ongoing. In the meantime, it certainly can't hurt to add luscious pineapple to your list of anti-cancer foods.

Pineapple Puts Out the Fire

Did last night's bowl of chili have your stomach in knots? Next time you overindulge, eat a few chunks of **PINEAPPLE** or sip a glass of 100 percent pineapple juice after your meal. The bromelain in the fruit aids digestion and will give you relief without the side effects of OTC antacids.

HOW'S THAT?

Q *I've heard that* **PINEAPPLE** *can soften a callus. How's that work? Do I need to soak my hand in pineapple juice?*

A There's no need to soak for this helpful healer. To soften a hard callus, simply apply a piece of fresh pineapple rind, with the inside of the rind touching the callus, and cover it with an adhesive bandage to hold it in place. Leave it on overnight. In the morning, remove the covering and your callus should be a good deal softer. You can repeat the procedure for several nights until you get the results you want. It's an enzyme in the rind that does the trick.

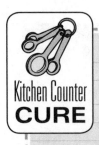

Quell Queasiness

When you're feeling green around the gills and can't even keep mild fluids down, reach for **WATERMELON**. Researchers at Brigham and Women's Hospital in Boston discovered that ice-cold chunks of watermelon went down easily—and stayed down— in pregnant women who had morning sickness. They still haven't figured out exactly why, but it does work!

Seeing Red

Red **WATERMELON** is rich in lycopene, a carotenoid that is being studied for its power to prevent various cancers. In fact, studies have found that men who ate the most lycopene and had the most lycopene in their prostate glands had the least chance of developing prostate cancer. While most of the men in the studies got their lycopene from tomatoes, cup for cup, watermelon delivers one-third more lycopene than fresh tomatoes do. These days, watermelon is available just about year-round. So, men, don't wait for a summer picnic to enjoy this healthful fruit.

A Natural Sports "Drink"

Absolutely nothing tastes as good as a big chunk of juicy, ice-cold **WATERMELON** after a long, hot afternoon of yard work. Watermelon is, after all, 90 percent water, so it goes a long way toward quenching your thirst. And the fruit's natural sugars boost your energy and get your blood sugar back to normal. What's more, like those sports drinks you can buy (but why bother?), watermelon contains potassium, which can help lower high blood pressure and is especially important for maintaining a normal heartbeat for people who take diuretics. The bottom line: Watermelon is a sweet, wonderful way to a healthy heart.

Make Mine Melon

The Chinese use **WATERMELONS**, cucumbers, and other members of the squash and melon families to reduce fluid retention. These foods— members of the cucurbit family—contain cucurbocitrin, which is said to increase the natural leakiness of tiny blood vessels in the kidneys. This means more water escapes into the kidneys for elimination.

The Broccoli Bunch

Like the Brady Bunch, **BROCCOLI** comprises at least six do-gooders: vitamin A, vitamin C, vitamin K, fiber, and the plant compounds lutein and sulforaphane. Many of these elements work together to provide broccoli's numerous health benefits. Chief among them: preventing cancer.

Prevent Prostate Problems

Studies have shown that eating three servings of vegetables a day can lower the risk of prostate cancer by an amazing 45 percent. But if some of those vegetables also happen to be **BROCCOLI**, men could drop their risk even further. So no more excuses, guys, go for the green!

Waylay Bladder Cancer

Here's more good news for men: An investigation of 50,000 men determined that those who ate a $1/2$-cup serving of **BROCCOLI** just twice a week reduced their chance of developing bladder cancer (the fourth-leading cancer, by the way) by 50 percent. In addition, research suggests that broccoli may cut the risk of colon cancer.

Broccoli Battles Heart Disease

Yep, that's right. Researchers found that women who ate **BROCCOLI** just once a week had half the risk of heart disease as those who didn't pile any on their plates. And you'll get these benefits whether you eat your broccoli raw, steamed, or in a stir-fry.

HEALTHY
Hint

BROCCOLI BONUS

As if fighting cancer and heart disease weren't enough, there's still more **BROCCOLI** benefits to shout about:

Prevent hip fractures. It's the vitamin K in broccoli that may help lower your chances of fracturing your hip.

Cancel cataracts. Since broccoli is high in lutein, which is important for eye health, eating this vegetable regularly may reduce your risk of developing cataracts as you age.

The Power of Kraut

Along with broccoli and kale, **CABBAGE** is a cruciferous vegetable. And while broccoli has gotten all the glory, cabbage is every bit as healthy. In fact, this much-maligned veggie is loaded with vitamin C—70 percent of the Daily Value! So don't shy away from putting cabbage on your plate.

Save Your Skin

Scientists have found that compounds extracted from **CABBAGE** may be a potent drug against melanoma, a type of skin cancer. The study found that when these compounds were paired with selenium, they target the proteins that trigger melanoma, and do so more safely than conventional drug therapy. While research is ongoing, it wouldn't hurt to add cabbage to your menu today.

Cabbage Cures Ulcers

For centuries, folk-medicine gurus have sworn by **CABBAGE** and cabbage juice as top-notch ulcer remedies. Well, recently, numerous medical studies have shown that drinking 8 ounces of 100 percent cabbage juice four times a day can heal both gastric and duodenal ulcers in anywhere from 2 to 10 days. Eating raw cabbage can perform the same miraculous feat. But if you'd rather not drink a quart of cabbage juice every day, you can substitute a wedge of raw cabbage, or about 1 cup of cabbage slices, for each 8-ounce cup of juice.

Back in the Day...

Whenever my Grandma Putt's arthritic knee started acting up, she went to the garden and cut a head of **CABBAGE**. Cabbage leaves have been used for centuries to soothe inflammation, and a sturdy outer leaf is just the right shape to place over a bent knee or elbow. Blanch a leaf (drop it into boiling water until slightly soft), then apply the leaf, either warm or cool, to your inflamed joint. Wrap it in gauze or an elastic bandage to hold it in place, and go about your business, pain-free.

Classic Help for Hemorrhoids

Remedies don't come much simpler than this old-time cure: Chop up a **CABBAGE**, lay the pieces on a towel, and sit on them for 30 minutes or so. And don't forget to take your pants off first!

Beat Back Boils

Boils can be as painful as all get-out, and hard to heal. Here's a simple cure: Cover the spot with a raw **CABBAGE** leaf. Hold it in place with a bandage or strip of cotton cloth, and leave it on for half an hour. Repeat several times a day, waiting two or three hours between treatments.

Keep Your Cool

As you baseball historians know, the great Babe Ruth had his share of superstitions and eccentricities, but at least one of them made a whole lot of sense: He stayed cool on the field and in the Yankees' non-air-conditioned dugout by wearing a **CABBAGE** leaf under his cap. He changed it for a fresh one every two innings. It still works—give it a try the next time you're puttering in the yard on a hot summer day.

Leaves Relieve Menstrual Cramps

Ladies, if you're prone to pain every month, do yourself a favor: Before and during your period, eat plenty of raw **CABBAGE**, lettuce, and other leafy greens. Not only will their nutrients help relieve your cramps, but their diuretic power will also help reduce bloating.

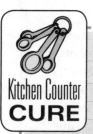

Kitchen Counter CURE

Cabbage Cools the Flames

Blanched **CABBAGE** leaves can reduce facial inflammation caused by burns, acne, or surgery. Once or twice a day, drop several leaves into a pot of boiling water for about a minute, or just until they soften. Cool, then apply the still-wet leaves to your face, and keep them on for 5 to 10 minutes. Since the leaves will be slippery, it's best to do this while you're slightly reclined.

You Can Count on Carrots

These bright orange veggies are packed with beta-carotene, which makes **CARROTS** tops for fighting cancer. Researchers have long known that folks who eat the most beta-carotene-rich fruits and vegetables have the lowest risk of lung cancer. Another plus: Beta-carotene helps build bones in children and keeps them strong in adults.

Develop a Drinking Habit...

For **CARROT** juice, that is—preferably made in your own home juicer or bought fresh from the machine at your local juice bar. Drinking an 8-ounce glass of carrot juice several times a week can work wonders for your health and well-being. Benefits include:

- Balancing your blood sugar levels

- Cleansing your liver

- Fortifying your blood and helping prevent anemia

- Guarding against the effects of secondhand smoke

- Helping fend off asthma attacks and other respiratory ailments

- Increasing the quantity and quality of a nursing mother's breast milk

- Nourishing your skin

- Preventing water retention

- Strengthening your immune system

Fresh Vegetables

HEALTHY Hint

COOK 'EM CRISP

Most folks think that to get the maximum health benefit from **CARROTS**, you should eat them raw. Not so! In fact, carrots are one of the few vegetables that release more of their important nutrients when they are either juiced or cooked whole (not sliced) until they are just tender-crisp. One example: A recent study at Newcastle University in England found that boiling carrots before slicing them increases their anti-cancer properties by 25 percent. Whatever you do, though, don't cook carrots longer than two to three minutes. If you overcook them (or any other vegetables), all their food value ends up in the cooking water.

Eradicate an Earache

If you've got an ache that just won't quit, grate a large **CARROT**, wrap the pulp in a piece of cheesecloth, and hold it against your ear for 15 minutes or so. The enzymes in the orange root will help draw out the infection that's causing the pain. Repeat every few hours until your misery is history.

Heal Bothersome Blisters

A blister is annoying enough at any stage, but when it's been punctured and becomes irritated, it's pure agony. Head to the kitchen, and grate a fresh **CARROT** or two. Apply the gratings to the afflicted area, and cover it with a warm, moist washcloth. Leave the carrots and cloth in place for 20 to 30 minutes. *Note: This remedy is also effective for clearing up weeping sores, skin ulcers, and cuts. But if the wound is already infected, get medical help ASAP.*

Back in the Day...

Grandma Putt—and even her grandmother—had no doubt that **CARROTS** can make your eyesight better. And now we know that's not just an old wives' tale, or a joke about rabbits not wearing glasses. Simply making carrots a regular part of your diet will indeed help keep your vision sharp. But to actually improve your faulty eyesight, do what country doctors have recommended for ages: Drink 5 to 6 ounces of 100 percent carrot juice twice a day for two weeks.

Douse Sore-Throat Flames

When a sore throat strikes, grate a **CARROT** and put it on a soft, clean cloth. Wrap it around your throat (with the gratings against your skin), and cover it with a scarf to keep it in place. To make the poultice even more effective, you can top it with either an ice pack or a hot compress.

Banish Bursitis Pain

When bursitis strikes, drink a 12-ounce glass of 100 percent **CARROT** juice with breakfast and lunch until you feel relief. The nutrients in the juice will help break down the sediment residue in your bursae that causes the inflammation.

Preserve Your Memories

Calling all ladies of, um, a certain age! During your childbearing years, your free-flowing supply of estrogen protects your memory by combating free-radical molecules that damage your brain cells. So what do you do when your estrogen levels wane during menopause? Feast on **CARROTS** and other veggies and fruits that are rich in antioxidants. You will soon find that you are better able to recall not only the names of your child-hood pals—but also where you put those darn car keys!

Prevent Gastrointestinal Worries

If you love beans, but you're not so fond of their infamous aftereffects, take an age-old tip from folks who live in the Appalachian Mountains: Whenever you cook your beans, toss a small whole **CARROT** into the pot or baking dish. Somehow, the orange root reduces the beans' gas production, so you can eat your fill of the healthful legumes without fear of polluting the air around you.

Calm Your Frazzled Nerves

After a long, hectic day, relax with a **CARROT** cocktail. Just mix equal parts of carrot and celery juice, and add honey to taste (plus a shot of Grand Marnier® if you'd like). Then sit back, relax, and drink up!

HOW'S THAT?

Q *Is it true that eating a lot of* **CARROTS** *will turn my skin orange? And is that dangerous?*

A Yes, consuming very large quantities of carrots or carrot juice over a prolonged period of time may cause your skin to turn orange. It's a perfectly harmless condition called carotenemia, and it will vanish when you cut back your intake. Unless you all but live on carrots and other orange or yellow veggies (like butternut squash and sweet potatoes), or you down more than 3 cups of carrot juice each day for months on end, you should have no problem.

Reduce with Cukes

CUCUMBERS aren't just something to slice into salads for a tasty crunch—they may help you lose weight. Researchers at Penn State University found that foods that take up a lot of room in your stomach yet have few calories can help you shed some pounds. Their theory is that when you eat these foods, you feel full, so you stop eating, even though you've eaten only a small amount of calories.

Soothe Sore Feet

When your feet feel so tired and achy that you don't think you can stand up for another minute, reach for three or four **CUCUMBERS**. Chop them up, toss the pieces into your blender or food processor, and whirl them into a thick pulp. Put an equal amount into each of two pans that are big enough to hold your feet. Then sit back in your chair, put a tootsie into each pan, and think lovely thoughts. You'll soon be ready to roll.

Relax and Smell the Cucumbers

Rather, I should say smell the **CUCUMBERS** and relax. Studies have shown that the scent of cukes helps you calm down during tense situations. The next time you're anticipating a stressful experience—say, a job interview or some medical tests—wash your hair with cucumber-scented shampoo, use cucumber-scented hand cream, and/or put a dab of it on a hankie or a piece of cloth to take with you.

Back in the Day...

Whenever I spent too much time at the ol' swimming hole and came home with a painful sunburn, Grandma Putt knew exactly what to do: She had me soak in a tepid bath with a few tablespoons of **CUCUMBER** juice added to it. (To make cucumber juice, just puree a cuke in the blender, strain out the seeds and pulp, and pour the juice into a bowl.) Cucumber juice also helps relieve the pain and itch of eczema. Just dab it onto your skin once a day with a cotton pad.

Spinach—A Sight for Sore Eyes

Because it supplies healthy doses of beta-carotene, vitamin C, lutein, and zeaxanthin, nothing can beat **SPINACH** for fending off three major eye problems: age-related macular degeneration (AMD), night blindness, and cataracts. Here's how it works:

■ **AMD and night blindness.** In a study of men with AMD who ate $1/2$ cup of cooked spinach four to seven times a week, most had improvements in night vision, contrast, and adjustment to bright light.

■ **Cataracts.** A Harvard study of 36,000 males found that those who ate the most spinach and broccoli had a lower risk of developing cataracts that were severe enough for surgical removal. And in a study of 50,000 females, those who most frequently ate spinach had a 22 percent decreased risk of severe cataracts.

Thanks for the Memories

When **SPINACH** isn't working overtime for eye health (see "Spinach—A Sight for Sore Eyes," above), it's busy tuning up other body parts like your brain. In fact, a diet high in spinach does your memory good. It's been found to boost memory in elderly rats, and more studies are ongoing. Spinach has also been found to improve motor learning—a skill that's especially important for stroke recovery.

HEALTHY Hint

EASE WOMANLY WOES

Ladies, when you eat your **SPINACH**, you can help battle these female health issues:

• **Fibroids.** Researchers in Italy found that women who ate less meat and more spinach and other green vegetables were the least likely to have painful benign uterine fibroids.

• **Ovarian cancer.** In German studies, spinach turned out to be one of the top veggies tested for their ability to prevent cells from turning cancerous. In a study at the University of Minnesota, women who ate the greatest amount of spinach and other green leafy vegetables had the lowest risk of developing ovarian cancer.

Fresh Vegetables

Fridge & Freezer Fixers

SPOTLIGHT ON
FATIGUE

If you toss and turn night after night, and struggle to stay focused during the day, you're not alone. More than 35 percent of Americans say they get fewer than six hours of sleep each night. In addition to the obvious dangers of chronic fatigue—nodding off while driving, industrial accidents, and difficulty performing daily tasks—people who don't get enough sleep are more likely to suffer from hypertension, diabetes, obesity, and depression. A healthy diet can go a long way toward sending you off to a good night's sleep, and helping you stay energized during the day. Be sure to eat plenty of these fatigue fighters:

◆ When you're tired and achy, whip up a salad with lots of **AVOCADO**. It's a great source of magnesium, which is the mineral used by your body to stave off fatigue and ease muscle pain.

◆ Fill your plate with **CARROTS**, **YAMS**, and other roots and tubers (along with grains, beans, fish, and poultry) to fight fatigue. Eating these nutrient-dense, unprocessed foods helps your immune system function at its optimal level, and gives you the energy to keep on truckin'.

◆ If you're stressed out and have a hard time falling asleep, eat more **CAULIFLOWER**. It provides lots of pantothenic acid, which is critical for keeping your adrenal glands in good working order whenever stress puts a strain on them.

◆ A steaming bowl of **GREEN BEANS** will help usher you into the Land of Nod. That's because they're an excellent source of potassium, which helps you fall asleep and stay asleep.

◆ Pass the **PEAS**. These little legumes are filled with protein, fiber, minerals, and vitamins—just what your tired body needs to get up and go again. Even a bowl of pea soup will give you the energy to get through your day.

CHAPTER 3

Pantry Pharmacy

Do you think your pantry shelves just hold the fixings for tonight's supper? Well, think again, because those jars, bottles, boxes, and cans contain ingredients that can clean your teeth, ease back pain, short-circuit a cold, discourage diabetes, hamper heart disease, help you lose weight, and much, much more!

BAKING SUPPLIES

Undermine Ulcer Pain

For decades, folks have turned to **BAKING SODA** to help ease indigestion. The same properties that make it work so well—namely, the ability to reduce your system's acidity—also make baking soda a natural for treating ulcers. The dose is 1 to 2 teaspoons in a glass of water whenever you feel discomfort.

Nix the Nicotine

Trying to quit smoking? Congratulations! Here's a tip that could help speed up your success: With each meal, drink a glass of cool water with 2 tablespoons of **BAKING SODA** mixed in it. The solution will reduce your cravings for those deadly cancer sticks.

Unstuff Your Nose

Does a nasty head cold have you all but glued to a vaporizer? Well, this simple additive will help clear things up in a hurry. Just pour 1 teaspoon of **BAKING SODA** into the water inside the unit. It'll unblock your nasal passages and keep your vaporizer clean, to boot!

Give Colds and Flu the Cold Shoulder

Old-timers knew a secret that the modern medical community has only recently rediscovered: Your body is best able to fend off health woes of all kinds, including infectious diseases, when your system is highly alkaline. In fact, back in the 1920s, doctors routinely prescribed a solution of 1/2 teaspoon of **BAKING SODA** mixed in a glass of cool water for patients who had come down with colds and flu (known in those days as the grippe). It works every bit as well today if you follow this schedule:

Day 1. Take one dose of the drink at roughly two-hour intervals for a total of six doses.

Day 2. Take one dose of the drink at roughly two-hour intervals for a total of four doses.

Day 3. Take one dose each morning and evening. Thereafter, drink a glass of the solution each morning until your symptoms are gone.

HEALTHY Hint

BAKING SODA CAUTION

Because of its high sodium content, **BAKING SODA** is not for everyone. To be on the safe side, if you are on a low-sodium diet, are over age 60, or are treating a child under the age of 5, be sure to consult your doctor before using any oral remedy that contains baking soda. On the other hand, topical potions are perfectly safe for use by people of any age.

Blast Body Odor

Stop the stench by dusting your underarms with **BAKING SODA**. It keeps your fridge odor free, and it'll do the same for you!

Conquer Cold Sores

When you're sick or stressed, out pops a cold sore. Try this old-time trick to clear them up in a hurry: Mix 2 tablespoons of **BAKING SODA** with enough water to make a thick paste, and cover the sore with a heavy coat of it. Reapply throughout the day as needed until your cold sore is gone.

Send Warts Away

Although they're harmless, warts sure are unattractive. The good news is that you don't have to use those smelly formulas from the drugstore aisle. Instead, turn to **BAKING SODA**. It will get the job done whether you're treating a single wart, or a whole passel of them. Here's how:

- **Single wart.** Make a paste of baking soda and water, apply it to the wart, let it air-dry, then cover it with a bandage. Repeat every day until the wart dries out and falls off.

- **Multiple warts.** Add a heaping teaspoon of baking soda to a quart of warm water and stir to dissolve. Wash your wart-plagued hand or foot with the potion, then let your appendage air-dry. Repeat several times a day until the ugly bumps have bugged off.

A Balm for Bug Bites

Ditch the itch and pain of bites and stings by dissolving 1 teaspoon of **BAKING SODA** in 1 cup of water. Then dip a clean cloth into the solution and hold it on the bite for 20 minutes.

Back in the Day...

All kinds of things can make your skin break out in hives and rashes. But no matter what caused the itchy red blotches, this old-time trick will send 'em packing in no time at all. Just add 1/2 cup of **BAKING SODA** to a tub of warm water, and settle in for a long, soothing soak (cool drink, glowing candle, and the latest best seller are optional).

SPOTLIGHT ON
GINGIVITIS

If your dentist has told you that you're at risk of having gingivitis—
or if you've already been treated for the disease and you want
to keep your gums in good health—these preventive potions
can help:

◆ Brush two or three times a day with a paste made from 3 parts
BAKING SODA and 1 part hydrogen peroxide. To perk up the
flavor, add a few drops of tasty extract, such as lemon, almond,
peppermint, or cherry.

◆ Mix ½ teaspoon of **BAKING SODA** with ¼ teaspoon of
goldenseal root powder (available in health-food stores and
online); then add the dry mixture to ¼ cup of warm water and
stir to dissolve. Swish the liquid around in your mouth and spit
it out. Use this remedy every day to keep gingivitis at bay.

◆ When your gums start bleeding, you need to see a dentist ASAP.
But while you're waiting for an appointment, **SALT** can help
stop the oozing. Just mix 1 part salt and 2 parts baking soda,
and stir in a few drops of tea tree oil. Then three times a day,
dip a damp soft-bristled toothbrush into the moist powder and
brush very gently.

◆ If your gums are sore, but not bleeding, **SALT** can still save
the day. The simple fix: Mix a pinch of salt into a tablespoon of
mustard oil, then dip your finger into the solution and gently
massage your sore gums in small, circular strokes. Gargle with
water. Repeat the treatment two to three times a day.

◆ To achieve your ultimate goal of having healthy gums and teeth,
turn to ground **CAYENNE POWDER**. Just add a pinch of the
fiery powder to your regular toothpaste each time you brush.
It may sting a bit or feel hot, but the cayenne helps to fight
bacteria in your mouth and put a stop to gum disease.

Starch Your Toes

If you frequently get blisters even though your shoes fit fine, it may be that your feet are too sweaty. To keep your dogs dry, splash a dash of **CORNSTARCH** into your socks before you put them on. Dust some between your toes, too, and you'll step a lot more lively! By the way, this same routine also helps to prevent athlete's foot.

Overcome the Ouch of Sunburn

Sunburn often strikes the areas at the edges of your bathing suit—the easy-to-forget, but oh-so-tender spots that you've neglected to smear with sunscreen or tanning lotion. Unfortunately, those burn spots will have to suffer daily irritation from bras and underwear. To reduce chafing, dust the area(s) thoroughly with **CORNSTARCH**. And whatever you do, don't mix the cornstarch with petroleum jelly or oil of any kind; that will only make the burn worse by blocking your sore pores.

Blissful Blister Relief

If your hands are prone to blisters—but you're not a fan of wearing gloves when you work in the garden—have I got the solution for you! Before you head out to do your chores, simply rub a generous tablespoon or so of **CORNSTARCH** onto your palms. The powdery stuff absorbs perspiration and will help prevent blisters from forming as you go about your garden tasks.

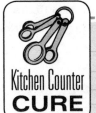

Kitchen Counter CURE

Take the Sting Out of Bites

If you spend much time working or playing in the great outdoors, you're bound to pick up your share of poison-plant rashes, bee stings, and insect bites. Regardless of which mishap befalls you, this remedy will ease your discomfort. Simply mix **CORNSTARCH** with enough lemon juice to make a paste (for a single insect bite, 1 or 2 teaspoons of cornstarch will do the trick). Rub the paste gently onto the problem spots. Presto—end of pain and itch! *Note: If the rash is from poison oak, ivy, or sumac, wash your hands thoroughly after applying to avoid spreading your trouble.*

Bust Blood Pressure Highs

Here's a routine that may help lower your blood pressure. Three times a day (with each meal), drink a potion made from ½ teaspoon of **CREAM OF TARTAR** mixed with ½ teaspoon of lemon juice in 8 ounces of water. *Note: This regimen is not meant to replace medical treatment. If you have high blood pressure, check with your doctor before you use this potion.*

A Hasty Halt to Hives

A friend of mine who is prone to breaking out in hives for no apparent reason swears by a remedy she found in her great-grandma's cookbook—you may want to give it a try for yourself or a loved one: Before breakfast, mix 1 teaspoon of **CREAM OF TARTAR** in an 8-ounce glass of water, and drink up. In no time flat, you should be itch-free. *Note: This trick works best if you use it as soon as the hives first appear.*

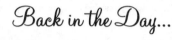

Back in the Day...

In the days before antibiotics, one popular "drug" for combating urinary tract infections was **CREAM OF TARTAR.** To ease your discomfort, dissolve 1 tablespoon of cream of tartar in 8 ounces of lukewarm water, and drink the potion three times a day. *Note: This formula is not meant to replace medical treatment. If you suspect that you have a urinary tract infection, see your doctor ASAP!*

Relaxing Bath Blend

Stress can not only ruin your day, but do some serious damage to your heath, too. So be sure to take some time for yourself. And nothing beats a long, relaxing bath to set you right. Make up a batch of this magical mixture, and keep it on hand for instant relief whenever you've had a stress-filled day. Simply mix 2½ cups of baking soda, 2 cups of **CREAM OF TARTAR**, and ½ cup of cornstarch. Store the blend in a covered container. When you feel the need, fill your bathtub with warm water, and stir in ¼ cup of the mixture. Then settle in, and soak your worries away. This makes enough for about 20 baths.

HEALTHY Hint

BAKING-SUPPLY BUDDIES

Baking soda and cornstarch aren't the only dry ingredients on your pantry shelves. Check out these homemade healers that use brewer's yeast, cornmeal, and more.

Vitamin-packed popcorn. Bet you never thought of popcorn as a health food. Well, it can be when you toss it with **BREWER'S YEAST**, which packs a hefty load of B vitamins, minerals, and essential amino acids. Just mix 1 tablespoon of brewer's yeast flakes with 1 teaspoon of dried onion flakes, 1 teaspoon of Old Bay® Seasoning, and 1 teaspoon of red-pepper flakes in a big bowl. Add your favorite popcorn and toss until thoroughly coated. Then dig in, and enjoy!

Diarrhea deterrent. If you've got a case of diarrhea caused by antibiotics, or have other intestinal distress, **BREWER'S YEAST** can provide relief. Take 1 to 2 tablespoons daily, either sprinkled on food, or mixed into water or juice.

Mealy cramp relief. The next time you're struck with a severe case of stomach cramps, use this folk remedy: Put 1 teaspoon of **CORNMEAL** in a mug, and add 1 cup of boiling water to it. Let it sit for five minutes, then stir in salt to taste, and drink the potion slowly.

Boil banisher. To relieve the pain and discomfort of boils, bring ½ cup of water to a boil, and stir in enough **CORNMEAL** to make a thick paste. Apply it to the boil, and cover it with a cloth or bandage. Repeat every one to two hours until the painful bump comes to a head and drains away.

Rolling sleep remedy. Here's a cure for sleeplessness that relies on a simple kitchen utensil—a wooden **ROLLING PIN**. Just lay it on the floor in front of your favorite chair, sit back, and take off your shoes (and your socks, if you like). Then put both feet on the pin, applying as much pressure as you can tolerate, and roll your tootsies back and forth for three minutes. Repeat each evening, within an hour or two of bedtime, and within a week you should be getting a full eight hours of shut-eye every night.

Relieve Skin Woes

If you have eczema or psoriasis, you know these conditions are rather annoying and unsightly, too. To moisturize scaly patches, gently wipe **VEGETABLE SHORTENING** onto the affected skin. You'll feel almost-instant relief from pain and roughness. Repeat the application every time after you wash your hands.

A Short(ening) Course on Wart Removal

There are more homegrown wart-removal methods than you can shake a stick at. And here's another: Mix 2 tablespoons of **VEGETABLE SHORTENING**, 1 chopped garlic clove, and ½ tablespoon of lemon juice in a bowl. Spread the mixture onto the wart, and cover with a piece of duct tape. Leave it on for 12 hours, then remove the tape and wash the cream off. Repeat daily until the wart is gone.

HOW'S THAT?

Q *I love cooking with my grandmother's cast-iron skillet, not only for the way it makes my food taste, but also because I know it adds iron to the food. But the pan's gotten rusty and I need to reseason it. Do you have any time-saving tricks?*

A I agree there's nothing better than a well-seasoned cast-iron pan. Did you know that it helps distribute heat better, so food cooks more quickly, preserving essential nutrients? But seasoning cast iron is not a quick job. Here's my no-muss, no-fuss method: Start by giving the pan a good, thorough cleaning with hot water, baking soda, and a nonabrasive plastic scrubbie. Then thoroughly rinse and dry the pan and immediately coat it with cooking oil to prevent the rust from reappearing.

To season, coat every inch of the skillet with a thin layer of **VEGETABLE SHORTENING.** Set the oven to 300°F and heat your pan for about an hour, or until the shortening is absorbed. Be sure to oil your pan after every use to keep rust at bay.

Bread Beats Diabetes

Whole-wheat **BREAD**, that is. Because whole-wheat—not white—bread retains the bran and wheat germ, it's loaded with vitamins, minerals, and fiber. And studies have shown that whole grains and cereal fiber appear to protect older women from developing type 2 diabetes. So pass the white and grab the wheat!

Put Mold to Good Use

When you have a cut that may be infected and you can't get to the drugstore for antibiotic ointment right away, try this stopgap measure: Soak a few slices of slightly moldy **BREAD** in condensed milk or half-and-half, apply the poultice to the wound, and fasten it on with a gauze bandage and adhesive tape. Change the dressing daily until the inflammation and redness are gone. If you don't see improvement after 48 hours, see your health-care provider.

A Dynamic Dietary Duo

Some food combos go together like, well, peanut butter and jelly. With a minor alteration to this lunchtime classic, you can add valuable nutrients to your diet. The simple fix: Nix the jelly, and spread your peanut butter on whole-grain **BREAD**. The payoff: This nutty, chewy sandwich packs all nine of the amino acids that your body needs to build muscles, bones, and hormones.

HEALTHY Hint

BURNT BREAD WILL MAKE YOU SMILE

Here's a goofy-sounding tip for whitening teeth, and it actually works! The next time you pop a piece of **BREAD** in the toaster and it comes out looking more like charcoal than toast, don't toss it in the trash. Instead, crush the charred bread into crumbs, mix them with about 1/2 teaspoon of honey, and brush your teeth with them. Yep, that's right, just put the concoction on your toothbrush and go to town. Then rinse your mouth thoroughly and admire your whiter, brighter choppers in the mirror.

Bet on Barley for BP Problems

Do you have high blood pressure? Are your cholesterol levels out-of-sight? If you said yes to either or both of these questions, it's time to make **BARLEY** your best friend. Researchers found that people who eat barley were able to significantly lower their blood pressure and cholesterol levels. The secret to barley's good works: It contains fiber and other nutrients that help lower blood pressure and cholesterol and limit the production of artery-clogging LDL cholesterol.

Balance Blood Sugar with Barley

Here's good news if you've got diabetes—researchers gave men meals made with regular pasta or pasta made with **BARLEY** flour. The men who ate the barley pasta didn't produce as much insulin (a hormone that plays a role in diabetes) as did those who had the regular pasta. You can find barley pasta and other barley products online, so get cooking!

Bar(ley) the Door on Ulcers

Soothe the pain of ulcers and help rebuild your stomach lining with **BARLEY** and barley water. To make barley water, boil 4 tablespoons of barley in 6 cups of water until the liquid is reduced by about half. Strain out the solids and set them aside. Drink the water, either warm or cool, throughout the day, adding honey and/or lemon if you like. Then eat the reserved barley plain, or add it to soup or stew.

Back in the Day...

As good as barley is at getting you going again (see Spotlight on Constipation, at right), it's also been used for decades as a cure for diarrhea. It works by slowing intestinal motion. Simply prepare pearl **BARLEY** (this type has the husk removed, so it has less fiber) according to the package directions, and add it to 1 cup of beef broth. The "soup" will replace lost fluids and electrolytes and tame your tummy's turmoil.

SPOTLIGHT ON CONSTIPATION

When your internal plumbing slows down, there are plenty of over-the-counter laxatives that can get things moving again. But if you prefer a more natural approach, try one of these. Just keep in mind that you'll most likely need to follow the routine for several days before you get relief.

◆ Eat a cup of cooked hulled **BARLEY**. It provides 14 grams of fiber—about half the daily recommended amount—and that will get things moving fast.

◆ Have a bowl of **OATMEAL**. It's loaded with a gummy fiber called mucilage, which soaks up water, softening stools and making them easier to pass. Just don't top your cereal with bananas, which are noted for their internal binding power, or you'll never get off the mark!

◆ Take 1 tablespoon of extra virgin **OLIVE OIL** first thing in the morning and a second tablespoon an hour after eating dinner.

◆ Mix 2 tablespoons of unfiltered **APPLE CIDER VINEGAR** in a glass of water or 100 percent apple or grape juice. Drink this mixture three times a day.

◆ Mix a tablespoon or two of raw **HONEY** in a glass of warm water, and drink it down. Things should start moving along within 24 hours. If they don't, you can take another dose.

◆ Eat one or two minced **GARLIC** cloves a day, mixed in milk or plain yogurt.

◆ Make a **GINGER** compress. Bring 2 gallons of water to a boil in a large pot. Tuck $4\frac{1}{2}$ tablespoons of grated fresh ginger into a cheesecloth bag, dunk it in the water, and remove the pot from the heat. Let the pouch steep until the water reaches a comfortably warm temperature. Then dip a clean towel into the brew, and lay it over your abdomen until the compress cools. Repeat the process four more times.

Bread & Grains

Pantry Pharmacy

Bran Battles Blood Sugar

Guess what? Chewy, high-fiber foods packed with **BRAN** not only make you eat more slowly, but they also enter your bloodstream in snail-like fashion, preventing your blood sugar from spiking and then dropping—along with your energy and resistance to chocolate bars. Put bran to work for you by choosing a bowl of steel-cut oat bran instead of sugary cereal, and hearty, whole-grain bread instead of white.

Wake Up Easier

All of the B vitamins can help improve energy levels, but vitamin B_1 is needed to break down and release energy from carbohydrates. To make sure you get enough B_1, eat a bowl of **RICE BRAN** cereal for breakfast to jump-start your day.

A Bran New Earache Remedy

There are few ailments more painful than an earache, and that's probably why so many folks have come up with ways to ease the agony. This is one of the best: Combine ½ cup of unprocessed **BRAN** (available

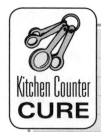

Kitchen Counter CURE

Trouble Prevention on the Double

If you're prone to indigestion and/or flatulence, this "aperitif" can help: Add 1 cup of **BRAN** and 1 cup of uncooked oatmeal to a gallon of water. Let it sit for 24 hours, then strain out the solids, and store the liquid in the refrigerator. Drink a cupful of the potion (either cold or warmed up) 15 minutes before each meal.

in health-food stores and most supermarkets) with ½ cup of kosher or coarse sea salt. Wrap the mixture securely in a generous-sized piece of cheesecloth so that the stuff doesn't spill out all over the place. Then heat the pouch in the microwave or an oven turned on low until it's as warm as you can comfortably handle. Lie down, place the poultice on the affected ear, and keep it there for 60 minutes or so. *Note: If your ear is discharging fluid, get medical help immediately. It could be that your eardrum has ruptured.*

Bread & Grains

Roll Back Cholesterol with Oats

Way back in the '90s, the Food and Drug Administration (FDA) approved the health claim that **OATMEAL** can help lower cholesterol. More than a decade later, that claim holds true. Study after study has shown that if you eat oatmeal regularly, you can lower your LDL ("bad") cholesterol without lowering HDL ("good") cholesterol levels. In addition, oatmeal eaters reduce their risk of developing high blood pressure, type 2 diabetes, and obesity. It's all the soluble fiber found in this grain that makes it so darn good for you. So be sure to enjoy a steaming bowl of oatmeal every day.

Banish Bronchitis

OATMEAL can reduce bronchial inflammation and relieve coughing spasms. Make it according to the directions on the package, just as though you were making a bowl for breakfast, but reduce the water by 1/4 cup per serving. Add honey to taste, and eat 1 cup of warm cereal four times a day and at the start of each coughing spell. *Note: For the sake of convenience, you may want to make your oatmeal in quantity ahead of time. If you do, then store it, covered, in the refrigerator, and warm up each "dose" before you eat it.*

HOW'S THAT?

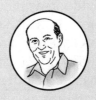

Q *Does it matter whether I eat instant OATMEAL or the slow-cooked kind? Is one type healthier than the other?*

A This may come as a surprise (I know it did to me), but the basic nutrient content of instant oatmeal is pretty much the same as it is for traditional, slower-cooking rolled oats. So when you're whipping up any of my health potions that contain oatmeal, feel free to use whichever type you have on hand, provided your instant oatmeal is plain. Steer clear of any oatmeal that contains sweeteners, fruit, flavorings, or other ingredients. Unless otherwise specified, use uncooked oatmeal.

Chewing Chases Heartburn

This isn't the most appetizing heartburn remedy in the world, but it sure does work! When you get that fiery feeling, slowly chew a teaspoon or two of uncooked **OATMEAL**, and then swallow it. The flames will flicker on out and die.

Ditch the Discomfort of Yeast Infections

An oat-filled bath of cool water can ease external itching (see Back in the Day, below), and this warm-water version can soothe the internal pain and itching of a yeast infection. Simply fill a cotton sack or panty hose leg with uncooked **OATMEAL**, and toss it into the tub as you run warm water into it. Squeeze the bag several times to extract the oaty goodness, and soak for 20 minutes or so. Repeat the procedure as needed until you're feeling better. *Note: Although this treatment will relieve your irritating symptoms, it will not cure a yeast infection. If you've contracted one for the first time, call your doctor.*

Super Sunburn Soother

Spent a bit too much time outdoors without proper sun protection? Ease the pain with **OATMEAL**. Wrap about 1 cup of dry, uncooked oatmeal in cheesecloth and run cool water through it. Wring out the excess liquid, and apply the poultice to your burned skin for 20 minutes every two hours until you feel relief. (You can use the same oatmeal sachet over and over. Just put it in a plastic bag, stash it in the fridge, and give it a cold shower before each treatment.)

Back in the Day...

Grandma Putt had a homemade remedy for just about everything under the sun. And when I was itchin' all over from bug bites or a run-in with poison plants, she sent me upstairs to take this soothing soak: Stuff a cotton drawstring bag or a panty hose leg with a cup or two of uncooked **OATMEAL**. Toss it into your tub as you run cool to lukewarm water, then settle in and relax for about 15 to 20 minutes. If possible, let yourself air-dry when you're finished.

Reduce with Rice

If you're trying to drop a few (or more) pounds, stock up on **RICE**. This gluten-free grain comes in thousands of varieties, though most of us are familiar with just a few. The most popular version is white rice, though brown rice is healthier because it still has the germ and bran, making it a whole grain (white rice has the germ and bran removed during refinement). Whole-grain brown rice contains more fiber, minerals, and phytonutrients, and in some studies, it has been shown to help lower blood glucose and spur weight loss. In addition, rice fills you up, so you'll eat less. The key is to pair it with healthy foods, so enjoy your rice with steamed or stir-fried vegetables and in soups and salads.

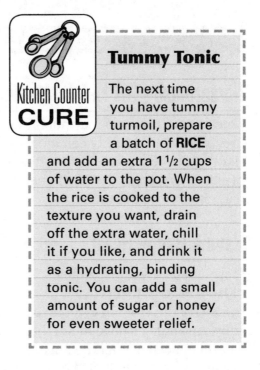

Kitchen Counter CURE

Tummy Tonic

The next time you have tummy turmoil, prepare a batch of **RICE** and add an extra 1 1/2 cups of water to the pot. When the rice is cooked to the texture you want, drain off the extra water, chill it if you like, and drink it as a hydrating, binding tonic. You can add a small amount of sugar or honey for even sweeter relief.

Rice Is Nice for Headache Relief

Headaches are an unfortunate fact of life—so add this simple tool to your first-aid kit. Mix about 1 1/2 cups of uncooked **RICE** with 5 or 6 drops of lavender essential oil. Stuff the mixture into a soft, clean cotton sock and sew it closed. Then, whenever that familiar throbbing starts, lie down and lay the fragrant sock over your eyes. The lavender scent will soothe you, while the weight of the rice will provide massage-like pressure against your eyes and forehead to help stop the searing pain.

Back-to-Back Rice

Need to relieve a backache? This trick will bring quick results: Fill a clean, thick sock with **RICE** (a wool kneesock is perfect), and warm it up in the microwave on a medium-low setting for 60 seconds, or until it's comfortably warm. Then lie facedown, lay the DIY heating pad over the painful area, and relax until your ache has eased.

CONDIMENTS

Horseradish—A Helpful Healer

Here's something you may not know: **HORSERADISH** increases your liver's ability to detoxify carcinogens. Not only does that help lessen your risk of developing cancer, but studies show it may suppress the growth of existing tumors. The recommended dose is as little as ¼ teaspoon a day, either fresh or bottled.

Have a Happy Heart

Fresh or prepared, just 2 tablespoons of **HORSERADISH** provide 12 percent of the vitamin C you need daily. And studies have found that vitamin C seems to fend off heart disease and cancer. It also helps speed wound healing, so you'll recover from minor cuts and oral surgeries a bit faster.

Don't Horse Around with Arthritis

The discomfort and stiffness of arthritis can make you want to head for the hills. Well, don't. Instead, make the pain gallop away with this: Boil ½ cup of milk, and mix 3 tablespoons of grated **HORSERADISH** into it. Pour the mixture onto a piece of cheesecloth, and lay it on your aching joint. By the time the poultice cools off, you should feel like hopping on your pony and movin' on down the trail!

HEALTHY Hint

WHEN THE FLOW IS SLOW

Having trouble urinating? Saunter over to your kitchen counter and grate ½ cup of fresh **HORSERADISH**. Add it to a pan with ½ cup of beer, and bring it to a boil. Let it boil for a minute or two, then remove it from the heat. When it's cool enough to drink, sip it down. Repeat two more times during the day, and the spigot should soon be functioning fine again. *Note: If this is a recurring problem, see your doctor to find out the cause. If you cannot urinate at all, call 911 or get to the emergency room pronto.*

A Hot Tip for Weight Loss

Recent studies have shown that adding just a few dashes of **HOT-PEPPER SAUCE** to your daily diet not only reduces your levels of the hunger-causing hormone called ghrelin, but also raises your level of GLP-1, a compound that naturally suppresses appetite. One of the tastiest ways to put this firepower to work: Add it to tomato juice.

Bring on the Heat

Capsaicin, the component that makes **HOT-PEPPER SAUCE** hot, can help ease the pain of arthritis. You can get your daily dose by applying a rub (see "How's That?," below) or by adding the sauce to your daily diet. If you're not used to using hot-pepper sauce, start with just a few drops on any one of these foods, then work your way up to more flavor: baked, roasted, or mashed potatoes; scrambled eggs; soups; tuna salad; baked beans; pork chops.

A Happy, Healthy "High"

When you're feeling low, perk yourself up with **HOT-PEPPER SAUCE**. Add enough drops—to your soup, stew, or whatever you're eating or drinking—to feel the heat. To counteract that heat, your brain releases chemicals called endorphins, which give you a sense of well-being.

HOW'S THAT?

Q *I work all day at my computer, and by quitting time, my neck is stiff and my shoulders are sore. I don't want to spend a small fortune on pain-relief ointments, so what's the alternative?*

A This one's a no-brainer. Grab a bottle of **HOT-PEPPER SAUCE** and concoct my peppery pain-relief ointment: Just combine 3 to 4 drops of the sauce with 2 teaspoons of olive oil. Then massage the mixture into your sore muscles. The heat will ease your aches, and you'll soon be saying "aaahhh."

Condiments

Mustard Cuts the Mustard . . .

When it comes to curing common health problems, nothing beats good ol' **MUSTARD**. Here's a terrific trio of treatments:

■ **Minor burns.** When your hand brushes up against a hot pan or the edge of the barbecue grill, run your singed skin under cold running water for about five minutes. Then slather on a nice thick layer of yellow mustard. The pain will vanish instantly.

■ **Migraines.** The minute you feel an attack coming on, open a jar of strong mustard—the hotter and spicier, the better. Slowly inhale the aroma three or four times, and your pain should be gone in a flash.

■ **Constipation.** Get your innards back on track with this tried-and-true method. First thing in the morning, on an empty stomach, drink ½ cup of cool water with ½ teaspoon of dry mustard mixed in it. Then follow up by eating your usual healthy breakfast. Do the same thing the following day, and before you know it, things will be moving smoothly again.

Back in the Day...

Before the days of antibiotics and other miracle drugs, folks treated chest colds, flu, bronchitis, and even pneumonia with this remedy. It still works like a charm—but use it with, not instead of, your doctor's prescription!

Have the patient put on a thick cotton T-shirt and lie down. Then mix ¼ cup of dry **MUSTARD** with ¼ cup of flour, and stir in 3 tablespoons of molasses. Add enough heavy cream or softened lard to get an ointment consistency. Dip a piece of cotton flannel into warm water, wring it out, and lay it on the patient's throat and upper chest, on top of the T-shirt. Apply the mustard mixture to the damp cloth, and leave it on for 15 minutes, or until the skin starts to turn red. *Caution: This stuff is hot, so wear rubber gloves as you work with it, and make sure none touches the patient's bare skin.*

Mustardy Muscle Relief

Attention, weekend warriors! Here's how to stop those muscle cramps you get on the golf course, tennis court, or jogging track—and make good use of the **MUSTARD** packets that come with take-out meals. Keep a supply in your golf or gym bag, and whenever you feel a cramp coming on, open the package, swallow the contents, and chase it down with water. Repeat every two minutes until the twinges stop. *Note: If you're at home, just take your medicinal mustard straight from the jar.*

Extinguish Aches and Pains

If you wouldn't dream of eating **MUSTARD** for your muscle cramps, that's okay. Just take a bath with 2 tablespoons of mustard and 1 teaspoon of Epsom salts added to the running water. Shower afterward so you don't smell like a hot dog!

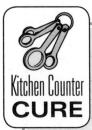

Kitchen Counter **CURE**

Reliable Mustard Rub

This versatile formula will clear up coughs and chest congestion and deliver fast relief to sore muscles and stiff, achy joints. For best results, administer this hot and spicy treatment just before you go to bed.

> 2 tbsp. of olive oil
> 1 tsp. of dry **MUSTARD**
> 1 tsp. of ground ginger

Mix the ingredients together, and rub a tiny dab on your inner arm. Then wait 10 minutes. If the skin shows no sign of irritation, rub the rest of the mixture onto the troubled area until you feel a warm, tingling sensation. Depending on what body parts you've massaged with the oily mix, either put on an old T-shirt, or cover the area with a soft, cotton cloth (thereby protecting your sheets). Then hop into bed and get a good night's rest. In the morning, wash off the residue with soap and water. Repeat as often as necessary.

SPOTLIGHT ON
THE COMMON COLD

Whether you're battling a stuffy or runny nose, a scratchy throat or one that aches, coughing, congestion, or any of the other miserable symptoms of the common cold, help is as close as your kitchen. So before you drag yourself to the drugstore to stare bleary-eyed at all the OTC cold remedies on the shelves, try one or more of these spicy homemade helpers:

◆ Drain clogged sinuses by taking 1 teaspoon of grated fresh **HORSERADISH** up to three times a day until your symptoms subside. Horseradish works wonders whether you add it to a sandwich, spread it on a cracker, mix it into tomato juice, or eat it straight from the spoon. After you're breathing freely again, a few teaspoons a month should help prevent future sinus woes.

◆ Fight back against cold germs by super-charging your chicken soup. Just add a generous splash of **HOT-PEPPER SAUCE** to the pot, and slurp your way to better health.

◆ Conquer cold symptoms with **HOT-PEPPER SAUCE**. Grab a bottle and shake it well. (Any brand that suits your taste buds will do the trick.) Then put 10 to 20 drops into a glass of water, and drink up. Repeat the procedure three times a day until you're rarin' to go again.

◆ To clear up congestion, rub a generous amount of spicy brown **MUSTARD** on your chest, and top it with a hot (but not burning hot!), damp cloth. The aroma of the hot mustard will clear your airways within minutes, and you'll be breathing freely again.

◆ Ease a sore throat with a combination of 1 tablespoon each of prepared **MUSTARD** (any kind will do), salt, and raw honey added to the juice of half a lemon in a heat-proof container. Then pour in 1/2 cup of boiling water, and mix thoroughly. Let the mixture cool to lukewarm, and gargle with it two or three times. Fair warning: This remedy won't win any awards for good flavor, but it'll put your throat back in the swing of things fast!

Fat Fights Fat

Yes, while it's true that **NUTS** are high in fat, much of it is mono-unsaturated (a.k.a. good) fat that fills you up without filling you out. In fact, studies show that folks who eat a handful of nuts each day are much less likely to be severely overweight than those who don't. The operative word here is *handful*—if you overindulge, you'll pack on the pounds.

How to Halt Heartburn

There is a natural chemical in **ALMONDS** that helps strengthen the sphincter separating your esophagus from your stomach. And the stronger that muscle is, the better able it is to keep acid in your tummy where it belongs, instead of letting it seep upward. Your "workout" routine: Eat 10 raw almonds after each meal.

A Nutty Headache Cure

The next time you feel that old familiar throbbing, grab a handful of **ALMONDS** and/or **WALNUTS**. Both are both packed with pain-relieving compounds that function much like aspirin—without any of the potential side effects. Of course, it should go without saying that if you are on a sodium-restricted diet, whatever you do, don't buy salted nuts! You'll find many no-salt and low-salt varieties in your local grocery store.

HEALTHY Hint

MIGHTY MIGRAINE MIX

As strange as this nut remedy may sound, it's powerfully effective for relieving the agony of a migraine attack. Put 2 tablespoons of **PECANS** and 2 tablespoons of **WALNUTS** in a blender, and mix them with just enough water to make a thick puree. (Add the water a teaspoon at a time until you get the right consistency.) Spread the mixture on two squares of gauze, and tape one to each of your temples. Then lie down in a comfortable spot for a few hours or until the throbbing stops—whichever comes first.

Beat the Blues

Feeling down in the dumps? Then reach for the nuts that are shaped like little smiles: **CASHEWS**. Natural health experts tell us that these tasty nuts may work just as well as prescription antidepressants. They contain an amino acid called tryptophan that helps boost your mood, stabilize your thoughts, and produce a general mellow feeling. The dose: a small handful of cashews a day.

Two Munchable Mood Boosters

Besides cashews (see "Beat the Blues," above), this dynamic duo is also highly effective at lifting low spirits:

1. **BRAZIL NUTS** are one of Mother Nature's best sources of selenium, a mineral that is likely to be lacking in your system if you're feeling depressed, anxious, irritated, and tired for no apparent reason. Simply eating three Brazil nuts a day will provide your recommended daily dose of this essential nutrient.

2. **WALNUTS** are high in serotonin, which has been shown to help brighten your mood when you're suffering from seasonal affective disorder (SAD) or simply battling a case of the blahs. The easy R$_X$: When you're going through a blue phase, eat a handful of walnuts every day or so. *Note: If you're suffering from severe depression, don't bother dosing yourself with nuts or any other homemade healer—get professional help ASAP!*

HOW'S THAT?

Q *I've heard that **NUTS** are good for my heart, but I've always thought they have too much fat and calories to really be healthy. What's the story?*

A The story is this: In moderation—a small handful (1^1/$_2$ ounces) per day—nuts help lower LDL ("bad") cholesterol and help reduce the risk of blood clots that can lead to a heart attack. For more good news, see "Spotlight on Heart Health" (at right).

SPOTLIGHT ON
HEART HEALTH

Nuts and seeds are packed with nutrients that keep your heart in good working order. They're loaded with monounsaturated fats, omega-3 fatty acids, fiber, and vitamin E, all of which contribute to a healthy ticker. And more good news—nuts are even part of the DASH (Dietary Approaches to Stop Hypertension) diet. The "dose" is a handful up to five times a week. Here's what you need to know:

◆ A handful of nuts (especially **ALMONDS, PECANS,** and **WALNUTS)** five or more times a week can cut your heart attack risk in half. How? All nuts contain vitamin E, which may help stop the development of plaques in your arteries. Plaques often narrow arteries, a condition that can lead to chest pain, coronary artery disease, or a heart attack.

◆ A tablespoon of ground **FLAXSEED** a day provides plant-based omega-3 fatty acids, which have been shown to normalize heartbeat and reduce inflammation throughout the cardiovascular system.

◆ Consuming 1 to 2 tablespoons of ground **FLAXSEED** per day may help prevent hardening of the arteries.

◆ **PUMPKIN SEEDS** are rich in monounsaturated fatty acids, which help lower LDL ("bad") cholesterol and increase HDL ("good") cholesterol levels. The R_x: $1^1/_2$ ounces a day.

◆ Eating just a handful of **SUNFLOWER SEEDS** every day can lower your LDL cholesterol levels. Just steer clear of roasted, salted seeds and stick to the raw, shelled, unsalted kinds.

Note: Keep in mind that nuts are high in fat and calories. So limit your daily portion to no more than $1^1/_2$ ounces, and cut back on the saturated fats in your daily diet—meats, eggs, and dairy products. If you eat nuts but don't cut back on the saturated fats, you won't be helping your heart or your waistline!

Nuts & Seeds

Flaxseed Fights Cancer

Is it possible to find one "superfood" that may protect against breast, prostate, and colon cancer? Meet **FLAXSEED**. This handy healer contains omega-3 essential fatty acids (the "good" fats that protect your heart); lignans, which have plant estrogen and antioxidants; and fiber. Here's a rundown of recent findings:

■ In animal studies, ALA, the omega-3 fatty acid that's found in flaxseed, inhibited tumor incidence and growth.

■ Flaxseed lignans may protect against cancers sensitive to hormones, such as breast cancer. Exposure to lignans during adolescence has been shown to help reduce the risk of breast cancer, and it may also help breast cancer patients live longer.

■ Other components in flaxseed have antioxidant properties, which may offer protection against cancer and heart disease.

Be sure to store your flaxseed properly to preserve its nutritional value. If you bought whole flaxseed, store it in a dark, cool place until you grind it. As long as it stays dry, flaxseed can be kept at room temperature for up to a year. Once you grind it, or if you bought pre-ground flaxseed, pour it into a ziplock plastic freezer bag and store in the freezer.

HEALTHY
Hint

FLAXSEED BUYER'S GUIDE

Now that you know the healthy benefits of adding **FLAXSEED** to your diet, you're probably ready to go online or run out to buy a bag. Here are a few pointers:

Whole or ground? You can buy flaxseed either way, but be aware that when eaten whole, flaxseed passes through your intestinal tract undigested, so you'll miss out on its healthful benefits. If you can't find ground flaxseed, buy it whole and grind it yourself in a coffee grinder or food processor. You'll find flaxseed in 1-pound bags in grocery and health-food stores and online. By the way, "milled" or "ground" flaxseed is the same as flaxseed "meal," so buy whatever is available.

Color doesn't matter. You'll find brown or golden flaxseed in stores. There is almost no nutritional difference between the two.

Flax vs. Diabetes

Studies have shown that a daily dose of **FLAXSEED** may be just what the doctor ordered for people with diabetes. Study participants who ate 1 tablespoon of ground flaxseed every day for a month had a significant drop in their fasting blood sugars, triglycerides, and cholesterol, plus a drop in their hemoglobin A1c levels—a prime measure of glucose. And that's not all the good news. Not only did the flaxseed eaters not gain any weight over three months, they actually lost inches in their waistlines! Researchers surmise that flaxseed may work by improving insulin sensitivity. *Note: If you're being treated for diabetes, be sure to check with your doctor before you use this remedy.*

Deflate Inflammation

Put the kibosh on your arthritic aches and pains with a spoonful of **FLAXSEED**. This potent seed contains compounds that help your body reduce the inflammation associated with both rheumatoid arthritis and osteoarthritis. All it takes is 1 tablespoon of seeds per day, and you can meet your quota in a couple of ways:

■ Grind the tasty seeds in a coffee grinder or food processor, and add the powder to a smoothie, mix it into yogurt or cottage cheese, or sprinkle it onto whatever you're having for breakfast, lunch, or dinner.

■ Take 1 teaspoon of flaxseed oil three times a day. Either sip it straight from the spoon, or mix it into food or beverages. (Keep the oil refrigerated to prolong its shelf life.)

Note: Like all natural remedies that go to the root of a problem rather than just masking symptoms, this one will take a little time to work. You can expect to wait at least a month for it to perform its pain-relieving magic.

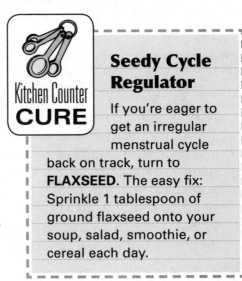

Kitchen Counter CURE

Seedy Cycle Regulator

If you're eager to get an irregular menstrual cycle back on track, turn to **FLAXSEED**. The easy fix: Sprinkle 1 tablespoon of ground flaxseed onto your soup, salad, smoothie, or cereal each day.

Pumpkin Prowess

If you're looking for a tasty snack that is actually good for you, reach for **PUMPKIN SEEDS**. These tiny treasures are packed with vitamins, minerals, antioxidants, and fiber. Here's a look at how they can help you:

- **Sleep well.** The seeds are loaded with the amino acid tryptophan, which is converted to serotonin and glutamate. Serotonin is often called nature's sleeping pill because it can help you relax, while glutamate helps reduce anxiety. The result? A good night's sleep.

- **Save your skin.** Pumpkin seeds are a very good source of vitamin E, which prevents injury to tissue cells and protects your skin from sunlight and pollution.

Shrink Your Prostate

Medical statisticians estimate that one out of every three men over the age of 60 has some kind of prostate problem. And according to natural health practitioners, an effective way to help relieve an enlarged prostate is to eat 1/2 cup of shelled, unsalted **PUMPKIN SEEDS** every day. One reason may be that the prostate gland contains 10 times more zinc than most other organs in your body, and pumpkin seeds are packed with that mineral. *Note: If you're being treated for an enlarged prostate, or suspect that you have one, be sure to check with your doctor before you use this remedy or the one below in Back in the Day.*

Back in the Day...

This bladder tonic comes from waaay back—an old Russian folk remedy calls on **PUMPKIN SEED** "tea" to relieve inflammation of the bladder and prostate. To make it, simmer 1/2 cup of whole (not shelled) pumpkin seeds in 1 quart of water for 20 minutes. Cool to room temperature, and pour it into a wide-mouthed jar with a tight-fitting lid. Don't strain out the seeds; let them settle to the bottom of the jar. Stir thoroughly before using the potion. Drink 6 to 8 ounces three times a day.

A Sunny Solution

Eating just a handful of **SUNFLOWER SEEDS** every day can help you quit smoking, relieve constipation, prevent tooth decay, and improve your memory. So make it a habit to munch on these super seeds.

Halt a Headache

The next time the throbbing starts, measure out 1/4 cup of **SUNFLOWER SEEDS** and chew them slowly. That should nip your headache in the bud.

Shell Out for an Asthma Antidote

Legions of chronic asthma sufferers swear by this classic prevention potion: Put 4 cups of shelled **SUNFLOWER SEEDS** in a pan with 2 quarts of water, and boil it until the water is reduced by half. Strain out the solids, add 8 cups of raw honey to the liquid, and boil it down to a syrupy consistency. Pour it into a sterilized glass jar with a tight-fitting lid (a clamp-top canning jar is perfect), and store it at room temperature. Then take 1 teaspoon of the syrup half an hour before each meal.

> # HEALTHY
> ## Hint
>
> ### SKIP THE SALT
>
> While the nutritional benefits of **SUNFLOWER SEEDS** are certainly something worth cheering about, the incredibly high sodium content of packaged, salted seeds definitely is not. So be sure to skip the salted kind and look for unsalted or raw seeds instead.

Turn Your Eyes to the Sun(flower)

For years, natural health experts have sworn by **SUNFLOWER SEEDS** for strengthening your eyes and improving your vision. Studies have found that people with high intakes of vitamin E (sunflowers provide 70 percent of the Daily Value) have a lower risk of developing age-related macular degeneration. The action plan: Eat a handful of the seeds (shelled, raw, and unsalted) every day.

OIL & VINEGARS

Boost Your Brain

To keep your mind healthy and your memory sharp, incorporate **OLIVE OIL** into your diet. Studies found that cognitive impairment was less common among elderly people whose diets included lots of olive oil, a monounsaturated fat (see "Help Your Heart," below). So splash olive oil on your salads, and try dipping crusty bread into a mix of olive oil and Italian seasonings.

Help Your Heart

Monounsaturated fats (MUFAs) can help lower total cholesterol levels and normalize blood clotting. And **OLIVE OIL** is one great MUFA source. Choose extra virgin olive oil, and use at least 4 tablespoons per day to help lower your risk of heart attack and stroke. Keep in mind that olive oil is high in calories, so use it in place of—not in addition to—butter and margarine.

Escape from Indigestion

If hot, spicy food gives you indigestion, about 15 minutes before you sit down to eat a "high-risk" meal, sip 1 tablespoon of **OLIVE OIL**. It'll provide a protective coating so you can indulge without setting your tummy on fire.

HOW'S THAT?

Q *Can a dose of OLIVE OIL before I go out on the town keep me from getting a hangover?*

A It sure can. Swallow 1 tablespoon before you head out. The oil can protect your stomach from the effects of alcohol, thereby helping to head off morning-after miseries. This treatment only prevents an upset stomach—it does nothing to counteract alcohol's ability to impair your reflexes and mental processes.

Joust a Java Jolt

When a gulp of steaming hot coffee or any other boiling beverage gives your throat a nasty burn, swallow 2 teaspoons of **OLIVE OIL**—it'll put out the flames fast! Then let the drink cool for a couple of minutes before you take your next sip.

Toss a Toothache

For all-but-instant relief, mix 3 drops of **OLIVE OIL** with 1 drop of clove oil, and use a cotton swab to gently dab the mixture onto your aching tooth. Leave it in place until the pain is gone (which should be within a minute or so), and then rinse your mouth with clear, lukewarm water.

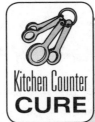

Kitchen Counter CURE

Bathe Psoriasis Bye-Bye

Unfortunately, there is no permanent cure for this nasty skin condition. But there are plenty of ways to ease the pain and itching of the unsightly symptoms and help you recover more quickly from flare-ups. One of the best—and simplest— is to mix ¼ cup of **OLIVE OIL** in a large glass of milk, and pour the mixture into a tub of warm water. Then settle in and soak for 20 minutes or so. Repeat as often as needed to relieve your discomfort.

Ease Eczema Flare-Ups

If you suffer from eczema or other skin irritations, make **OLIVE OIL** your new best friend. Why? Because it's loaded with antioxidants that reduce inflammation. For that reason, it's a key ingredient in many commercial products that are designed to relieve eczema and other skin woes. But you don't have to spend your money on those over-the-counter concoctions. In fact, olive oil is just as effective all by its lonesome, plus it has none of the chemicals you often find in those store-bought creams. The simple R_X: Gently rub on about 1 teaspoon of extra virgin olive oil per square inch of affected skin, and let the oil penetrate before you put on any clothing. For an extra-intensive treatment, cover your oiled skin with plastic wrap, and leave it on overnight. Just make sure you wear old pajamas and/or put a large towel over your sheets to protect your bedding.

SPOTLIGHT ON
SINUSITIS

At one time or another just about everyone I know has had a bout of sinusitis. You know, the kind that makes you want to slam your head against the wall to break up what feels like concrete in there. Well, don't charge at the plaster just yet. Check out these kinder, gentler alternatives:

◆ Pour 1 tablespoon of extra virgin **OLIVE OIL** into a bowl, and mix in 3 or 4 drops of peppermint, eucalyptus, lavender, or rosemary oil. (Whichever oil you choose, if you haven't used it before, test a drop or two on your wrist to make sure you're not sensitive to it.) Then massage the mixture onto your nose, cheekbones, temples, and forehead. Almost immediately, you should feel your sinuses beginning to clear up. Repeat two or three times a day, as needed, until you're breathing freely again.

◆ Two or three times a day, use one of these **APPLE CIDER VINEGAR** remedies—or, if you like, try them both and see which one works best for you: Drink a glass of warm water with 2 teaspoons of unfiltered cider vinegar mixed in; or mix 2 tablespoons of unfiltered cider vinegar and 1 tablespoon of raw honey in 8 ounces of lukewarm water, and drink it down.

◆ Steam your sinuses clear with this potion: Mix 1 cup of unfiltered **APPLE CIDER VINEGAR** and 1 cup of water in a pan. Heat it on the stove, then bend over the pan and inhale the steamy vapors while keeping your mouth and eyes closed. Have tissues at hand because this should get things flowing fast. Just be careful not to burn yourself!

◆ Give chicken soup's cold-fighting powers a boost and get your clogged sinuses draining by adding unfiltered **APPLE CIDER VINEGAR** to the pot. The recipe: Heat 1 cup of soup or broth, and stir in 1 tablespoon of the vinegar, 1 crushed garlic clove, and a dash of hot-pepper sauce. Pour it into a bowl or mug, and sip slowly.

Make a Dent in Diabetes

Medical research shows that **APPLE CIDER VINEGAR** (ACV) may help control blood sugar for folks with diabetes. The vinegar appears to block the digestion of starch, thus lowering blood sugar levels. The R_X: Mix 1 to 2 tablespoons of unfiltered apple cider vinegar in a glass of water, and drink it once a day. If you have diabetes and want to try this approach, speak with your doctor first. *Note: For this and any other medicinal purpose, always use raw, organic, unfiltered apple cider vinegar (available in health-food stores and in the health-food sections of most supermarkets). The clear, filtered kind that's generally found with the salad dressings in the grocery aisles has been stripped of the enzymes and friendly bacteria that give apple cider vinegar its healing power.*

ACV + H$_2$O = RELIEF

Unfiltered **APPLE CIDER VINEGAR** and water can help solve a myriad of nagging health problems. Reach for this classic combo whenever one of these conditions strikes.

HEALTH PROBLEM	THE R_X
Bladder infection	2 tsp. of ACV in a glass of water three times a day*
Dizzy spell	1/2 tsp. of ACV in a glass of water
Facial neuralgia	1/2 tsp. of ACV in a glass of water once an hour for seven hours
Hot flashes	1 tbsp. of ACV in 8 oz. of ice water as needed
Indigestion	2 tsp. of ACV in a glass of water once an hour until you feel better
Morning sickness	1 tsp. of ACV in a glass of water as soon as you get up*

* Get your doctor's okay first.

Give Bursitis the Boot

Ease the ache and discomfort of this painful condition by boiling 1 cup of unfiltered **APPLE CIDER VINEGAR** in a saucepan over high heat, then stirring in 1 teaspoon of cayenne pepper when the vinegar starts to simmer. After it comes to a full boil, remove from the heat and let it cool to a comfortably warm temperature. Soak a soft cloth in the warm vinegar, and apply it as a compress to the affected area. The heat from the cayenne pepper should bring almost-instant relief. The area should feel nice and warm, but not burning. If it's uncomfortable, remove it immediately, and wait until the compress has cooled down before trying again.

Take the Edge Off Arthritis Pain

It seems that every arthritis sufferer either has a favorite remedy or is searching high and low for one that really works. Well, according to everyone I know who's tried it, this one's a jim-dandy: Combine equal parts of unfiltered **APPLE CIDER VINEGAR** and raw honey, and store the mixture in a lidded glass jar at room temperature. Then once a day, stir 1 teaspoon of the combo and 1 teaspoon of unflavored Knox® Gelatine into 6 ounces of water, and drink it down. Before you know it, your joints should be jumpin'!

HEALTHY Hint

A TRIUMPHANT TRIAD

Worldwide studies show that a mixture made of **APPLE CIDER VINEGAR**, honey, and garlic can cure or help prevent almost every ailment under the sun, including arthritis, asthma, high blood pressure, obesity, and ulcers, as well as ease muscle aches and colds. The simple formula: Mix 1 cup of unfiltered ACV, 1 cup of raw honey, and 8 peeled garlic cloves in a blender on high speed for 60 seconds. Pour the blend into a glass jar with a tight-fitting lid, and let it sit in the refrigerator for five days. Then every day (ideally before breakfast), take 2 teaspoons of the tonic stirred into a glass of water or fruit juice. Researchers especially recommend using fresh-squeezed orange or 100 percent grape juice. Now, I can't guarantee that this will cure what ails you, but it's worth a try!

Vinegar Clobbers Coughs and Colds . . .

And sore throats, too, when you use it in this classic triple-threat combo: Mix equal parts of unfiltered **APPLE CIDER VINEGAR**, raw honey, and warm water, and stir in about 1/4 teaspoon of mashed fresh ginger per cup of the mixture. Store it at room temperature in a covered glass jar, and take 1 teaspoon three times a day. Before you know it, your colds and coughs will be history!

A Tangy Sore-Throat Solution

If your painful throat is not associated with a cold, give this trick a try: Mix 2 teaspoons of unfiltered **APPLE CIDER VINEGAR** in 8 ounces of warm water, and proceed as follows: Gargle a mouthful of the solution, and spit it out. Then swallow a mouthful. Keep it up, alternating gargling and swallowing, until the glass is empty. Wait 60 minutes, and perform the routine again. Continue as needed until you've put your pain to rest. *Note: If your throat is still sore after a week or so, and you have no other symptoms, see your doctor to rule out a more serious condition.*

Back in the Day...

Grandma Putt was a firm believer in the healing power of **APPLE CIDER VINEGAR**. One of her favorite recipes was for this delicious, sweet-tart super juice. It's a powerful cold killer, crackerjack hangover cure—and an efficient delivery mechanism for all the health-giving benefits of ACV. And it's super easy to make: In a pitcher or large jar, mix 1/2 cup of unfiltered apple cider vinegar, 1/4 cup of 100 percent organic grape or apple juice, 1 tablespoon of lemon juice, 1 teaspoon of raw honey (or more to taste), 1/2 teaspoon of ground cinnamon, and 2 cups of water. Store it, tightly covered, in the refrigerator. Serve it in ice-filled glasses anytime you want a super-refreshing and super-healthy pick-me-up. This makes about five servings, but you can double or even triple the recipe if you like because it'll keep for several weeks in the fridge.

Stop a Headache in Its Tracks

As kooky as it sounds, the old-timers in my family swore by this headache remedy, and I still do today. Here's all there is to it: Dip a large white cotton cloth—an old T-shirt is perfect—in a large bowl filled with **VINEGAR** (either white or apple cider), and wring it out well. Put it against your forehead, and tie it tightly in the back. Keep it there until the pain disappears, which should be within 30 minutes. If your head is still pounding after half an hour, repeat the process.

Battle Chronic Fatigue

We all get tired every now and then. But if you feel constantly fatigued, the reason may be that lactic acid has built up in your system. (That tends to happen during periods of stress or strenuous exercise.) If that's the case, this simple trick may help: At bedtime each night, take 3 teaspoons of unfiltered **APPLE CIDER VINEGAR** mixed into 1/8 cup of raw honey. Continue the routine until your old vim and vigor return. *Note: If that doesn't happen within a few weeks, call your doctor.*

HEALTHY Hint

A WORD TO THE WISE

VINEGAR is strong stuff, so to avoid upsetting your stomach, never drink it straight. Always mix it with a milder carrier such as water, fruit juice, or raw honey. Also, over time, the acid in vinegar can do some serious damage to your tooth enamel, so whenever you use it as a gargle or dental aid, rinse your mouth thoroughly with clear water immediately afterward.

Like many healers (homemade and otherwise), vinegar interacts with some medications, including digoxin (Lanoxin®), insulin, and diuretic drugs. So if you're taking any of those meds, check with your doctor before you use vinegar in medicinal quantities. Finally, if you are pregnant or think you might be pregnant, ask your obstetrician how much vinegar is safe for you to consume.

Balsamic Blasts Belly Fat

If you're struggling to lose that "spare tire" around your middle, reach for **BALSAMIC VINEGAR**. This tastiest of all vinegars can help eliminate the fat around the belly that can lead to such conditions as heart disease, sleep apnea, and type 2 diabetes. It works by activating genes that cause your body to distribute fat more evenly, rather than store it at your waist. The jury is still out on exact dosages, but a good amount to aim for is 5 teaspoons a day, which is the amount that researchers have found to increase insulin sensitivity in diabetics (see "Make a Dent in Diabetes" on page 133).

Great Grapes Alive!

Thanks to the Trebbiano and Lambrusco grapes that it's made from, **BALSAMIC VINEGAR** is loaded with compounds that fight cancer, strengthen your immune system, and destroy the free radicals that cause premature aging and hardening of the arteries. So here's a hot tip for all you pasta fans: The next time you order a big dinner at your favorite Italian restaurant, make sure you include balsamic vinegar on your salad. It'll keep your blood sugar from spiking, thereby preventing the sudden fatigue (a.k.a. "sugar crash") that can set in a few hours later. By the way, this trick works just as well for runners who load up on carbs before a big race.

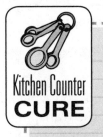

Kitchen Counter CURE

Stomp Stomach Acid

It probably shouldn't surprise you that more than 40 percent of Americans suffer from heartburn at least once a month. It seems that just about everyone has experienced that uncomfortable burning in the chest. If you're one of them, try this before you reach for an antacid: Sprinkle **BALSAMIC VINEGAR** on your salads, vegetables, and fruit. Why? Because it can help neutralize stomach acid. In fact, in Italy's Modena region where balsamic vinegar is produced, people take a spoonful or two of the vinegar before meals to aid digestion and help avoid heartburn.

The Fountain of Youth?

Folks throughout Japan drink *Tamago-su,* or egg vinegar, to maintain good health and slow down the aging process. The recipe has been around since the days of the famous samurai warriors, who claimed they owed their strength and power to this potion. Of course, the samurais didn't know why it worked, but we do: It prevents both the formation of damaging free radicals and the buildup of LDL ("bad") cholesterol in your body. Here's how to make your own supply of this ancient Japanese beverage:

1. Immerse a whole raw egg in 1 cup of **RICE VINEGAR**, and let it sit, covered, for seven days.

2. When the week is up, you will find that everything has dissolved into the vinegar except the transparent membrane that was just inside the shell. Discard the membrane, and stir the egg-infused vinegar thoroughly. Store the tonic in a glass jar that has a tight-fitting lid (a mason jar works well for this).

3. Three times a day, take a break and stir 1 or 2 teaspoons of the vinegar into a glass of hot water, put your feet up, and drink to a long, healthy life. When you have used up your supply of *Tamago-su,* mix up a new batch and keep on truckin'!

HOW'S THAT?

Q *I don't like to drink milk or eat yogurt, so I worry about getting enough calcium in my diet. I've heard that vegetables like kale, collard greens, and Swiss chard are all good sources of calcium. Is this true?*

A It sure is. These dark, leafy greens do have a decent amount of calcium in them, but it's not in a form that your body can readily absorb. The good news is that you can solve that problem easily by splashing your cooked greens with **RICE VINEGAR**. The acetic acid in the vinegar helps your body absorb the calcium, so you don't have to fret about not devouring dairy.

Can Cancer with Chocolate

Studies show that compounds called polyphenols slow the growth of cancer cells. And 1 ounce of dark **CHOCOLATE** contains almost as many polyphenols as a cup of green tea does and twice as many as a glass of red wine does (two widely touted sources of the compounds). Remember—the operative word is *dark*. So look for chocolate that consists of more than 70 percent cacao.

I Heart Chocolate

Here's another reason to reach for this sweet treat— **CHOCOLATE** offers a ton of antioxidants, compounds that battle heart disease as well as cancer. In fact, dark chocolate packs a whopping 5,700 anti-oxidant units per 1 1/2 ounces. Compare that to five whole strawberries, which contain about 2,400 antioxidant units. Now, there's nothing wrong with eating a bowl of berries, but I'll take a piece of yummy dark chocolate anytime!

Too Much of a Good Thing

Please don't rush to the candy aisle and scoop up every tasty

Back in the Day...

Long before the medical community put a name to it, lots of folks had trouble digesting milk. What did they do to ease the bloating and gas brought on by what we now call lactose intolerance? They stirred a few teaspoons of **COCOA POWDER** into their milk. Of course, they didn't know why it worked, but today we do. It turns out that cocoa helps stimulate an enzyme that breaks down lactose, the compound in milk that's responsible for the intestinal discomfort.

CHOCOLATE treat in sight! Instead, limit yourself to the equivalent of 1 1/2 to 4 ounces of dark chocolate per month. This translates to a full-size chocolate bar two or three times a month, or a mini one every day. Choose solid chocolate candies, or those with nuts. Steer clear of creamy fillings, which contribute calories but very few antioxidants.

Honey, I Shrunk My Waistline!

Seems just about everyone I know is on a diet. They lose a few pounds, and gain them back a month or two later. Then they move on to the next great meal plan. If this sounds familiar, I'm here to tell you to just forget about elaborate diets or expensive weight-loss products. Instead, half an hour before each meal, mix 2 teaspoons of raw **HONEY** in a glass of water, and drink it down. It'll naturally suppress your appetite, so you won't be as tempted to overeat.

Bounce Back Fast

Diet alone isn't going to make the pounds melt. You've got to move to burn calories. Whether you walk, ride a bike, or lift weights, after your workout, reach for a spoonful of raw **HONEY**. It'll help your muscles recuperate quickly by replacing the carbohydrates your body burned during your exercise routine.

Sleep Tight

Sleepless nights are no fun—and they're not good for your health either. So if you find yourself tossing and turning when you should be cuttin' some z's, try this time-tested remedy: At bedtime, mix 1 teaspoon of raw **HONEY** in warm milk or lukewarm water, and drink it down. In no time flat, you should drift off to dreamland. *Note: If you continue to have trouble falling asleep or staying asleep through the night, see your doctor to rule out any serious health issues.*

HEALTHY Hint

OUT OF THE MOUTHS OF BABES

Although **HONEY** supplies heaping helpings of health benefits, it should *never* be given to babies under one year of age. That's because honey contains the spores of *Clostridium botulinum*, which causes infant botulism. While adults and children can digest the spores with no harm at all, the human gastrointestinal tract is not fully operational until an infant reaches 12 months of age. And to play it extra safe, consult with your doctor before you give honey to a child under the age of two.

Soothe Acid Indigestion

When you're bitten back by the foods you love to bite, take 1 to 3 teaspoons of raw **HONEY** for instant indigestion relief. To ease a chronic problem, take 1 tablespoon each night at bedtime, on an empty stomach, until you feel better. *Note: If your discomfort continues for more than a week, or if you experience other symptoms, call your doctor.*

Foil a Migraine

Fast action can often stop a migraine in its tracks. The minute you feel the early warning signs, swallow a tablespoon of raw **HONEY**. If your headache isn't gone within 30 minutes, take another tablespoon of honey, and chase it down with three glasses of water. That should be all she wrote!

HOW'S THAT?

Q *I really like* **HONEY** *and use it to sweeten my tea and on my toast just about every morning. But is the kind I buy at the grocery store just as healthy and good for me as the kind I see at my farmers' market?*

A Good question! To get the health benefits of honey, you should always use the pure, raw (a.k.a. unprocessed) kind, not the brands you find next to the peanut butter and jelly in your supermarket. The commercial types of honey have been put through a heating and filtering process that kills off the health-giving enzymes and nutrients. So while these may taste fine, they aren't worth beans for treating ailments. Fortunately, the good stuff is easy to come by: You already know you can find it at your local farmers' market; it's also in health-food stores, in the organic/natural-food sections of most major supermarkets, and (of course) on scads of websites. And keep in mind that studies have shown that dark-colored honey, like that made from buckwheat and blueberry pollen, contains more antioxidants than lighter types and therefore offers the most protection against debilitating diseases.

Head Off a Hangover

If you're going to enjoy a night on the town, take a tip from the experts at the National Headache Foundation: Before you start drinking, eat a piece of toast or a few crackers slathered with a generous layer of raw **HONEY**. It helps break down the by-products of alcohol in your bloodstream that make you feel so awful. *Note: If you don't remember to take your preventive "medicine" before you start to imbibe, take it as soon as possible after the party's over. You'll still avoid most, if not all, of the typical morning-after miseries.*

Give Hay Fever the Slip

When seasonal allergies have you sneezing up a storm, go to the nearest farmers' market, or independently owned health-food store. Buy a jar of locally produced, raw **HONEY**, and start taking 1 tablespoon a day in whatever form(s) you like. Your immune system will become accustomed to the neighborhood pollen contained in the honey, and your body will stop kicking up such a fuss. You may not feel 100 percent better, but it's highly likely that you'll be a lot more comfortable.

Plan Ahead for Sneeze-Free Days

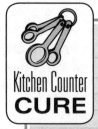

Kitchen Counter CURE

Clear Up Cold Sores

Cold sores (a.k.a. fever blisters) are caused by the herpes virus. Although they have no direct relation to either colds or fevers, they do hurt like crazy. Never fear, **HONEY** can help relieve the pain. Mix 3 tablespoons of raw honey with 1 tablespoon of unfiltered apple cider vinegar, and store it in a jar with a tight-fitting lid. Then dab the mixture onto your sore(s) in the morning, in the late afternoon, and just before bedtime.

Next year, two to three months before allergy season starts, begin taking 1 to 3 teaspoons of locally produced, raw **HONEY** a day (see "Give Hay Fever the Slip," above). By the time the pollen starts flying, your immune system will have built up enough resistance that your symptoms should be greatly lessened, if not eliminated entirely.

SPOTLIGHT ON
COUGHS

No matter what brought on your cough—a cold, the flu, or a nasty case of postnasal drip—you want to get rid of it ASAP. Here are a few sweet and simple cures:

◆ Mix a full cup of raw **HONEY** with ¹/₂ cup of olive oil and 4 tablespoons of fresh-squeezed lemon juice. Heat the mixture on low for five minutes, then stir vigorously for two minutes. Pour the potion into a jar with a tight-fitting lid, and keep it at room temperature. Take 1 teaspoon every two hours, as needed. If you prefer to take your medicine straight, sip 1 teaspoon of raw honey at bedtime, and let it trickle down your throat. Before you know it, your hacking will be history!

◆ If you're prone to bronchitis in the winter months, mix up a batch or two of this potent syrup and keep it close at hand. Put 6 tablespoons of raw **HONEY** in a clean bottle with a tight-fitting lid, and add 3 drops of anise oil and 3 drops of fennel oil (both available in health-food stores and online). Store it at room temperature, and take 1 teaspoon of the syrup whenever you start to feel the wheezing coming on.

◆ Peel two large sweet **ONIONS**, cut them into thin slices, and spread them out in a single layer in a large shallow bowl or baking dish. Pour 2 cups of dark, raw honey evenly over the slices, and cover the container with plastic wrap or anything else that fits (for instance, a pot lid or a wooden cutting board). Let it sit for eight hours or so, strain off the syrup, and mix it with 2 ounces of brandy. Pour the mixture into a glass jar with a tight-fitting lid, and store it in the refrigerator. Take 1 teaspoon every two to three hours, or as needed, to halt your cough.

◆ To clear your airways and ease the hacking, eat an **ONION** every day. How you use it is up to you—add it raw to a tossed salad, stir-fry it with other vegetables, or make a big bowl of steaming hot onion soup.

Sweeteners

The Miracle of Molasses

If you're looking for a sweetener that actually has nutritional value, meet blackstrap **MOLASSES**. This thick syrup is a by-product of sugar refining, and it contains antioxidants, calcium, magnesium, potassium, copper, and other trace minerals. Here's what this alternative to sugar can do for you:

- **Regulate blood pressure.** A 3 1/2-ounce serving of blackstrap molasses provides a whopping 61 percent of the Daily Value of magnesium. This mineral works with copper to maintain muscle contraction and help regulate blood pressure.

- **Keep your heart healthy.** A 3 1/2-ounce serving of blackstrap molasses provides 42 percent of the Daily Value of potassium. This important mineral helps maintain a steady heartbeat.

- **Build strong bones and teeth.** A 3 1/2-ounce serving of blackstrap molasses contains 21 percent of the Daily Value of calcium, which is vital to bone and tooth growth and maintenance.

- **Restore your hair to health.** A mere 2 tablespoons of blackstrap molasses contains 14 percent of the Daily Value of copper, which helps support healthy hair. Some studies suggest that long-term consumption of blackstrap can improve hair quality, regrow hair in men, and even restore your hair's original color!

Look for organic, unsulfured blackstrap molasses. Two popular brands are Grandma's® and Brer Rabbit®. One way to incorporate blackstrap molasses into your daily diet is to mix 1 to 2 tablespoons of it in boiling water, wait for it to cool down a bit, then drink it through a straw to avoid having the sticky sweet cling to your teeth.

HEALTHY Hint

EAT YOUR IRON

A 2-tablespoon serving of blackstrap **MOLASSES** contains about 13 percent of the Daily Value of iron, which our bodies need to carry oxygen to our blood cells. People who are anemic (including pregnant women) can boost their iron levels by eating 1 to 2 tablespoons of blackstrap molasses per day.

Beets Can Keep Your Heart Beating

In addition to being a good source of vitamin C, iron, and fiber, the good ol' **BEET** (and its greens) contains a healthy dose of folate. Why should you care? Because folate helps lower homocysteine levels in your blood. A buildup of this inflammatory compound can lead to severe artery damage, so decreasing the amount of it in your body can help reduce your risk of cardiovascular disease.

Can They Curb Cancer?

The beautiful, deep-red color of **BEETS** comes from a phytochemical called betacyanin. Research is under way to study the effects of this compound in beet juice and its ability to inhibit cancer-cell growth. Specifically, studies are looking at its possible role in preventing cell mutations in breast, prostate, and pancreatic cancers, so stay tuned.

Beat Blood Sugar Spikes

Contrary to popular belief, **BEETS** do not rapidly raise blood sugar. In fact, a full cup of cooked beets packs about the same amount of carbohydrates as a slice of whole-wheat bread—and raises your blood sugar even more slowly. That's good news for people with diabetes who also happen to be true-blue beet lovers. So eat your beets!

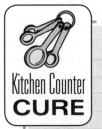

Kitchen Counter
CURE

Best Beet Prep

If the only way you eat **BEETS** is out of a jar, stop! Those veggies have been cooked, and heating decreases their antioxidant power. Instead, wash and peel raw beets; then either slice them thinly or grate them, and toss with a tablespoon of olive oil, a pinch of freshly ground black pepper, and a dash of vinegar or lemon juice. And don't forget the greens—you can eat them raw in salads, or sauté them in a bit of olive oil and fresh garlic until they're wilted, then serve them hot with a sprinkling of crumbled feta or Parmesan cheese.

Vegetables

A-OK for Arteries

These power-packed bulbs are just what the doctor ordered. **ONIONS** are loaded with quercetin, a flavonoid that is also found in red wine, tea, and apples. Quercetin prevents "bad" LDL cholesterol from gunking up your arteries. This and other compounds found in onions keep your blood platelets from clumping together and forming clots that can trigger a heart attack or stroke. So go for onions!

Onion Eaters Have an Edge . . .

Even if their breath is a bit, um, *fragrant*. That's a small price to pay when you consider the overwhelming health benefits of adding **ONIONS** to your daily diet. Whether you eat them raw or cooked, onions can:

- Reduce the risk of stomach and respiratory tract cancers

- Slow cell growth in colon and renal cancers

- Reduce the risk of lung, bladder, ovarian, and brain cancers

- Deter diabetes

Kick a Kidney Infection

Eating plenty of fresh **ONIONS** will help prevent kidney problems. But when you're battling an infection, wrap a cup of grated onions in a piece of cheesecloth, and place the poultice over your kidney area (on your back, just under your rib cage). Leave it on for an hour and repeat as needed. *Note: If you're being treated for a kidney infection, check with your doctor before using this or any homemade healer.*

HEALTHY Hint

WHEN TO PUT THE BRAKES ON BULBS

The very things that make **ONIONS** so good for most of us—they lower blood sugar and slow blood clotting—can have some less than healthy effects on folks who take either diabetes medications or anticoagulant drugs (including prescription doses of aspirin or ibuprofen). If you're in this group, be sure to check with your doctor before you increase your intake of onions. Also, the compounds in onions interact with lithium, so speak with your doc if you are on any drugs containing that chemical.

Quell the Common Cold

For centuries, **ONIONS** have been used to relieve cold symptoms. Here's how:

- At bedtime, put a slice of raw onion on the sole of each foot, and hold the slices in place with thick wool socks. Overnight, the curative compounds in the onion will draw out the infection and lower your fever.

- Slice an onion in two, and set one half on each side of your bed so that you can breathe in the healing aroma as you sleep.

- To break up congestion as you sleep, eat a whole onion just before you go to bed. It's fine to add the onion to a salad and/or sandwich—you don't have to munch on it like an apple.

Onion Juicing 101

ONION JUICE is one of the most powerful, and versatile, healers you can find. It's a snap to make your own supply. Just grate a raw onion, or chop it finely in a food processor, squeeze the pieces through some cheesecloth, and pour the liquid into a jar with a tight-fitting lid. You can store it in the refrigerator for up to 14 days. For best results, make only as much as you'll use within a day or two.

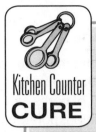

Kitchen Counter CURE

Juicy Solutions

Some health issues are more convenient to treat using **ONION JUICE** rather than the bulbs themselves. You can extract the fluid following the simple procedure outlined in "Onion Juicing 101" (at left). And here are juicy remedies for a handful of common problems:

Athlete's foot. Massage the juice into your tootsies. Wait 10 minutes, rinse your feet in warm water, and dry them thoroughly before you put on your footwear. Repeat three times a day until the fungus is no longer among us.

Laryngitis. Mix 2 parts onion juice with 1 part raw honey in a jar with a tight-fitting lid. Take 3 teaspoons of the mixture every three hours until you're warbling normally again.

Tinnitus. Put 2 drops of onion juice in each ear three times a week until the bells stop ringing.

You Say Potato . . .

I say, eat one soon! One medium baked **POTATO** delivers 24 grams of carbohydrate. While this could be a problem for those with diabetes, for the rest of us, that jolt of carbs can actually soothe jangled nerves and elevate mood. In addition, potatoes have vitamin B_6, which is needed to boost serotonin, the natural brain chemical that makes you feel happy.

Reach for the Reds

There are particular kinds of **POTATOES**, specifically red and russet, that contain high levels of flavonoid antioxidants and vitamins A and C, which may offer protection against the devastating effects of cancer. In addition, potatoes contain a compound called quercetin, which has been proven to have anti-cancer and anti-tumor properties.

Soothe a Sour Stomach

When you've overindulged in tummy-troubling food, grate a raw **POTATO**, and squeeze it through cheesecloth into a bowl. Mix 1 tablespoon of the juice with ½ cup of warm water. Drink the potion slowly, and you'll soon be feeling right as rain!

Send a Headache on Hiatus

To stop the throbbing: Soak four thin **POTATO** slices in vinegar. Then, tie a bandanna around your head, and tuck the potato slices into it at your temples and forehead. Leave it on for a few hours. When you take it off, the spuds will be hot and dry—and your head should be ache-free!

Back in the Day...

Got a young'un who's in bed with a fever? Take a tip from Grandma Putt and put a **POTATO** to work. Tape a slice of raw potato on the bottom of each of the child's feet. Besides lowering his or her temperature, the unconventional footgear should give both of you some hearty chuckles— and, after all, laughter is the best medicine! *Note: Just make sure the patient doesn't try to walk around in his or her slippery "slippers"!*

Vegetables

SPOTLIGHT ON
HIGH BLOOD PRESSURE

If you have high blood pressure, reach into your pantry and pull out these pressure-busting veggies:

◆ Eat a **POTATO**. Just one spud packs more potassium than a banana. Potassium helps lessen the effect that sodium has on your body, thereby helping to control blood pressure. Spuds are also a good source of magnesium, a mineral many older adults don't get enough of, and one that also helps reduce high blood pressure. If you have diabetes or insulin resistance, check with your doctor before you indulge in potatoes.

◆ Shave raw **BEETS** into your salads. These red veggies contain nitrates, which convert to nitric oxide in your body. That, in turn, can help relax and open up blood vessels, improving blood flow and reducing pressure.

◆ Set your sights on **ONION** skins. They contain massive amounts of quercetin, a compound that has almost miraculous power to lower blood pressure (and LDL cholesterol), reduce inflammation, fight allergies, relieve depression, treat some forms of cancer…the list goes on and on. A simple way to tap into this medicinal gold mine: Toss a whole, unpeeled onion or two into a pot of stew, soup, or rice, and fish the bulb out before you serve the dish. Or, whenever you peel onions, save the skins in a paper bag. Then stuff a handful of the peels into a cheesecloth pouch, and put it into the cooking pot. At serving time, discard the skins.

◆ Fit **FIGS** into your diet. One serving of dried figs (about four) provides more potassium than a banana does. This mineral helps lower your blood pressure. For more about the healthy benefits of figs, see page 150.

Note: High blood pressure is a serious condition. Be sure to monitor your numbers and see your doctor regularly for checkups.

Pantry Pharmacy

Go Fig-ure!

Never tried a **FIG**? You don't know what you're missing. Figs supply a boatload of nutrients that benefit your body. For instance, each serving of dried figs (three Calimyrna or four Mission figs) contains about 5 grams of fiber. And we all know we need our fiber! Plus, recent studies have found that the soluble fiber found in figs can reduce cholesterol levels.

Don't Give a Fig...

Eat one instead, especially if you're trying to lose weight. That soluble fiber found in **FIGS** (see "Go Fig-ure!," above) just might help you drop a few pounds. When overweight women were given a soluble-fiber supplement, they began eating fewer calories and reported feeling fuller. So stock up on figs, and munch three or four before each meal to help curb your appetite and eat less.

More Fig-Fiber News

In addition to the soluble fiber found in **FIGS** (see "Go Fig-ure!," above), these mighty morsels provide fiber in the insoluble form as well. Insoluble fiber helps thwart constipation and may even drop your risk of getting colon cancer.

HEALTHY
Hint

STAY IN FIGHTING FORM WITH FIGS

It's not easy to eat the recommended five servings of fruits and vegetables every day. Make a dent by enjoying dried **FIGS** (about four figs). Here's why:

Calcium. A single serving provides 20 percent of the Daily Value of calcium. They're an excellent alternative for folks who are lactose intolerant or who don't eat much dairy.

Phenols. The polyphenols in figs may be able to curb cancer, head off heart trouble, and more. One serving packs twice as much as most of us get from vegetables in a day!

Coumarin and benzaldehyde. Studies have linked coumarin and benzaldehyde consumption with a reduced incidence of prostate cancer.

A Prune by Any Other Name . . .

Is now called a dried plum. But we know a **PRUNE** is still a prune. And that's okay because prunes are perfect packages of antioxidants— those natural compounds that fight free radicals in our bodies and keep our cells healthy. Ounce for ounce, prunes pack more than twice as many antioxidants as raisins do. And antioxidants are valuable compounds because they help fight cancer and heart disease.

The Power of Prunes

Research suggests that the good ol' **PRUNE** is a powerhouse when it comes to lowering cholesterol levels. Antioxidants in prunes have been shown to prevent LDL ("bad") cholesterol from clogging the arteries. In one trial, men with slightly high cholesterol who ate about a dozen prunes a day significantly lowered their bad cholesterol levels. If you give this a try, just be prepared for their laxative effect (see Back in the Day, below).

Prune Juice Is a Plus

While eating whole **PRUNES** ensures you get plenty of fiber, prune juice does have one advantage—just 1 cup kicks in about 17 percent of the iron you need in a day. Five prunes offer only about 4 percent. Look for juice brands without added sugar to avoid packing on the pounds. One cup of unsweetened prune juice already has 70 more calories than a cup of orange juice.

Back in the Day...

Old-timers have passed down this constipation corrective for generations: When you're all backed up, eating about five **PRUNES** will have you on the go again in no time. And even after all these years, researchers still aren't sure just what it is that gives prunes their laxative effect. But who cares, as long as they get the job done!

CHAPTER 4

Spice Rack Relievers

The next time you sprinkle zesty cinnamon on your oatmeal, or tuck a few aromatic cloves into a ham before putting it in the oven, here's something to keep in mind: Many of the herbs and spices you have in your spice rack can be called on to do double duty. Yes, they liven things up in the kitchen, but they make handy healers, too. Read on to discover why herbs, spices, and seasonings should take their rightful place in your first-aid kit.

HERBS & SPICES

Dodge Diabetes

It's no secret that type 2 diabetes is rapidly reaching epidemic proportions all across the country. But here's good news: Numerous studies show that adding 1/2 to 1 teaspoon of ground **CINNAMON** to your daily diet could be enough to help control your blood sugar levels and avoid this dreaded disease. That's because it can improve the ability of your body's cells to recognize and respond to insulin—a process that goes haywire in diabetics. *Note: If you already have either type 1 or type 2 diabetes, consult your doctor before you start dosing yourself with cinnamon—or anything else!*

The Cinnamon Solution

Protecting you against diabetes isn't the only healthful benefit **CINNAMON** has to offer (see "Dodge Diabetes," at left). New research shows that consuming ½ to 1 teaspoon of this tasty ground spice each day can lower your LDL ("bad") cholesterol, lessen your risk for chronic diseases, and may reduce the growth of leukemia and lymphoma cancer cells. And it's a snap to get your daily dose of cinnamon. Just sprinkle it on cereal, toast, or English muffins; add it to coffee, tea, or cocoa; or stir it into yogurt or applesauce. Now that's what I call an easy and delicious way to stay healthy!

Alleviate Arthritis Pain

Thanks to its very potent anti-inflammatory power, **CINNAMON** has proven to be remarkably effective for relieving joint pain and stiffness. The recommended dose (according to a study at the University of Copenhagen in Denmark) is ½ teaspoon of ground cinnamon mixed with 1 tablespoon of honey every morning before breakfast. Arthritis sufferers who swallowed this tasty medicine faithfully reported noticeable relief within the first week. And by the end of the first month of continued use, they were walking with no pain whatsoever!

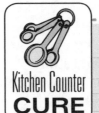

Kitchen Counter CURE

Spicy Flu Potion

The next time you start coming down with a cold or flu, show those germs the door with this powerful (and quite pleasant) potion.

- **3–4 whole cloves**
- **1 CINNAMON stick**
- **2 cups of water**
- **2 shots of whiskey**
- **1 ½ tbsp. of blackstrap molasses**
- **2 tsp. of lemon juice**

Put the cloves, cinnamon stick, and water in a saucepan, and bring the mixture to a boil over medium heat. Let it boil for three minutes or so. Remove the pan from the stove, and mix in the whiskey, molasses, and lemon juice. Cover the pan, and let it sit for about 20 minutes. Drink ½ cup of the tasty toddy every three to four hours (warm it up each time). Before you know it, you'll be back in full swing again!
Yield: About 5 doses

Cure Your Cold

Sore throats, coughs, and stuffy noses are no match for **CINNAMON**! To put its power to work, pour 1 cup of water into a saucepan, add a cinnamon stick, bring the mixture to a boil, and continue to boil for two minutes. Remove the cinnamon stick, and use the freshly boiled water to brew a cup of your favorite tea. *Note: If your cold symptoms last longer than a week, consult your doctor.*

Ease Indigestion

If you regularly suffer from heartburn or indigestion after meals, **CINNAMON** can help ease the discomfort. Simply drink a freshly brewed cup of cinnamon tea after every meal. If your indigestion persists after a few days, make an appointment to see your doctor.

Control Cold-Weather Woes

The natural warming power of **CINNAMON** can help relieve a couple of problems caused by low-digit temperatures:

HEALTHY Hint

VERSATILE INFECTION FIGHTER

A spicy **CINNAMON** brew can clear up yeast infections and also alleviate athlete's foot. The simple recipe: Bring 4 cups of water to a boil in a medium saucepan, and add 10 broken cinnamon sticks. Reduce the heat to low, and simmer for five minutes. Remove the pan from the stove, cover, and steep for another 45 minutes. When it's cooled to lukewarm, use it as a vaginal douche to get rid of the notorious vaginal infection *Candida albicans*.

To cure athlete's foot, after the brew has steeped, pour it into a basin, and soak your feet for 30 minutes. Repeat daily until the fungus has fled.

- **Cold feet.** Warm up your chilly toes by mixing ½ teaspoon of ground cinnamon into 8 ounces of hot water, letting it steep for 15 minutes. Drink three times a day, and it's all but guaranteed that your "hind paws" will be better able to tolerate the frigid temperatures.

- **Headaches.** When a heavy dose of cold air makes your head start pounding like a kettle drum, mix 2 to 3 teaspoons of ground cinnamon with just enough water to make a fine paste. Smooth it onto your temples and forehead, and you should feel almost-instant relief.

Stop the Runs

When it comes to curing diarrhea, **CINNAMON** is a champ. How you put it to work is your call. Here's a trio of tried-and-true prescriptions:

1. Mix 2 pinches of ground cinnamon per cup of warm milk, and sip it slowly. Drink as much of the beverage as possible throughout the day. This is an old—and delicious—Pennsylvania Dutch folk remedy that's especially helpful to children. (Stir in $1/2$ teaspoon of sugar if your young patient balks at drinking this spicy cure.)

2. Add 1 teaspoon of ground cinnamon and 1 teaspoon of sugar to 1 cup of hot water. Stir, let it cool to room temperature, and gulp it down as quickly as you can. One or two doses should get your inner workings back to normal.

3. In a saucepan, bring 2 cups of water to a boil, and add $1/4$ teaspoon of ground cinnamon and $1/8$ teaspoon of cayenne pepper. Reduce the heat, simmer for 20 minutes, then remove the pan from the burner. When the liquid is cool enough to drink, start sipping $1/4$ cup of the brew every 30 minutes or so until the runs have run their course.

HOW'S THAT?

Q *Jerry, I've heard that* **CINNAMON** *can make me a better driver. That's preposterous! Please tell me it's not true.*

A My friend, it is indeed true. Good ol' cinnamon can actually help you drive more safely. If you're like most folks I know, a traffic-clogged, rush-hour commute can send your stress level soaring off the charts. But cinnamon can make you feel more at ease—and therefore safer—behind the wheel. In a recent study, participants who chewed cinnamon-flavored gum during simulated traffic-jam scenarios significantly decreased their frustration, increased their alertness, and even said their ride seemed shorter. Not a gum chewer? Not to worry: You can achieve the same safety improvement by hanging a cinnamon-scented air freshener in your car. Now that's what I call a no-brainer!

Cloves Nix Nicotine

If you think you've tried every stop-smoking ploy under the sun, and you're still reaching for the cancer sticks, give this old-time trick a try: Always keep a whole **CLOVE** in your mouth. Suck on one for a couple of hours, then toss it out and put in a fresh one. The cloves neutralize the taste of nicotine in your mouth, which (according to the experts) is a major reason a smoker always feels the need for another cigarette.

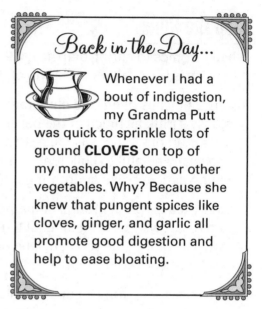

Back in the Day...

Whenever I had a bout of indigestion, my Grandma Putt was quick to sprinkle lots of ground **CLOVES** on top of my mashed potatoes or other vegetables. Why? Because she knew that pungent spices like cloves, ginger, and garlic all promote good digestion and help to ease bloating.

Clobber Pain with Cloves

CLOVE oil is a natural painkiller that works well for just about any kind of oral pain. Dip a cotton swab into the oil, and dab a little on the sore areas of your gums. Don't have clove oil? Then tuck a whole clove between your cheek and gum. It's not as effective as the concentrated oil, but it will turn the throbbing down a notch. *Note: Clove oil is available in health-food stores, herbal-supply stores, and online.*

Cloves Cut Back Coughs

To relieve a nagging cough, pop a whole **CLOVE** into your mouth and suck on it. The oil in the clove helps numb the tickle in your throat better than flavored cough drops or sweetened syrups.

Fast Help for Kitchen Cuts

Yikes! You were slicing a tomato for sandwiches, got distracted for a second, and sliced into your finger instead. Well, at least it happened within reach of a quick cure! Grab a jar of ground **CLOVES**, and pour a thin layer over your cut. It'll stop the pain and help prevent infection.

SPOTLIGHT ON
BAD BREATH

While bad breath won't kill you, it can make the people you're speaking to ready to keel over! Bad breath is certainly better than no breath at all, but you (and those around you) don't have to suffer with halitosis—the polite term for dragon breath. Here's a handful of easy ways to sweeten your breath, courtesy of your spice rack:

◆ Clear up bad breath and brighten your teeth at the same time. In a small dish, mix 1 tablespoon of baking soda, ½ teaspoon of ground **ALLSPICE**, ½ teaspoon of ground **SAGE**, and ½ teaspoon of sea salt or kosher salt. Sprinkle the mixture onto your toothbrush and brush your teeth with it, or stir 1 teaspoon into a cup of warm water and use it to gargle.

◆ Dissolve 1 tablespoon of ground **ALLSPICE** in 1 cup of hot water, let it cool to a comfortable temperature, and use it as you would any other mouthwash.

◆ Pop a pinch of **ANISEED** or a few whole **CLOVES** into your mouth, and chew on them to freshen your breath.

◆ Dilute 5 to 10 drops each of **CAYENNE** (red pepper) tincture and myrrh tincture (both available in health-food stores, herbal-supply stores, and online) in half a glass of warm water and use it to rinse your mouth. It'll kill germs and leave your breath spicy fresh, to boot.

◆ Spicy **CARDAMOM**, **CORIANDER**, and **MACE** are three excellent breath savers. Chew a few seeds of any one of these seasonings for a few minutes to release their breath-refreshing goodness.

◆ Suck on a **CINNAMON** stick to keep your breath naturally clean and fresh. You can also make a cinnamon mouthwash by simmering several sticks in boiling water for 10 minutes; let cool, then use the liquid as a breath-freshening rinse.

◆ Make your own odor-fighting mouthwash with whole or ground **CLOVES** steeped in hot water. Then swish, swish, swish.

◆ Chew a few **FENNEL** seeds after each meal. They'll help freshen your breath and promote healthy digestion.

Herbs & Spices

Count on Cumin

The folks who study such things tell us that **CUMIN** is the second-most-popular spice in the world (black pepper ranks number one). We love it most for the zing it adds to tacos and other Mexican food, as well as Indian, Middle Eastern, and North African cuisines. But it also packs a powerful load of health benefits. It boosts your energy, fights the free radicals that cause cancer and other diseases, and improves your kidney and liver function. To make this superstar part of your health-care team, simply work it into your diet a few times a week.

Blast Gas

If you suffer from bouts of gas every time you eat beans, sprinkle them with ground **CUMIN** before you dig in. This tasty spice helps diminish legumes' gas production, so you won't pollute the air around you.

Don't Tolerate Tummy Trouble

The next time you indulge in a rich dinner and end up with an upset stomach, reach for this quick fix: Dilute a tablespoon of ground **CUMIN** in a cup of hot water and sip slowly. The essential oils, sodium, and magnesium in cumin help to aid digestion, and will bring fast relief for your sour stomach.

HEALTHY Hint

CONK OUT WITH CUMIN

While there are no scientific studies to back this up, many folks have relied on **CUMIN** to take them off to the Land of Nod. About a half hour before your normal bedtime, simply pop a few cumin seeds into your mouth and chew on them to release their stress-reducing oils. Or, boil a cup of water and pour it into a mug containing 2 tablespoons of ground cumin. Stir, let the brew cool to a comfortably warm temperature, sip slowly, then toddle off to bed.

Breathe Easy

When you've got a nasty chest cold, you know how every breath is labored. You can ease your inhalations with **CUMIN**. Simply chewing on several cumin seeds will release their spicy heat, allowing cumin's expectorant properties to loosen up the mucus that's causing you so much effort to breathe.

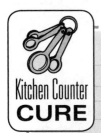

Kitchen Counter CURE

Spicy-Hot Cold Remedy

Spicy foods like jalapeño peppers and chili contain capsaicin, a substance that can help you reduce your nasal and sinus congestion. And the pungent spices in **CURRY POWDER** have a similar effect. Add a generous helping of the powder to a bowl of steaming-hot chicken soup. Your eyes will tear up, and your clogged-up nose will start running, and before you know it, you'll be breathing freely!

Curry Up to Good Health

Turmeric, the spice that gives **CURRY POWDER** its yellow color, is a potent cancer crusader. Studies suggest that turmeric and curcumin (the active ingredient in turmeric) may inhibit production of an enzyme found in certain types of cancers, including bowel and colon. It may also help fight prostate cancer. So sprinkle curry powder on your food regularly to boost your immune system and keep cancer at bay. *Note: Turmeric can slow down blood clotting, so if you are taking aspirin or any other anticoagulant, check with your health-care provider before using large amounts of curry.*

Defy Diabetes

When you have diabetes, your body doesn't make enough insulin, the hormone that delivers blood sugar to your cells. Turmeric and other spices found in **CURRY POWDER** can help regulate your body's insulin levels.

Bolster Bone Density

Studies are under way to test the effects of **CURRY POWDER** on bone density. Animal tests show that turmeric, one of the spices in curry powder, increases the speed of bone regrowth, connectivity, and repair, while reducing signs of bone loss by up to 50 percent. While we're waiting for human studies to show the same results, it sure doesn't hurt to add curry to your meals. Here are a few tasty ideas: Sprinkle the powder on air-popped popcorn or low-fat chips; stir a teaspoon into scrambled eggs; add 2 teaspoons to plain low-fat yogurt and use it as a dip for veggies; season chicken with it before baking or broiling instead of using salt and pepper.

Nip Nausea with Nutmeg

You probably sprinkle ground **NUTMEG** in eggnog and mix it into pumpkin when you're making a pie. It's the perfect ingredient that'll enhance those flavors! Ever since way back when, nutmeg and its oil have been used in Chinese and Indian traditional medicines to help cure digestive woes. In fact, one popular R_X is to mix a teaspoon of nutmeg with a tablespoon of honey to relieve nausea, gastritis, or indigestion.

Be Good to Your Heart

NUTMEG is a good source of minerals, such as calcium, copper, iron, magnesium, manganese, potassium, and zinc. Potassium is an important component of cell and body fluids that help control heart rate and blood pressure. It's also rich in many vital B-complex vitamins and anti-oxidants, like beta-carotene, that are essential for optimum heart health.

Zap Zits

Okay, a breakout isn't exactly a dire health emergency, but it sure can make you feel awfully self-conscious when you need to be out in public! And let's face it, even adults get an occasional pimple or two. Here's a super-quick fix: Mix a little milk with ground **NUTMEG** to form a paste, then apply it to your trouble spot to help reduce redness.

Back in the Day...

It should come as no surprise that my Grandma Putt and her friends knew all the tricks and tips when it came to relieving tooth pain. And well they should, because dentists were few and far between a couple of decades ago, and mighty expensive to visit, too. Just about everyone back then turned to home remedies to ease their pain. Here's one of the best: Rub a generous spoonful of **NUTMEG** oil on your gums around the sore tooth. The oil contains eugenol, which has a long history of use in dentistry for toothache relief. *Note: Nutmeg oil is available in health-food stores, herbal-supply stores, and online.*

Thyme to Get Healthy

THYME has been used for centuries to treat hypertension. Now animal studies have found that thyme lowers LDL ("bad") cholesterol levels and increases HDL ("good") cholesterol levels. So be good to your health and use thyme instead of salt in your diet.

Curtail a Cough

Halt the hacking with a soothing cup of hot **THYME** tea. Simply stir 1 tablespoon of chopped fresh thyme (or 2 teaspoons of dried) in a cup of boiling water. Let the fresh thyme steep for three to four minutes; if you're using the dried herb, let it steep for up to 10 minutes. Strain, then sip and enjoy!

HEALTHY Hint

THYME TO NIX NIGHTMARES

Are scary dreams waking you (or your spouse) up in the middle of the night? Well, don't take that sleep-depriving nonsense lying down. Instead, drink a cup of **THYME** tea before you go to bed. It's an old-thyme, er, old-time trick for banishing bad dreams, and it works like a charm! See the brewing instructions in "Curtail a Cough" (at left).

Curb the Surge

To control excessive menstrual bleeding, steep 2 tablespoons of fresh **THYME** in 2 cups of freshly boiled water for five minutes. Strain out the herb, and drink 1 cup of the tea. Pour the other cup into a bowl, and add an ice cube or two. Soak a washcloth in the cold brew, then wring it out and lay it across your pelvic area. *Note: If your periods are consistently heavy, get a medical checkup just to rule out any serious problems.*

Scratch No More

No matter what has you scratching up a storm, **THYME** can be a timely cure. Just make a pint of thyme infusion (use the recipe in "Curb the Surge," above), and pour it into your bathwater. The herb contains a substance called thymol, which has antiseptic and antibacterial properties that can make your itch vanish in a flash.

Quell Cancer

Recent studies suggest that **BLACK PEPPER** may help ward off breast cancer. A chemical compound in peppercorns called piperine may be able to prevent a breast cancer tumor from developing. And here's more good news about this spicy seasoning: Black pepper's cancer-preventing heroics are heightened when it buddies up with turmeric, so season your food with a cancer-bashing combo.

Tame a Cold

Like other pungent spices, **BLACK PEPPER** is a natural decongestant. So the next time you're stuffed up, sprinkle a generous portion of pepper onto your food and dig in. It'll loosen up mucus and make your nose start running, which is just what you need to clear your head.

Exit, Earwax!

Earwax may not be a major health problem, but if you've got an accumulation, it sure is annoying. To send the wax on its way, warm 1 tablespoon of corn oil to a comfortable temperature, and sprinkle in a little ground **BLACK PEPPER**. Dip a cotton ball into the mixture, and put the soaked blob in your ear. Wait five minutes, and remove the wax-covered cotton ball. You should feel instant relief.

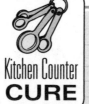

Kitchen Counter CURE

Black Pepper Tea

Got a cough that won't quit? Or a scratchy, sore throat? Or a nasty head cold? Whatever has you down for the count, this spicy-sweet **BLACK PEPPER** tea will pick you up and get you going again in no time.

- **1 tbsp. of honey**
- **1 tsp. of freshly ground black pepper**
- **1 tsp. of ground ginger (optional)**
- **1 tsp. of lemon juice**
- **2 cups of cold water**

Bring the water to a boil. While it's heating, put the remaining ingredients in a mug. Then pour the boiling water into the mug, stirring well. Sip the tea slowly, keeping it in your mouth for a few seconds before swallowing so the heat penetrates your sinuses.

A Red-Hot Heart Healer

In order to stay in good working order, your heart needs to receive a steady supply of blood. One of the best ways to ensure an ongoing flow of that life-giving fluid is to drink ⅛ teaspoon of ground **CAYENNE PEPPER** in a glass of water, herbal tea, or 100 percent fruit juice every day. *Note: Cayenne pepper is widely used to dissolve blood clots, but it also interacts with antacids, aspirin, and blood thinners. So if you take any of these medications on a regular basis, consult with your health-care provider before you use any cayenne remedy.*

Attack Arthritis Aches

Here's a simple way to ease the pain in your joints: Twice a day, mix ⅛ teaspoon of ground **CAYENNE PEPPER** in a glass of water or fruit juice, and drink up. The capsaicin in the pepper will block the debilitating pain.

Block Back Pain

Almost every adult on the planet gets a backache at one time or another. No matter what caused the problem, **CAYENNE PEPPER** liniment will send the pain packin' pronto. To make it, mix 2 tablespoons of ground cayenne pepper in 2 cups of boiling water. Reduce the heat, and simmer for 30 minutes. Remove the pan from the heat, and stir in 2 cups of rubbing alcohol. Let the potion cool, and store it at room temperature in a glass bottle with a tight-fitting lid. Then, whenever you feel the need, rub the liniment into your sore back. *Note: With any topical cayenne pepper remedy, test the potion on a small patch of skin first. And wash your hands thoroughly after applying it.*

HOW'S THAT?

Q *Jerry, is it true that I can use **CAYENNE PEPPER** to stop a toothache?*

A Yep, it sure is! Just press a few grains of ground cayenne pepper onto your painful tooth and gum. Yes, I know that it will sting like the dickens at first—but only for a second or two. As soon as the "fire" goes out, your toothache should be gone.

Make Ulcers Say "Uncle"

Doctors advise ulcer sufferers to avoid spicy foods because they can further irritate your stomach's lining. But there is one major exception to this rule: **CAYENNE PEPPER**. Studies show that it can actually help heal ulcers and prevent them from forming in the first place. It works in three ways:

- **Kills bacteria.** Cayenne pepper kills harmful bacteria in your stomach—including *Helicobacter pylori*, which is the prime cause of ulcers.

- **Regulates stomach secretions.** The capsaicin in cayenne pepper not only acts as a natural pain reliever, but it can also stop your stomach from producing acid, which irritates ulcers.

- **Relieves common side effects.** This versatile spice can relieve heartburn, indigestion, and other gastrointestinal discomforts that often accompany an ulcer. *Note: If you're under medical care for an ulcer, consult with your health-care provider before you embark on a cayenne pepper treatment routine.*

Back in the Day...

If you suffer from migraines, here's an old-time tip that could help end your agony: At the first sign of symptoms, dip a flat-ended toothpick into a jar of ground **CAYENNE PEPPER**, and sniff a tiny bit into each nostril. This remedy works for two reasons: Hot pepper contains both magnesium, which can help ward off migraines, and capsaicin, which blocks pain impulses from traveling to your brain. Remember to use only a few grains—even a midsize dash of pepper in your nose will deliver a very HOT surprise!

Conquer Carpal Tunnel

No one can deny that the computer age has given us many benefits, but it has also produced its share of unpleasant "side effects"—including carpal tunnel syndrome. If too much time at the keyboard has landed you with this painful affliction, reach for a jar of ground **CAYENNE PEPPER**. Mix 1 teaspoon of the red-hot powder into ¼ cup of skin lotion (any kind will do), and rub 1 teaspoon of the mixture—no more!—on the sore area. *Note: Be careful not to get the sizzling mixture on any broken skin or near your eyes, and wash your hands thoroughly after you've performed the procedure.*

Fabulous Fever Reliever

It might seem odd that something as hot as **CAYENNE PEPPER** could reduce your body's temperature when you're sick, but it does just that in this healthy helper. And making the tonic is a simple three-step process:

Step 1. Boil ½ teaspoon of ground cayenne pepper in 1 quart of water.

Step 2. Let the potion cool until it's comfortably warm, but not hot.

Step 3. Pour 1 cup of the "tea" into a bowl or measuring cup. Mix in ¼ cup of orange juice and 1 teaspoon of honey, and drink the potion slowly. Store the remaining cayenne-water solution in the fridge, and drink the remaining 3 cups throughout the day, heating it up each time, and adding the orange juice and honey to each cup.

HEALTHY Hint

LOWER YOUR STRESS LEVEL

No matter what has you all hot and bothered, let **CAYENNE PEPPER** help you reduce tension and supply a pleasant burst of energy, to boot. Start by drinking ⅛ teaspoon of the ground pepper in 8 ounces of warm water once a day. Stick with that dosage until you've gotten used to its firepower, then increase the amount of pepper to ¼ teaspoon, then ½ teaspoon. Continue this "drinking habit" until you're feeling calm, cool, and collected.

Tame Strain and Sprain Pain

Whether you're a weekend warrior who overdid it on the tennis court, or you just slipped on a patch of ice and twisted your ankle, **CAYENNE PEPPER** can come to your aid. Just mix a pinch of the fiery stuff in a cup or so of apple cider vinegar, dampen a cloth with the solution, put it on your sore body part, and leave it on for about five minutes. Repeat as often as necessary until the pain is gone and you're back to normal.

Rub Away Bruises

The next time you have a run-in with your coffee table or any other body-bashing object, mix 1 part ground **CAYENNE PEPPER** with 5 parts petroleum jelly, and rub the ointment onto your bruise. Repeat the procedure every day or two until the black-and-blue patch vanishes.

Warm Up Your Tootsies

If you're one of those people whose feet go into ice cube mode the minute you go outdoors in cold weather, this tip has your name written all over it: Before you pull on your boots or shoes, put on a pair of thin socks. Then grab a second, thicker pair, and sprinkle 1 teaspoon of ground **CAYENNE PEPPER** into each sock and pull 'em on over your stockinged feet. Your dogs will stay toasty warm.

Stay Cozy All Over

To rev up your circulation, thereby helping to keep your whole body warmer in cold weather, use either, or both, of these surefire remedies:

- Once a day, drink a glass of warm water with about 1/4 teaspoon of ground **CAYENNE PEPPER** stirred into it.

- Stir 1 or 2 teaspoons of ground cayenne pepper into a tub of warm bathwater, and settle in for a nice hot soak. Just beware that the oils in the pepper will heat up the water, so start off cautiously, and add more hot water from the tap if you need to.

Note: It goes without saying (I hope!) that these preventive measures are not substitutes for bundling up when you go outdoors!

HOW'S THAT?

Q *Jerry, I recently started drinking CAYENNE PEPPER "tea," and while I figured it might burn my mouth and throat at first, I got an unpleasant surprise when I urinated and felt the heat. Is that normal?*

A Not everyone is accustomed to eating spicy foods so, as you've discovered, when you first start drinking cayenne pepper in water, it will burn when you swallow it *and* when it comes out the other end. Over time, your body should adjust to the heat, but in the meantime, you can minimize the discomfort by taking your cayenne in capsule form.

If you want the more direct impact of the ground pepper mixed in water, start with no more than 1/8 to 1/4 teaspoon, and work your way up to bigger doses if the situation calls for that.

Salt of the Earth

Long before commercial pain relievers came along, folks swore by hot, dry **SALT** for treating a trio of common woes. It works wonders by drawing out pain quickly, safely, and inexpensively. Here's all you need to do: Heat a few tablespoons of salt in a dry frying pan until the salt is hot, but not too hot to touch. Either pour the salt into a clean cotton sock or wrap it up in a clean, dry dish towel. Then proceed as follows, depending on the location of the pain:

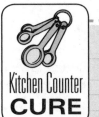

Kitchen Counter CURE

Sore-Throat Soother

Everybody on earth gets a sore throat now and then. So, of course, Grandma Putt knew all sorts of remedies to nix that nastiness and get back to her song-singin' self. This was the simplest: Just mix 1 teaspoon of **SALT** in about 2 cups of warm water. Then tip your head back and use it to gargle that sore-throat pain away!

■ **Arthritis.** Lay the poultice on your aching joint until you feel relief. To keep the salt comfortably warm, put a hot-water bottle or heating pad on top of it.

■ **Earache.** Hold the salty sock or towel against your sore ear. By the time the salt cools off, your pain should be gone. If not, repeat the treatment.

■ **Headache.** Hold the sock or pouch to the back of your head (even though you feel the throbbing in the front), and rub it over your scalp.

Clear Out Your Sinuses

Whether your stuffed-up airways are caused by a head cold or allergies, this trick will get the air flowing again: Mix 1/4 teaspoon of **SALT** and 1/4 teaspoon of baking soda in 8 ounces of warm, distilled water, and fill a bulb (a.k.a. ear) syringe with the mixture. (You can find bulb syringes in the baby products section of most drugstores.) Then lean over a sink, hold one nostril closed with your finger, and gently squirt the fluid into your open nostril. Blow your nose, and repeat the procedure on the other side. Bingo—you should be breathing freely again!

If you suffer from sleep apnea, a potentially dangerous condition in which your breathing is interrupted while you're sleeping, using this treatment at bedtime may help to keep your nasal passages open.

Sayonara, Psoriasis!

Legions of psoriasis sufferers have found that frequent dips in the ocean can send the crusty, itchy patches packin' pronto. If you're not lucky enough to live by the sea, here's your best alternative: Dissolve 1/2 cup of sea **SALT** per gallon of water in your bathtub, and soak your affected skin in the briny brew several times a day.

A Briny Bonanza

Psoriasis (see "Sayonara, Psoriasis!", above) is far from the only health condition that **SALT** water can cure. Just cast your eye on this list of remarkable remedies:

- **Athlete's foot.** Toss about 1/2 cup of salt into a basin filled with warm water, and mix it well. Then soak your feet for 5 to 10 minutes.

- **Heat exhaustion.** Mix 1 teaspoon of salt in a glass of water, and sip.

- **Ingrown nails.** Soak your afflicted fingers or toes for 30 minutes in a solution of 1 tablespoon of salt per quart of warm water.

- **Itchy skin.** Whether it's caused by poison ivy, insect bites, food-allergy rashes, or post-sunburn peeling, mix 1/2 cup of salt in a tub of warm water, and soak for as long as you like.

- **Jock itch.** Pour a cup or two of salt into the tub, and soak for 15 to 30 minutes. Repeat two or three times a day until the itch is history.

Back in the Day...

When I was a kid, I was always on the run, and sometimes things ran into me (like wayward baseballs!). When I came home with a shiner, my Grandma Putt knew just what to do to help fade it fast. She mixed 2 tablespoons of **SALT** with 2 tablespoons of vegetable shortening, then she spread the mixture on a soft cotton cloth and had me lay it against my black eye. Try it the next time you get a bruise—it'll stimulate blood circulation, which helps to eliminate those battered and blackened skin cells in no time flat.

HEALTHY Hint

CAN CANKER SORES

Canker sores do not pose a serious threat and, unlike cold sores, they are not contagious. But they sure can hurt like crazy! A simple way to solve the problem: Mix 1 teaspoon of baking soda, 1 teaspoon of **SALT**, and 2 ounces of 3% hydrogen peroxide, and rinse your mouth with the mixture four times a day until the sores disappear. If you find the tingle uncomfortable or the taste too strong, add 2 ounces of water to the formula.

A Salty Mouthful

Good old NaCl is just about the best friend your mouth and throat ever had. Here's a trio of fast fixes to get you in fine fettle again:

- **Laryngitis.** Gargle every few hours with a solution made of 1/2 teaspoon of **SALT** in 1 cup of warm water. Don't use any more salt than that, or it may increase your throat irritation rather than relieve it.

- **Mouth or tongue bites.** Mix 1 teaspoon of salt in 1 cup of warm water. Swish it around in your mouth until the wound feels better, which shouldn't take more than a minute.

- **Uncomfortable new dentures or braces.** Rinse with a solution of 1 to 2 teaspoons of salt in a glass of warm water. If your discomfort persists, call your dentist or orthodontist.

Ring Out Ringworm

Contrary to its name, ringworm is not a worm; it's a fungus that causes circular, scaly patches on the skin. Unfortunately, it can also spread like wildfire. But there's a simple two-step way to douse the flames:

Step 1. Soak a gauze pad in a solution made from 1 teaspoon of **SALT** dissolved in 2 cups of distilled water, and put it on the affected area for about 30 minutes.

Step 2. The next day, repeat the process using a gauze pad soaked in a solution made from 1 part apple cider vinegar mixed with 4 parts distilled water.

Alternate these compresses—salt one day, vinegar the next. In a week or so (depending on its severity), the foul fungus should be gone.

SPOTLIGHT ON
BLEEDING

Now I'm not talking about treating serious, gushing wounds. Those need immediate medical attention. Instead, I'm offering a handful of tips for stanching the blood when it's coming from a minor cut, your nose, your gums, or from menstruation.

◆ Quickly heal kitchen cuts with **BLACK PEPPER**. Simply pour a generous amount of ground black pepper onto the wound and apply pressure (and a bandage, if needed). Finely ground black pepper works best, and no, black pepper does not sting when put on a cut! This treatment is so effective that soldiers carried black pepper in their first-aid kits during World War II. Black pepper has antibacterial properties and makes blood coagulate quickly to stop the bleeding.

◆ There are a number of reasons your nose can start bleeding— because of allergies, a sinus infection, cold weather, or a bump on the schnozz. Regardless of what started the bleeding, you can stop it by drinking a glass of warm water with 1/8 teaspoon of ground **CAYENNE PEPPER** mixed into it. *Note: If you have recurrent nosebleeds, it may signal an underlying ailment, so make an appointment to see your health-care provider.*

◆ When your gums start bleeding, you need to see a dentist ASAP. But while you're waiting for your appointment, **SALT** can help stop the oozing. Just mix 1 part salt and 2 parts baking soda, and stir in a few drops of tea tree oil. Then, three times a day, dip a damp, soft-bristled toothbrush into the moist powder and brush very gently.

◆ Almost every woman of childbearing age knows that excessive menstrual flow is a major inconvenience—to put it mildly. Well, here's good news: **CAYENNE PEPPER** can help regulate your profuse bleeding. Just mix 1/8 teaspoon of the ground pepper into a cup of warm water or your favorite herbal tea. Drink a "cuppa" as often as needed throughout the day until the raging stream has slowed to a healthy trickle. *Note: If you're not sure whether your bleeding is due to extreme menstrual flow or hemorrhaging, don't take any chances—call your health-care provider pronto!*

Deal With Diarrhea

When you're suffering from the runs, it's important to replace the sodium, potassium, and chloride your body loses with each trip to the bathroom. One simple way to do that is to dissolve 1/2 teaspoon of **SALT** and 4 teaspoons of sugar in 1 quart of water. Stir in a tablespoon or two of orange, lemon, or lime juice for flavor and potassium. Then drink the whole quart over the course of the day.

Tackle a Toothache

Got a tooth that hurts like the dickens? Reach for **SALT**. Then mix up 2 tablespoons of apple cider vinegar, 1 tablespoon of salt, and 4 ounces of warm water. Swoosh the solution around the sore tooth and spit it out. Repeat until you've used up all of the rinse. That should ease the pain until you can get to the dentist's office. *Note: Use unfiltered apple cider vinegar, available in health-food stores and in the health-food sections of most supermarkets.*

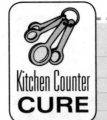

Kitchen Counter CURE

Singed Skin Soother

Whether it's a slight sunburn or very minor burn (nothing blistering), you can help heal the damaged skin with **SALT**. First, run cold water over the area for about five minutes. Then mix 1 to 2 teaspoons of salt (preferably sea salt) in a glass of ice-cold milk, and sponge the solution onto your skin once or twice a day, or as needed, until the pain is gone. *Note: If the burn is any more severe than a normal sunburn or very minor burn, or if your skin shows signs of becoming infected, don't hesitate—get medical help pronto.*

Fight Off Food-Borne Bacteria

Wooden cutting boards are more hygienic than plastic ones, which collect disease-causing bacteria by the zillions in the nicks and cuts that knives leave behind. Still, wooden versions can pick up their fair share of bacteria. To avoid trouble, it's important to follow routine maintenance: Every two to three weeks, cover the board's surface with a layer of coarse kosher or sea **SALT**, then rub it thoroughly with the cut side of a lemon half. Then rinse the board with hot water, dry it, and wipe on a light coat of mineral oil. (Avoid vegetable oil, which may turn rancid.)

CHAPTER 5

Healing Plants

Parsley, sage, rosemary, and thyme. We've all heard that refrain from Simon & Garfunkel's "Scarborough Fair." And while you may already use herbs like these to enhance your cooking, what you may not realize is that many cooking herbs (along with tomatoes and roses) are equally useful for medicinal purposes. So whether you're tending small pots of herbs on your windowsill or have a full-fledged kitchen garden, here's how to make the most of your health-giving bounty.

ON THE WINDOWSILL

Better Health with Basil

Researchers have been testing the oil from **BASIL** leaves and, according to their findings, these are some of the wonders that basil can work:

- Dampen the ulcer-producing activity of aspirin and alcohol
- Fight inflammation and swelling
- Battle infection-causing bacteria

Cancel Out Colon Cancer

Eugenol, a compound in **BASIL**, can increase the production of antioxidants in your intestines. The antioxidants help your body get rid of toxic substances that may cause cancer in the colon.

Basil Builds Bones

A handful of **BASIL** leaves provides a small amount of the minerals calcium, copper, magnesium, and manganese, all of which are important for a sturdy skeleton. So sprinkle the herb—fresh or dried—into soups, sauces, and salads.

Battle Bloat

Did you overindulge just a tad last night? **BASIL** can help reduce the resulting bloating and flatulence. Steep 2 tablespoons of chopped fresh basil leaves or 2 teaspoons of dried leaves in 1 cup of just-boiled water for 15 minutes. Then strain and sip slowly.

Back in the Day...

When you're battling a headache that just won't go away, try this old-time remedy: First, put a bottle of witch hazel in the refrigerator to chill for an hour or two (better yet, keep a bottle stashed there). Then put 1 teaspoon of dried **BASIL** into 1 cup of hot (not boiling) water, and let it sit for 10 minutes. Strain it into a large bowl, let it cool, and add 2 tablespoons of cold witch hazel. Soak a cotton washcloth or hand towel in the tea, wring it out, and lay the compress over your forehead and temples. Before you know it, you'll feel blessed relief! If, no matter what you do, your headache persists for more than a few days, or if it comes on suddenly and the pain is severe, get yourself to the emergency room.

On the Windowsill

Start the Flow

If your period is running late (and you know you're not pregnant), a cup of **BASIL** tea can get the show on the road. Just steep 1 tablespoon of the chopped fresh herb in 1 cup of just-boiled water for five minutes. Then strain, sip, and get ready for regularity. But first, make sure that you have a supply of tampons or sanitary pads on hand!

Kitty Knows Best

CATNIP may turn your lazy feline into a rowdy cat, but it actually has the opposite effect on us humans. In fact, sipping a cup of catnip tea after dinner may be just the ticket for winding down after a long, hard, stressful day. The simple recipe: Steep 1 teaspoon of the dried herb in just-boiled water for 15 minutes, then strain and enjoy. Just a word of warning: Be sure to stash your catnip out of the reach of all cats!

Ease Stomach Distress

The mellow, sedating quality of **CATNIP** calms the intestinal tract and decreases cramping. So the next time you have tummy troubles, make some catnip tea by adding 1 teaspoon of the dried herb to 1 cup of just-boiled water. Steep for 10 minutes, strain, and drink. *Note: Before using catnip in any form, be sure to read "Catnip Caveat" on page 13.*

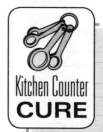

Kitchen Counter CURE

Easy Eye Soother

When a cold, flu symptoms, a night on the town, or an allergy attack leaves your eyes swollen and inflamed, treat those puffy peepers to a **CATNIP** eyewash. To make this restorative elixir, bring 3 cups of water to a boil, and add 2 tablespoons of fresh catnip leaves. Reduce the heat setting to low, and simmer for three minutes (no more!). Remove the pan from the burner, and let the brew steep for another 50 minutes. Then strain out the solids, pour the liquid into a clean glass jar with a tight-fitting lid, and store it in the refrigerator. When the need arises, soak a terry-cloth towel in the solution and put it over your eyes for half an hour—repeating the process until you feel relief.

Countless Cures

CATNIP tea is famous for its ability to do everything from reducing fevers to relieving nausea and nasal allergy symptoms—and, of course, to help you relax and get a good night's sleep. But catnip can also provide those same benefits in other forms, and it's delicious to boot. So give yourself a healthful treat by cutting up fresh leaves and tossing them into salads, or adding dried leaves to soups or stews. They're also great simply sprinkled over meats.

Calm a Nervous Stomach

When you feel like you're about to toss your cookies, add $\frac{1}{4}$ teaspoon of dried **OREGANO** and $\frac{1}{2}$ teaspoon of dried marjoram to 1 cup of just-boiled water. Let it steep, covered, for 10 minutes. Then strain the tea into a mug, and sip it slowly. Two hours later, if your tummy still feels queasy, make another cup and drink it to get your system back on an even keel.

Go, Oregano!

If you're always on the go until you're ready to drop, **OREGANO** is just what you need to relieve your aching body. The simple R_X: Put 1 cup of fresh oregano leaves into a cheesecloth pouch or an old panty hose foot, and toss it into a steaming-hot bath. Then slip into the water and breathe deeply, inhaling the aromatic herb to lift your spirits and ease your aches.

No More Labored Breathing

A nasty head cold can sure knock you for a loop. Here's a quick way to break up the congestion and get your nose flowing again: Put a handful of fresh **OREGANO** leaves into a medium-size heat-proof bowl and pour boiling water over them. Cover the bowl with a towel and let the mixture steep for about five minutes. Then carefully raise one end of the towel, lower your head over the bowl, and breathe in the healing vapors.

HOW'S THAT?

Q *Help, Jerry! Mosquitoes are eating me alive! I've heard that OREGANO can help stop the itching. But how?*

A This is an easy one: For centuries, folks have used oregano as a poultice for easing bug bites and stings. Just put $\frac{1}{4}$ to $\frac{1}{2}$ cup of fresh leaves in a blender with a small amount of water and puree until it's a sticky paste. Apply the paste to the affected area, wrap a piece of gauze around it to hold it in place, and secure with tape. Change at least once during the day, making a fresh batch of poultice each time (it does not store well). That's all there is to it!

Stand Tall with Parsley

Attention, ladies of, um, a certain age! If you're taking calcium supplements to help fend off osteoporosis, here's something you should know: Those high doses of calcium can impair your body's ability to absorb manganese, which is a crucial bone-building compound. But that doesn't mean you should give up the calcium. Instead, simply include 1 tablespoon or so of fresh **PARSLEY** in your daily diet to enhance manganese absorption.

Axe Arthritis Aches

The potent anti-inflammatory compounds in **PARSLEY** can make quick work of reducing pain and stiffness in your joints. Steep 1 fully-packed cup of fresh parsley in 1 quart of just-boiled water for 15 minutes. Strain out the solids, and refrigerate the liquid in a covered container. Drink 1/2 cup before breakfast, 1/2 cup before dinner, and 1/2 cup whenever your pain is especially severe.

HEALTHY
Hint

HELP FOR THE FREQUENTLY BRUISED

Some folks seem to attract bruises the way dark clothes attract lint. If that sounds like you or the youngsters in your household, keep a supply of anti-bruise cubes on hand. To make them, just mix 1 cup of finely chopped fresh **PARSLEY** with 2 tablespoons of water, and pour the slurry into an ice cube tray. Then, whenever someone bumps into a table or gets a black eye from a wayward tennis ball, pop a cube out of the tray, and gently glide it over the victim's bruise. The healing power of icy parsley will send it packin'.

Keep Your Liver Lively

Your liver performs more than 200 crucial functions, including eliminating toxic substances from the blood, and producing bile, which is essential for digestion. Simply making fresh **PARSLEY** a regular part of your diet will help keep that vital organ running smoothly. But every once in a while, give it an extra boost with a cocktail made from 1/2 cup of finely chopped fresh parsley leaves and the juice of a medium-size carrot and half a raw beet. *Note: If you don't have a juicer, substitute 1/2 cup each of organic carrot juice and beet juice.*

A Juicy Way to Relieve Asthma

A highly recommended blend for easing asthma symptoms is 2 ounces each of **PARSLEY**, carrot, and onion juices. Drink it twice a day—but keep in mind, this is not a substitute for professional medical care.

To make parsley juice, puree the fresh herb in a food processor or blender, then strain it through cheesecloth or a fine sieve to extract the juice. Use 4 to 5 cups of fresh parsley to give you 2 to 3 ounces of juice. You can purchase organic carrot juice if you're not making your own. To get onion juice, grate a raw onion, or mince it finely in a food processor, and squeeze the pieces through cheesecloth to extract the juice.

Drink Green for Good Health

Like many other herbs, **PARSLEY** makes a tea that can perform a passel of health-care feats. To make it, steep 1 teaspoon of dried or (even better) 2 tablespoons of chopped fresh parsley per 8 ounces of freshly boiled water for 10 minutes. When the tea is ready to drink, it'll be a vibrant green color. Strain it, and (presuming you made it in quantity) store it, covered, in the refrigerator. Then drink 3 or 4 cups of the tea a day, either cold or warmed up, to work any of these wonders:

■ Detoxify your kidneys, liver, and bladder

■ Reduce prostate swelling

■ Relieve urinary tract infections

Note: Consult with your doctor before you use parsley tea (or other homemade healers) to treat any of these conditions.

Back in the Day...

Nothing puts a damper on a good meal like a bout of indigestion. But you can nip your discomfort in the bud with this trick that Grandma Putt swore by. Simply nibble on a few sprigs of fresh **PARSLEY** (now you know why it's used as a garnish on dinner plates around the world). If you're fresh out of fresh parsley, just stir ¼ teaspoon of dried parsley into a glass of warm water and drink up. Your tummy will feel better in no time.

On the Windowsill

Can the Cramps

When your indigestion cramps your stomach as well as your style, steep 1 teaspoon of dried or 1 tablespoon of chopped fresh **PARSLEY** in 1 cup of just-boiled water for five minutes. Strain, and sip the tea slowly. *Note: Parsley is a potent diuretic, so don't stray too far from a bathroom!*

Reduce Your Gas Emissions

You say your digestive problems tend to express themselves outwardly? Steep 1 teaspoon of **PARSLEY** seed per cup of just-boiled water for 5 to 10 minutes. Drink 1 cup of the tea half an hour before each meal. (Find parsley seed in herbal-supply stores or online.)

Fast-Acting Sting Relief

You're puttering around in your yard on a fine summer morning when …OUCH! An insect plants its stinger (or its mouth parts) in your skin. What do you do? Well, if you grow **PARSLEY**, just pluck a few of the leaves, and rub them on the bite site. The plant's compounds will instantly relieve the pain.

Scram, Skeeters!

Don't let disease-spreading vampires spoil your warm-weather fun. Make yourself some liquid "armor" by mixing 1 tablespoon of dried **PARSLEY** per ¼ cup of apple cider vinegar in a large jar that has a tight-fitting lid. Shake the jar to blend thoroughly, and keep it where you can get at it easily. Then, before you venture outdoors, rub the lotion generously onto your exposed skin using a cotton pad.

HEALTHY
Hint

PARSLEY PERIL

If you are pregnant or think you might be pregnant, do not drink **PARSLEY** tea or juice, or use parsley seeds or essential oil. All of these contain high concentrations of the plant's volatile oils, which can cause serious problems. It's usually fine to eat either fresh or dried parsley in normal food portions. But just to be safe, ask your obstetrician how much of the herb is safe to consume. Once the baby arrives, if you're nursing, bypass parsley because it can slow the flow of breast milk. And steer clear of it entirely if you have kidney disease, high blood pressure, or edema.

Rah-Rah for Rosemary!

The next time you reach for **ROSEMARY**, you could be protecting your body against cancer. This aromatic herb is packed with carnosol, a compound that fights cancer by interrupting inflammation so that those evil cells can't get a toe-hold and grow. Carnosol also appears to boost your liver's production of several cancer-fighting substances. Rosemary is being explored for its ability to relax you when it's inhaled, so make sure that you breathe deeply whenever you cook with it.

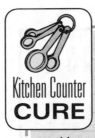

Kitchen Counter CURE

Anti-Arthritis Tea

ROSEMARY is a potent pain reliever, and just what you need to soothe aching arthritic joints. So get your joints jumpin' again! Place 2 tablespoons of fresh rosemary (or 2 teaspoons dried) in 1 cup of just-boiled water; steep for five minutes. Strain out the herbs, and enjoy. Sip 2 cups a day for maximum relief.

Savor the Flavor

Talk about an herbal superstar! In addition to fighting cancer (see "Rah-Rah for Rosemary!," above), **ROSEMARY** offers up a boatload of anti-aging antioxidants, and can (among other feats) improve memory and concentration, lift your spirits, aid digestion, relieve muscle pain, and boost your immune system. The simple R_X: Sprinkle ground rosemary, or place a whole branch of it on pork, chicken, or beef while it's cooking to infuse flavor and reap the healthy rewards.

Quick Fix for Dizziness

Feeling like the room is spinning? Make your own smelling salts by crushing dried **ROSEMARY** leaves inside a tissue or handkerchief. Then take a good long whiff.

Say "Ta-Ta" to Ticks

ROSEMARY does a dandy job of keeping ticks and fleas away from you (and your four-footed pals). To make the repellent powder, dry the leaves and grind them up in a blender. Sprinkle the powder around your patio and outdoor areas. For Fido, simply rub the powder into your pets' fur.

On the Windowsill

HEALTHY Hint

CURB CHOLESTEROL

If you're on the front lines in the war against high cholesterol, add **SAGE** to your arsenal. Studies have found that drinking sage tea three times a day for two months helped lower LDL ("bad") cholesterol and triglycerides and raise HDL ("good") cholesterol levels in participants who had high cholesterol. *Note: If you are currently on medication for high cholesterol, check with your doctor before using any herbal teas.*

Dodge the Itch...

Of mosquito bites and—more importantly—the dastardly diseases they can deliver. How? Just put rosemary and **SAGE** to work. Skeeters hate the smell of both herbs, and any of these terrific tricks will keep the little buggers at bay:

- At your next barbecue, toss some fresh sage or rosemary sprigs on the coals.

- Make insect-repelling candles. Melt grated white wax in a heat-proof container, and mix in a handful each of dried rosemary and sage. Pour the wax into molds (clean tuna cans are perfect), and insert a wick in the center of each one. When they're dry, set them around your outdoor gathering areas, and light them to keep biting bugs at bay.

- Brew a strong cup (or more) of rosemary or sage tea (see the recipe for Anti-Arthritis Tea on page 179). Let it cool, then pour it into a spray bottle. Then spritz it on your exposed skin whenever you venture into skeeter territory.

A Sage Choice

While **SAGE** may not make you any smarter, it just may help you recall what you already know. Research is under way to determine whether sage can improve memory in people with mild to moderate Alzheimer's disease. But there's no need to wait for the results: Get a head start by making a tea with 1 teaspoon of dried (or 2 tablespoons fresh) leaves, steeped for five minutes in just-boiled water. Drink up to 2 cups per day to help keep your mind sharp. Talk about sage advice!

SPOTLIGHT ON
STOMACH TROUBLES

We've all been there—feeling green at the gills, from either a too-rich meal, a scary roller-coaster ride, or general anxiety and stress. But no matter why your stomach is roiling, there's an easy fix. Brew up a tea made from any of the herbs on this list, and you'll be taming your tummy troubles in no time. The simple recipe, unless otherwise noted: Steep 2 teaspoons of dried (or 2 tablespoons of fresh) leaves in 1 cup of just-boiled water for five minutes. Strain, then sip slowly.

◆ A cup of **BASIL** tea can aid digestion and expel gas. Herbalists also recommend basil for easing stomach cramps and vomiting.

◆ If you're feeling bloated and gassy, sip **BAY** tea. Bay has long been used to soothe the stomach and relieve flatulence.

◆ Relax those cramped stomach muscles with **CATNIP**. It also helps to ease the pain of menstrual cramps.

◆ **CHAMOMILE** is a strong antispasmodic, relaxing the digestive tract. It's been used for thousands of years to relieve stomach cramps, bloating, and indigestion.

◆ **CORIANDER** comes to the rescue when your stomach is doing flip-flops. You can make a tea from steeping the seeds, or simply chew on a few seeds themselves whenever your stomach is acting up.

◆ **FEVERFEW** helps relieve upset stomach and bloating.

◆ **LAVENDER** infusion soothes stomachaches. To make lavender tea, use the same proportion of dried or fresh flowers and just-boiled water as you would for herb leaves.

◆ From the **MINT** family, peppermint, spearmint, and wintergreen all help relieve stomachache, heartburn, and indigestion.

◆ Cut down on gassiness and ease indigestion with **ROSEMARY**.

◆ Nix nausea with **SAGE**. Sip the tea hot or cold to relieve your queasiness and improve digestion.

◆ **THYME** is a time-honored digestive aid. Use the tea to relieve gassiness and stomach distress.

On the Windowsill

Comforting Calendula

If you grow **CALENDULAS** (*Calendula officinalis*), a.k.a. pot marigolds, in your kitchen garden, you have the makings of a powerful, gentle—and versatile—healer. It's terrific for treating minor cuts, burns, and insect bites, and even massaging achy muscles. Here's how to make a supply:

1. Put 5 cups of fresh calendula blossoms in a pan, and pour in just enough extra virgin olive oil to reach 2 inches above the flowers.

2. Heat the mixture on low until it almost simmers. Continue to heat on low, uncovered, for six to eight hours, or until the oil has turned a golden-orange color and has a strong herbal aroma. (Test every hour, and make sure it doesn't simmer.)

3. Remove the pan from the heat, and cool to room temperature. Strain it through cheesecloth, and store in a tightly capped bottle in the refrigerator. It'll keep for six months to a year.

Paint Away the Pain

For a speedy end to a raw, sore throat, "paint" it with **CALENDULA**. Dip a cotton swab into the Classic Calendula Infusion (at right), and apply it to the back of your throat, paying attention to the sides. If you don't relish the thought of poking a swab down your throat, gargle with the infusion instead. Repeat the procedure up to three times a day.

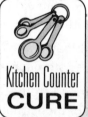

Kitchen Counter CURE

Classic Calendula Infusion

An herbal infusion is simply a strong tea. This **CALENDULA** recipe can be brewed, then refrigerated for up to two days.

2 tsp. of dried calendula flowers (or 4 tsp. of fresh flowers)

1 cup of water

Place the herbs in a teapot or large mug. Heat the water until it just reaches a boil. Pour the water into the teapot or mug, cover, and steep for 20 minutes. Strain out the solids, and use the liquid infusion as called for in your healing recipe. Store any leftover infusion tightly covered in the refrigerator, and use or dispose of it within 48 hours.

End Eye Irritation

When your eyes are itching or watering from allergies or exposure to cigarette smoke, a **CALENDULA** compress can bring quick relief. Start by making an infusion (see the Classic Calendula Infusion, at left). Let it cool to room temperature, then soak a clean cotton cloth in the infusion for one minute. Wring out the cloth so that it's still wet, but not dripping, and fold it over to be small enough to cover your eyes. Recline in a comfortable chair, or lie down, place the compress over your eyes, and relax for 10 minutes. Repeat throughout the day until your bleary eyes are better.

Calendula Cure for Cuts

Help heal a cut with a **CALENDULA** poultice. Simply saturate a piece of sterile gauze or cotton cloth with a calendula infusion (see the Classic Calendula Infusion, at left). Place the soaked cloth on your injury, and leave it on for about an hour to help soften the skin and make any debris easier to remove. Afterward, put a drop or two of the infusion directly onto the wound to keep it germ-free and to minimize scarring.

Back in the Day...

If you spend any time in the kitchen, you've probably experienced a few minor burns. So do what Grandma Putt did, and use a tincture of **CALENDULA** for minor-burn first aid. The herb is an anti-inflammatory, astringent (cleanser), and antiseptic all rolled into one. Here's the simple R_x: Combine 1 ounce of dried calendula flowers and 5 ounces of vodka in a glass jar with a tight-fitting, non-metallic lid. Put the jar on a sunny windowsill for two weeks, shaking the contents every few days so that the alcohol can extract the herb's active ingredients. After two weeks, strain the liquid into another clean jar with a tight-fitting lid. It will keep in the pantry for up to two years.

To treat a minor burn, first wait a day or two after the mishap so the tincture won't sting. Then add several drops of the tincture to a cup of room-temperature water. Dip a clean cloth into the mixture, and carefully dab it on the burn several times each day.

The Many Charms of Chives

We're all familiar with the culinary uses for **CHIVES**, but did you also know that these powerful little onions can help lower cholesterol in addition to its other health benefits? That's because whether you're choosing chives that are related to onions or those related to garlic, either type has the ability to head off heart disease, curb cancer, and more. So what's their magic ingredient? A compound called allium, which has been shown to have antibacterial and antifungal properties that can prevent infections. This compound also helps to reduce cholesterol and protect against cancers of the stomach and colon. So what are you waiting for? Snip some chives over your baked potato, stir them into your scrambled eggs, and toss 'em in your salad to crunch into their health-giving goodness.

Unstuff with Chives

When the congestion of a cold or flu gives you a headache from you know where, **CHIVE** tea will end your misery fast. To make it, put 1½ tablespoons of finely chopped chives and ½ tablespoon of finely shredded fresh ginger into a mug or teapot, and pour 1 cup of boiling water over them. Cover the top, and let the mixture steep for 30 minutes. Strain out the solids, and drink the tea lukewarm. Your head should stop throbbing in 20 minutes or less. Repeat as often as needed during your illness.

HOW'S THAT?

Q *Hey, Jerry, I'm not a huge fan of* **CHIVES,** *but my wife says they'll help me sleep better at night, so she insists on sprinkling the darn things on just about everything we eat! Can you give me some ammunition to fire back, so I can stop this chive madness?*

A Sorry, pal, but your wife is right. Chives contain, among other nutrients, choline, which helps maintain a healthy nervous system and induces sleep. Those chives she's adding to your meals just may help you snooze more soundly, so eat up and stop your complaining!

Comfrey Comforts Sprains

Sprained ligaments are no bed of roses. But a stroll (or hobble) into your kitchen garden can speed up the recovery process. Just blanch two to four fresh-picked **COMFREY** leaves, and put them over your sprained body part. Cover the leaves with an elastic bandage, and go about your business. Renew the dressing every day, and you'll be back in the running before you know it.

Banish a Bruise

Did your kneecap meet up with the corner of your coffee table? Or did your hip say "hello!" to an opened kitchen drawer? However you got bruised, **COMFREY** can bring relief. This herb's leaves contain allantoin, which helps skin repair itself and helps reduce inflammation. To get comfrey's bruise-busting benefits, start by boiling some water in a medium saucepan. Then use tongs to dip one fresh-picked comfrey leaf at a time into the boiling water just until the leaf is soft. (The number of leaves you'll need is based on how large the bruise is. Use enough to cover it with some overlap.) Lay the hot leaves on paper towels until they are comfortably cool. Wrap the leaf or leaves around your bruised body part and hold it in place with a strip of gauze. Leave the poultice on for three hours, then start again with fresh leaves. By the way, this same comfrey poultice works well for minor cuts and scrapes.

Put a Halt to Hemorrhoids

These swollen anal veins really are a pain in the keister. Here's a quick way to get relief: Boil about 1 teaspoon of chopped-up **COMFREY** root in 3 cups of water. Strain out the solids and soak a soft, clean washcloth in the liquid, then gently hold it against your tender tush. Repeat the treatment throughout the day until you're sitting pretty again.

Put the Kibosh on Colds and Flu

Research has shown that regularly taking **ECHINACEA** may keep you from getting sick—and if you do come down with a cold or flu, your symptoms will be less severe. Place 2 teaspoons of dried echinacea root in a saucepan. Add 1 cup of water and bring to a boil. Lower the heat, cover the pot, and simmer for 30 minutes. To drink immediately, strain the liquid into a mug. To make a larger batch to store for use later, increase the amount of dried root and water, keeping the same proportions. After boiling and simmering, turn off the heat and leave the mixture in the pot, with the cover on, until it reaches room temperature. Then strain the liquid into a large glass jar or pitcher. Store, tightly covered, in the refrigerator for up to two days. Drink 1 cup, hot or cold, two to three times a day during cold and flu season. *Note: Do not use echinacea if you're pregnant or nursing, or if you have an autoimmune disease such as lupus, rheumatoid arthritis, or multiple sclerosis.*

Echinacea Evicts Cold Sores

ECHINACEA can battle cold sores by boosting the immune fighters in your mucous membranes. The simple routine: Mix ¼ teaspoon of echinacea extract in water or fruit juice, and drink it three times a day.

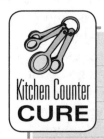

Kitchen Counter CURE

Sore-Throat Solution

When your throat feels like it's on fire, douse the flames with the antiviral power of this **ECHINACEA** gargle.

1 tablespoon of dried echinacea root

2 cups of water

Place the dried root in a saucepan and cover with water. Bring to a boil, lower the heat, cover, and simmer for 30 minutes, checking occasionally to be sure the water hasn't cooked away. Turn off the heat and leave the mixture in the pot, covered, until cooled to room temperature. Strain out the solids and pour ¼ cup of the liquid into a glass; this is enough to allow you to gargle and swish it around your mouth, spit out, and repeat. Store the remaining solution tightly covered in the fridge for up to two days.

Feverfew Flattens Migraines

In numerous studies, **FEVERFEW** has proven effective in lessening the duration, severity, and frequency of migraine headaches as well as related symptoms such as dizziness, nausea, and vomiting. If you're a chronic migraine sufferer, then you can take your preventive medicine in one of two ways:

- Eat two to four leaves of fresh feverfew each day.

- Steep two to eight fresh leaves per cup of freshly boiled water for five minutes or so, and sip 1 or 2 cups of the tea each day.

The downside is that this herb has a bitter taste, and some people develop mouth sores after chewing on the leaves, so for them the tea is a better option. Sweeten it by adding a teaspoon of honey. *Note: Women who are pregnant should not use feverfew because it may cause the uterus to contract, increasing the risk of miscarriage or premature delivery.*

Alleviate Arthritis

Studies suggest that **FEVERFEW** can reduce inflammation. Research is under way to determine whether this can help those who suffer from rheumatoid arthritis. In the meantime, it can't hurt to give it a try. Make a tea as described in "Feverfew Flattens Migraines" (above), and sip a cup, warm or cold, twice a day.

Back in the Day...

Here's some folklore that has stood the test of time: More **FEVERFEW** equals fewer bee stings. Make that *no* bee stings, according to Grandma Putt. So whether you're allergic to bee venom, or you simply want to keep the buzzers from spoiling your summertime fun, do as she did and grow plenty of feverfew *(Tanacetum parthenium)* in your outdoor living areas. It'll make your backyard a safer and more pleasant place to hang out because bees won't go anywhere near it.

From the Kitchen Garden

Take Tea and See...

How quickly and effectively **LAVENDER** tea can perform heaping helpings of healing feats. The basic formula is the same as it is for any other herbal tea: 1 to 2 teaspoons of dried flowers or double the amount of fresh per cup of just-boiled water, with honey and/or lemon added to taste. Or make a batch of brew (by the quart) ahead of time. Then put it into the refrigerator, where it'll keep for three to four days, or freeze it in ice cube trays or plastic cups. When teatime rolls around, warm it up, drink it cold, or eat it like an ice pop. Use it to:

- **Ease anxiety.** Drink 2 or 3 (or more) cups a day as needed to calm your nerves.

- **Heal cuts and scrapes.** Clean the wound, then dip a cotton ball or pad in lavender tea, and apply it to the "owie."

- **Quell migraines and headaches.** Sip the brew as needed throughout the day to tame the pain.

- **Relieve heartburn and indigestion.** Take 1 cup in the morning and at bedtime.

- **Strengthen your gums.** Swish room-temperature tea around in your mouth every day or two. It'll sweeten your breath, too!

- **Vanquish vertigo.** When a dizzy spell strikes, drink 3 or 4 cups a day until you're feeling steady on your feet again. *Note: If you suffer from vertigo frequently for no apparent reason, it could indicate the presence of a serious health problem, so see your doctor ASAP.*

HEALTHY Hint

HOMEGROWN ONLY

When using **LAVENDER** for health purposes, always use homegrown flowers, unless you know that the lavender you buy was organically grown. Never consume flowers that came from a florist or the supermarket's floral section—they've been sprayed with insecticides, fungicides, and/or chemical fertilizers.

Relieve Body Aches

When you go a little overboard at the gym or yank a few weeds too many out of your flower beds, don't pop pills to ease your pain. Massage **LAVENDER** oil into your sore joints and muscles. The oil's anti-inflammatory compounds will deliver deep-down relief. As a bonus, the lavender scent will relax you and might even take your mind off your aching body.

Inhale Asthma Away

At the first sign of asthma symptoms, fill a pot with water, and for each quart, add 2 tablespoons of **LAVENDER** flowers (fresh or dried). Boil the water, and inhale the rising steam to open your respiratory passages. *Note: If you're having what you think is an asthma attack, and you are not already under medical care for the condition, call your doctor.*

Heal Burns from the Inside

Toss fresh or dried English **LAVENDER** *(Lavandula angustifolia)* leaves, petals, or flower tips into salads, soups, and vinegars to help reduce the pain and speed the healing of burns. *Note: To retain the health-giving volatile oils of dried lavender, always store it in an airtight container in a cool, dark place (but not the fridge).*

Soothe Inflamed Skin

This lovely **LAVENDER** lotion will heal red, raw hands in a jiffy. To make it, put 1/2 cup of dried lavender flowers and 1/2 cup of finely chopped fresh sage in a pan with 2 cups of water. Simmer, covered, on low heat for 20 minutes. Strain the liquid into a glass jar with a tight-fitting lid, let it cool, and add 8 drops of lavender oil. Put the lid on the jar, and shake it thoroughly to mix in the oil. Then gently smooth the lotion onto your skin with cotton pads or a soft cotton cloth. Repeat as needed until your hands are sore no more.

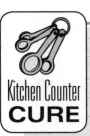

Kitchen Counter CURE

Blister Dust

You never know where you'll be when blisters erupt on your hands or feet. So stash containers of this remarkable remedy where you can grab it quickly for instant relief.

Buds from 1 sprig of dried LAVENDER, crushed
4 tbsp. of cornstarch
4 drops of lavender oil

Mix all of the ingredients together, and store the mixture in an airtight container, where it will keep indefinitely. Dip a cotton ball or swab into the mixture and dab it onto your blister(s). Yield: About 1/4 cup.

From the Kitchen Garden

Healing Plants

Fight Finger Infections

Splinters, insect bites, and even hangnails can all result in finger infections, but no matter what causes them, they're a lot like toothaches: The pain they cause is way out of proportion to the size of the afflicted body part. The simple remedy: Boil 2 tablespoons of fresh or 1 tablespoon of dried **LAVENDER** flowers in 1 quart of water for 10 minutes. Strain out the solids, let the potion cool to a comfortable temperature, and soak your sore digit for 5 to 10 minutes. Repeat the procedure several times a day until the problem is gone. *Note: If you don't start to see progress after a few days, or if the infection reaches deep into your skin or the joints of your finger, get medical help.*

Back in the Day...

As all you mothers and mothers-to-be know, your sense of smell becomes much more acute during pregnancy. Odors that you never even noticed before, like those from your dog's bed or a basket of dirty laundry, can send you rushing for a bucket. The solution: Arm yourself against trouble by carrying this old-time aromatic antidote with you wherever you go. Fill a small tin with dried **LAVENDER** and keep it in your pocket or purse. Then, whenever you catch a whiff of something that turns your stomach, pull out your fragrant defense mechanism, open it up, and breathe in deeply.

Sock It to Stress

Looking for quick stress relief? It's in your sock drawer. At least it can be if you try this terrific trick: Mix up equal parts of dried **LAVENDER**, dried rosemary, and broken cinnamon sticks, all of which have aromas that are highly effective in lowering anxiety levels. Stuff a handful or so of the mixture into a clean sock until you have a wad that's about the size of a baseball, and tie the top closed with yarn or ribbon. Then, anytime you feel on edge, repeatedly squeeze the ball to release a blast of calming scent. And if you keep this stress buster in your sock drawer, it'll remind you to start off every morning on an easygoing foot!

Call It a Night

Studies have shown that consistently poor sleep can reduce your life span by a whopping 8 to 10 years. We know that even a few nights of tossing and turning can make you feel (and act) like a zombie. No matter what's keeping you awake at night, the calming scent of **LAVENDER** will beckon the Sandman in a hurry. Here are a few simple options:

■ Keep a vase of fresh or dried lavender on your bedside table.

■ Fill a small fabric pouch with dried lavender, and tuck it under your pillow. Replace it when the scent fades.

■ On laundry day, put some dried lavender into a small zippered pillowcase, and toss it into the dryer with your bed linens.

■ Pour cooled, strong lavender tea into a plastic spray bottle, and spritz your pillowcase and sheets. (Allow them to dry before hitting the sack.)

STRIKE OIL

No medicine chest should be without **LAVENDER** oil, and if yours is, just take a gander at some of the healing heroics it can perform.

HEALTH PROBLEM	HOW TO SOLVE IT
Blister	Apply 2 drops of lavender oil to a bandage and cover the blister with it.
Headache	Put a drop of lavender oil on the tip of each index finger, and massage your temples with your fingertips for a minute or two.
Heat rash	Apply a drop or 2 of lavender oil directly onto the rash three or four times a day.
Stuffy nose	Put a drop of lavender oil under your tongue.
Weeping sore	Apply several drops of lavender oil to the sore throughout the day.*

If your sore doesn't heal within a week, see your doctor.

From the Kitchen Garden

Keep Yourself in Mint Condition

We don't often think of **MINT** (both peppermint and spearmint) as healthy, especially when we equate it with gum, candy, and those delicious Girl Scout Thin Mints®! But mint actually packs a wealth of healthy benefits. This herb contains limonene, a powerful anti-cancer agent that may be able to block the growth of breast tumors and even shrink them. Mint also packs another breast cancer fighter, luteolin, which may help inhibit the production of inflammatory compounds linked with the development of cancer. So toss a few tablespoons of chopped spearmint into salads, on berries, and in place of basil in the pesto for your favorite pasta.

Wake Up and Smell the Peppermint!

Why? Because sniffing **MINT** in any form, whether it's fresh or dried leaves, extract, essential oil—or even candy or chewing gum—can do a couple of things for you:

- **Increase your energy level.** The aroma of peppermint works directly on your sensory nerves to increase alertness and get-up-and-go.

- **Help you lose weight.** In a study by the Smell & Taste Treatment and Research Foundation, 3,193 volunteers who regularly sniffed the scent of peppermint, green apples, or bananas lost an average of 30 pounds in six months.

HOW'S THAT?

Q *When I was a kid, I got carsick during every long trip. My granddad would hand me a roll of* MINT *candies to calm the nausea, and it always helped. Was it just the power of suggestion, or can mint really cure a queasy stomach?*

A You had one smart granddad! Peppermint contains menthol, which helps prevent spasms in the digestive tract, lessening cramps and easing nausea. So if you've happened to pass your green-at-the-gills trait on to your kids, be sure to bring along plenty of peppermint on family road trips.

Prevent the Hurt of Heartburn

Research has shown that good old **PEPPERMINT** can relieve gas, stop spasms in the digestive tract, promote stomach secretions, and kill bacteria. So if you tend to suffer from heartburn after meals, whip up a batch of mint tincture and take 1 teaspoon three times a day. The simple R$_X$: In a glass or ceramic jar, combine 7 ounces of dried mint leaves in about 4 cups of vodka. Close tightly with a non-metallic lid. Set the jar in a cool, dark place for two to six weeks, shaking the jar periodically to extract the herb's active ingredients. Then strain out the solids and store the liquid, tightly closed, for up to two years.

> # HEALTHY
> ## Hint
> ### MIND YOUR MINT
>
> Do not give **MINT** tea to children under the age of 2 because the menthol can cause a choking sensation. For children up to the age of 12, try a very diluted tea of just 1 teaspoon of dried mint leaves per cup of boiling water. Let the tea cool down to warm before serving.

Unclog Your Schnozz

The next time you have a stuffed-up nose, get things flowing with a **MINT** decongestant. Fill your bathroom sink with steaming hot water, and add a handful of fresh or dried mint leaves. Then drape a towel over your head and bend over, breathing in the fragrant fumes. Stay there as long as you can, or until the vapors dissipate and the water cools. Repeat as needed throughout the day.

Aid an "Ouchie"

MINT can help numb pain, and it is often used in commercial first-aid creams for sunburn and wounds. You can harness mint's anesthetic powers by making a simple poultice from the leaves. Start by chopping 1/4 to 1/2 cup of fresh leaves (or put them in a food processor). Add a bit of water to make a paste. Then apply the paste to the injured skin, and wrap a clean cloth or strip of gauze over the area.

Send a Headache Packin'

No matter where you're from, a headache is a major pain in the, well, head. In two far-flung places, old folk remedies use **MINT** as a surefire cure for the throbbing:

■ In Mexico, folks say to paste or (in more modern times) tape a fresh mint leaf on the part of your head where the ache is most severe, and leave it there until the pain is gone.

■ Our English friends juice their mint leaves and use the fluid as ear drops (yes, you read that right). To try this trick, liquefy a few mint leaves in a blender or food processor, and mix in enough water so the fluid will flow easily through a medicine (a.k.a. eye) dropper. Tilt your head and put a few drops into each ear, and before you know it, your headache should be history.

Fight Fatigue

The next time you need to crank up your workout—or you need more get-up-and-go power—and you're just not in the mood, take a whiff of **PEPPERMINT**. One study has shown that sniffing peppermint boosts exercise performance, making workouts seem easier to complete. So whether you're pumping iron or pulling weeds, mint can give you the energy you need to get the job done.

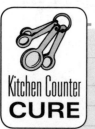

Kitchen Counter CURE

Mighty Mint Tea

While **MINT** can energize you (see "Fight Fatigue," above), it can also calm you down (go figure!). So ditch the coffee and soothe your frazzled nerves with a cup of peppermint (or spearmint) tea. Here's the simple how-to: Just steep a small handful of fresh-picked peppermint or spearmint leaves in 1 cup of freshly boiled water. After three minutes, sample for taste; keep steeping if you want a stronger flavor. Then strain and, if desired, sweeten your tea with a spoonful of honey, sit back, and enjoy.

Roses Ride to the Rescue

Pretty **ROSE** petals are packed with enough healing power to tackle a trio of common health problems. And here's more good news: The petals' medicinal power increases as the flowers fade, so you can use blooms that you'd otherwise toss in the compost bin. Here's the scoop:

- **Ease joint pain.** Toss the petals from four over-the-hill roses into your bathwater, and settle in. Put a piece of cheesecloth over the drain before pulling the plug, or you'll clog your plumbing!

- **Soothe a sore throat.** Make a concentrated tea by steeping ¼ cup of fresh petals in 1 quart of boiling water for 15 minutes. Strain, and drink 2 or 3 cups a day until you're feeling better.

- **Strengthen weak, tired eyes.** Throw a handful of faded petals into a pot, cover with water, and bring to a boil over medium heat. Remove the pot from the stove, let it cool, and strain out the petals. Soak a washcloth in the solution, and put it on your closed eyes for 30 minutes.

Back in the Day...

Do you toss and turn night after night? Then take a tip from Grandma Putt and let roses lead you to dreamland with this old-fashioned sleepy-time syrup: Make a strong tea by steeping 3 tablespoons of dried **ROSE** petals in 1 cup of freshly boiled water for 15 minutes. Strain, and pour the liquid into a small saucepan. Add 1 cup of honey or granulated sugar, stir well, and heat over low heat, stirring until the sweetener has completely dissolved. Pour the syrup into a glass or ceramic container with a non-metallic lid. Take 1 to 2 teaspoons before bedtime.

Defeat Diarrhea

Stop the runs with this **ROSE**-petal tincture. Combine 1 ounce of dried rose petals with 5 ounces of vodka in a glass or ceramic jar and cover with a non-metallic lid. Put the jar in a cool, dark place for six weeks, shaking it occasionally. Then strain the liquid into another jar and store, tightly sealed, for up to two years. Take 1 teaspoon up to three times a day for several days, or until you're back to normal.

SPOTLIGHT ON
HEALING WITH HERBS

Throughout this chapter I've talked about the healing properties of teas, tinctures, syrups, and poultices, all made with herbs or flowers from your garden. Here's a rundown of those techniques, plus more, that will ensure you make the most of your herbal healers. The proportions here are for dried herbs; if you are using fresh herbs, double the herb amount but keep the other ingredient amounts the same.

◆ A **COMPRESS** is made with a liquid solution, and is usually used hot to ease a headache or sore muscles. Start with an herbal decoction or tea. Soak a clean washcloth or piece of old T-shirt in the liquid. Wring it out, fold it over several times, and apply the damp compress to the injured area. Repeat with hot liquid once it has cooled.

◆ A **DECOCTION** is an herbal tea made from the tough plant parts— bark, roots, or dried berries. Add 1 tablespoon of the dried herbs to 2 cups of water in a saucepan. Bring to a boil, then lower the heat and simmer, covered, for 30 minutes, or for the time specified in your recipe. Check occasionally to make sure the water hasn't boiled off. Strain and use immediately, or allow to cool in the saucepan, then strain and pour into a glass or ceramic container with a non-metallic lid. Store for up to two days in the refrigerator.

◆ You can make herbal massage **OIL** with heat, which is quicker, or cold, which is best if you are using delicate flowers. For either method, you need 8 ounces of dried herbs and 3 cups of extra virgin olive oil. Heat process: Combine the herbs and oil in the top of a double boiler, filling the bottom pan with water. Cover, and heat on low for two to three hours, checking occasionally to make sure the water hasn't evaporated. Strain the oil into a dark-colored bottle and store in the refrigerator for up to one year. Cold process: Pack a clear glass jar with the herbs and pour the oil over them. Put a lid on the jar, and place it on a sunny windowsill for two weeks. Shake the jar once every day. After two weeks, strain the oil into a dark-colored bottle and store it in the refrigerator for up to one year.

- Herbal **OINTMENT** can provide antibacterial or antifungal healing benefits. Stir 1/2 to 1 teaspoon of tincture into 1 ounce of commercial hand lotion, mixing well. Spoon it into a clean jar, and use it up within four months. Or combine 2 ounces of dried herbs with 16 ounces of petroleum jelly in a double boiler, filling the bottom pan with water. Heat on low for two hours, checking occasionally to be sure the water hasn't evaporated. Remove from the heat and cool slightly. While it is still warm, put on a pair of rubber gloves and use a cloth to strain out the herbs and squeeze the ointment into a clean jar. Store for up to four months in the refrigerator.

- A **POULTICE** is similar to a compress, but you start with whole herbs. Put 1/4 to 1/2 cup of herbs into a blender or food processor and puree, adding water to make a sticky paste. Apply the paste to the affected area, and cover with a strip of gauze or a clean cloth. Or dip large fresh leaves into boiling water to soften them, then place the warm leaves over the affected area, holding them in place with a gauze strip.

- Herbal **SYRUP** makes healing herbs easier to ingest. Use 1 part herbal tea or decoction to 1 part honey or granulated sugar. Combine in a saucepan. Heat on low, stirring frequently, until the sweetener is completely dissolved. Pour into a clean glass or ceramic container with a non-metallic lid. Store up to six months in the refrigerator.

- An herbal **TEA**, also called an infusion, is made from the stems, leaves, or flowers of an herb. Place 1 to 3 teaspoons of dried herbs in a teapot or mug. Boil 1 cup of water, pour it over the herbs, and let steep for 10 to 20 minutes, or as specified in your recipe. Strain out the herbs and drink the tea, or pour it into a glass or ceramic container with a non-metallic lid. Refrigerate for up to two days.

- **TINCTURES** are made with alcohol, usually vodka, but you can use rum or brandy to sweeten the taste. Combine 1 ounce of dried herbs with 5 ounces of alcohol in a glass or ceramic jar with a non-metallic lid. Put the jar in a cool, dark place for two to six weeks, shaking it occasionally. Strain the liquid into another clean jar with a non-metallic lid, and store in a cool, dark place for up to two years.

From the Kitchen Garden

Terrific Tomatoes

Red **TOMATOES**—especially the foods made with them—are brimming with lycopene, an antioxidant that has been found to protect against prostate cancer. In fact, researchers found that men who eat tomato products (sauce and even pizza!) twice a week could lower their risk of prostate cancer by as much as 40 percent. Now that's what I call terrific news!

Lycopene Lessens Cancer Risk

When Harvard researchers pored through 72 studies regarding the relationship of lycopene (see "Terrific Tomatoes," above) to the prevention of *any* type of cancer, they discovered that a huge percentage of the studies found that frequently eating **TOMATOES** and tomato products reduced the risk of cancer, especially cancers of the prostate, lung, and stomach. Lycopene may also help ward off breast, cervical, and colon cancers. Researchers are currently investigating whether eating more tomato products will improve the outcomes of breast cancer patients or those at high risk for the disease because of genetic susceptibility. So stay tuned.

Go Red for Heart Health

Go for red **TOMATOES**, that is. Researchers are investigating whether having one to two daily servings of tomato products can keep heart disease at bay. Preliminary results indicate that the lycopene in these red fruits may lower LDL ("bad") cholesterol levels, and that's nothing but good! To get your daily dose of lycopene, you need only drink ¾ cup of tomato juice and eat a single tomato, or have a bowl of pasta with tomato sauce and some chopped fresh tomato mixed in.

HEALTHY Hint

DITCH THE ITCH

Brushing up against poison ivy or poison oak is no fun. But you can prevent a rash from breaking out if you act quickly. Simply dash to your garden and pluck a green **TOMATO**. Then cut it open and squeeze the juice onto the affected skin. That should do the trick.

CHAPTER 6

Countertop & Cupboard Appeal

Mushy, ripe bananas, a single clove of garlic, a few drops of vodka in the bottom of the bottle—toss 'em on the compost pile or pour 'em down the drain? Not a chance! These leftover "throwaways" are actually part of a bountiful beauty bonanza that help you look your best. Don't believe me? Take a peek at the tips and formulas here. I'm guessing you'll never consider your countertop and cupboard staples again without wondering, how can they make me look so darn good?

ON COUNTERTOPS

Whip Wrinkles with Bananas

Chances are your face has already collected some signs of "experience." While that's nothing to be ashamed of, there's also no harm in discouraging more fine lines and wrinkles from joining the crowd. So make an anti-aging treatment by mashing a ripe **BANANA**, and mixing in a few drops of peanut oil. Smooth it onto your face using an upward and outward motion, and leave it on for at least 30 minutes. Then rinse it off with lukewarm water and gently pat your skin dry.

Smooth Rough Lips

When harsh wind or sizzling sunshine leaves your lips parched, dry, and sore, intensive care is right in your kitchen. Just mash a few slices of ripe **BANANA** with a couple teaspoons of extra virgin olive oil to make a thick paste, and rub it onto your lips. Leave the salve on for 15 to 20 minutes, and rinse it off with warm water, then gently pat your lips dry.

Boot Blemishes the Banana Way

Got unsightly spots that you'd like to clear up and a **BANANA** that's too ripe to eat? Then this is your lucky day! Just before bedtime, mash the banana, and smooth it thickly over the affected skin. Cover the mush with gauze, and tape it in place. Then toddle off to dreamland. While you're snoozing, the sugar and enzymes in the fruit will draw out the impurities and help clear up the infection.

Sweet Treat for Skin

Here's a super-simple skin treatment that will leave your face glowing. Just mash one **BANANA** in a bowl and stir in 1 tablespoon of honey. Cover your face with the mixture, let it sit for 15 minutes, and rinse off with warm water. Pat dry and follow up with a moisturizer, if needed.

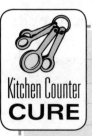

Kitchen Counter **CURE**

Intensive Care for Hair

Here's an extra-strength treatment that's tailor-made for dry, frizzy, or damaged hair.

1/2 ripe avocado
1/2 ripe BANANA
1 tbsp. of extra virgin olive oil
3 drops of lemon oil

Mash the avocado and banana in a bowl, then add the olive and lemon oils and stir well. Scoop up the mixture with your fingers and work it into your dry hair. Cover your hair with a shower cap, wait 60 minutes or so, then shampoo as usual. For badly damaged hair, repeat this treatment up to three times a week until the bounce and shine return.

Coffee Conquers Cellulite

Are you concerned about cellulite on your hips and thighs? Well, wake up and smell the **COFFEE**! Then (after you've drunk a cup or two), let the grounds cool off, and massage them into the problem areas, working in a circular motion. They contain the same active ingredient—caffeine—as most cellulite creams, without the exorbitant expense.

Café au Lips

Just can't get enough of that java taste? No problem. Make **COFFEE**-flavored lip gloss to keep the joe flowing. The simple recipe: Put 1 tablespoon of petroleum jelly in a microwave-safe dish and nuke it, checking every 10 seconds, until it's just melted. Stir in a spoonful of finely ground coffee (mocha- or vanilla-flavored is especially yummy), nuke again for another 20 to 30 seconds, remove from the oven, and let it cool. Then store the gloss at room temperature in a covered container and use within two weeks.

> # BEAUTY
> ## Bonus
> ### OBLITERATE ODOR
>
> We've all had occasions when no matter how frequently or ferociously we've scrubbed, we smell more foul than fresh, and the lingering odor has turned our favorite sweaters into instant castoffs. Some body odor is caused by what you eat; the notorious smells of garlic and onions come right through your pores. But you may not realize that **COFFEE** can also be a culprit because it increases the activity of your sweat glands. So try eliminating your usual cup (or cups!) of joe and see if your foul funk fades.

Get to the Root of the Issue

If you're like most Americans, you use your fair share of hair products on a daily basis. Over time, those conditioners, sprays, gels, and serums can really build up in your scalp. The good news is that **COFFEE** grounds can help clear them out. Once or twice a month, massage a handful of grounds into your wet scalp and hair to wash away flakes and remove unwanted product buildup. Then shampoo as usual. *Note: Coffee can stain lighter hair, so forget this treatment if you're a blonde.*

Pungent Pimple Treatment

Send a pimple packing with this aromatic fix: Peel a fresh **GARLIC** clove, slice it in two, and rub one of the cut sides onto your blemish. It should vanish within a day or so.

Axe Acne with a Mask

To treat widespread acne, peel and mash five **GARLIC** cloves, and mix them with 1 tablespoon of honey. Spread the mixture over the trouble spots, and leave it on for 10 minutes. Then rinse it off with lukewarm water, pat dry, and apply your usual toner and moisturizer. *Note: The mask may sting a little when you first apply it, but don't worry—that feeling is normal and should vanish within a minute or two.*

Pore-Perfect Pair

GARLIC and tomatoes are a dynamic duo at the dinner table. Their combined antiseptic properties also team up to clear out clogged pores. Mash a peeled garlic clove and a medium-size tomato, and mix them together. Spread a thin layer onto your face, and leave it on for 20 minutes. Rinse it off with lukewarm water. Splash your face with cold water to seal your pores, and follow up with your usual moisturizer.

HOW'S THAT?

Q *Jerry, it seems that just about everyone has a favorite home remedy for getting rid of warts. What's yours?*

A There are a ton of DIY wart-removal methods out there, but this may be the simplest (and it's certainly the cheapest!), which makes it my all-time favorite: Just before you go to bed, cut the tip off a fresh **GARLIC** clove, and rub the cut side directly onto the wart for a few seconds, then hop in the sack, without washing the area. (You can put on a pair of clean cotton gloves or socks if you don't want to offend your significant other with garlic odor.) Repeat the procedure each night until the beastly bump vanishes.

Reinforce Your Fingernails

Nail down a plan to stop peeling, splitting fingernails with this remarkable remedy: Add a finely minced **GARLIC** clove to a bottle of nail polish (either clear or your favorite shade), and let it sit for a few days. Then simply paint the potent polish onto your nails in the usual way. Once the polish has dried completely, remove any lingering garlic odor by washing your hands with fresh-squeezed lemon juice. Repeat the procedure once a week, and your nails will stay strong and healthy, even in the coldest winter months.

Derail Dandruff on the Double

Are you suffering from dandruff or shedding hair? A super-simple **GARLIC** treatment can solve your problem. Just pulverize two peeled garlic cloves in a food processor, and massage the mush into your scalp using small, circular motions. Wait 60 minutes, then work 2 tablespoons of olive oil into your scalp, massaging it in right over the garlic. Cover your head with a shower cap, and leave it on for at least three hours (enough time to watch a movie or dive into a good book). Wash with a gentle shampoo, and follow up with conditioner. Repeat once or twice a week until your tresses are healthy again.

More Pepper, Less Salt

Just about all of us develop gray hair over time, but the color change is most obvious in folks whose hair is naturally black. Here's an easy—and inexpensive—way to cover up the unwelcome gray strands:

Step 1. Gather up the peels from three or four **GARLIC** bulbs.

Step 2. Heat the peels in a frying pan over low heat until they're thoroughly dry and black.

Step 3. Grind the blackened peels into a fine powder, using a coffee grinder, food processor, or a mortar and pestle.

Step 4. Mix the grindings with enough olive oil to reach a consistency that's similar to commercial hair dye. Pour the potion into a stop-pered glass bottle, and store it in a dark place for a week or so.

Step 5. After a week, work the dye into your wet hair just before bedtime. Then cover your head with a shower cap, and hit the sack. (The longer the dye stays on your head, the deeper it will penetrate into your hair shafts—and the longer the color will remain.) Come morning, rinse your hair, and shampoo as usual. Repeat the treatment when the color begins to fade, which is generally after three to four weeks.

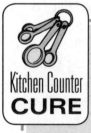

Kitchen Counter CURE

Hair's to Garlic Taming Treatment

When your hair is so dry that it feels like it's about to split all the way up the shafts, replace the moisture with this sweet and pungent potion.

> **2 tbsp. of GARLIC oil***
> **1 tsp. of honey**
> **1 egg yolk**

Mix the oil and honey together, then beat in the egg yolk. Rub the mixture into your hair one small section at a time. Cover your head with a shower cap or a plastic bag, and wait 30 minutes. Rinse thoroughly, and shampoo as usual. * *Available in health-food stores.*

Dial Down the Oil

Is your skin shinier than an oil slick? Don't sweat it! Your road to radiance couldn't be simpler. Just put 1 teaspoon of **BLACK TEA** in a mug, fill it with boiling water, and let it steep for 15 minutes. Strain out the tea leaves, dunk a soft washcloth in the brew, squeeze it out, and cover your face with the compress. Leave it on for 20 minutes, then rinse with lukewarm water, and apply your usual moisturizer. Repeat the procedure every three or four days.

Tame Inflamed Skin

One of the most effective remedies for a painful pimple is to cover it with a tea bag because **BLACK TEA** contains tannins, which help pimples drain. Soak a tea bag in hot water just long enough to soften it. Let it cool slightly, then hold it on the pimple for 10 minutes or so. Repeat up to three times a day until the offender has dried up and disappeared.

BEAUTY
Bonus

LET YOUR DARK HAIR SHINE!

If your black or dark brown locks are looking a little lackluster, try this trick to bring back the high-wattage shine and rich color. Steep two **BLACK-TEA** bags in 2 cups of boiling water for 10 minutes. Let the tea cool to room temperature, wash your hair, and immediately pour the tea over your wet head, rubbing it through your hair as you would shampoo. Leave the rinse on for 10 minutes, then shampoo again and apply your usual conditioner. The result: soft, shiny, and more manageable hair. Repeat the process once a week, or whenever you feel in need of a shine boost.

Banish Black Eyes

Here's an easy way to soothe a black eye—use a tea bag. Those tannins that help clear up acne (see "Tame Inflamed Skin," above) also work to reduce swelling. Brew a cup of **BLACK TEA**, let the tea bag cool, then squeeze out the excess moisture. Lie back, close your eyes, and hold the tea bag against the injured area for 10 minutes.

On Countertops

Stinky-Toe Tea

The tannic acid in **BLACK TEA** helps close sweat glands, thereby starving the bacteria that cause foot odor. Brew two tea bags in 1 pint of boiling water for 15 minutes, add the tea to 2 quarts of cool water, and soak your feet for 20 to 30 minutes. Dry them without rinsing. After 10 days your stinky feet will smell sweet!

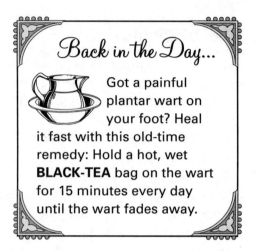

Back in the Day...

Got a painful plantar wart on your foot? Heal it fast with this old-time remedy: Hold a hot, wet **BLACK-TEA** bag on the wart for 15 minutes every day until the wart fades away.

Bad Breath Buster

Scientists tell us that the polyphenols in **BLACK TEA** can stop the growth of microbes that cause halitosis, as well as the bacteria's production of odiferous gas. Don't believe me? Then try tea and see!

Oust the Odor

If you like to cook, you know how smelly your fingers get after you've been cutting onions for salads, or chopping garlic to toss into tomato sauce. To get rid of any lingering aromas, just rinse your hands with brewed **BLACK TEA**, or rub your skin with a couple of used tea bags. It removes odors left by onions, garlic, fish, or other strong-smelling foods.

Slash Rash Pain

A painful rash from razor burn or poison ivy can quickly be conquered with **BLACK TEA**. Here's the how-to:

- **Razor burn.** Soak a tea bag in hot water until softened. Let it cool, then hold it against the tender area for 10 minutes. Let your skin air-dry, and try to keep fabric from rubbing against it.

- **Poison ivy.** Brew a tea bag in a cup of boiling water until it's very strong (about 15 minutes). Refrigerate the tea for a half hour, then dip a cotton ball into it and gently dab it on the affected areas, letting your skin air-dry. Repeat several times a day until the rash has dried up.

Rejuvenate Dry Skin

This intensive-care facial routine will invigorate dry skin, leaving your complexion soft and radiant: Mix ¼ cup of brewed **GREEN TEA** and two crushed vitamin C tablets. Apply the mixture to your face using a cotton ball or pad, and smooth on a thin layer of petroleum jelly to lock in the moisture. Leave the mask on for 20 minutes or so, and rinse it off with warm water. Then look in the mirror and admire the "new" you!

Teatime Toner

Tone and firm any type of skin with this simple trick: Pour 1 cup of boiling water over 4 teaspoons of loose **GREEN-TEA** leaves or two green-tea bags. Let it steep for 10 to 15 minutes to get a nice strong brew. When the tea has cooled to room temperature, pour it into a bottle with a tight-fitting lid, and keep it in the refrigerator. Once or twice a day, dab some toner onto your face and neck with a cotton pad or ball, and follow up with your usual moisturizer.

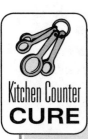

Kitchen Counter CURE

Forever Young Facial Cleanser

GREEN TEA contains compounds called polyphenols that protect your skin from the sun's destructive rays and flush out cell-damaging free radicals. Sugar sloughs off dead skin cells and attracts moisture that keeps your skin hydrated. Putting this age-defying duo to work for you is a snap!

> ½ cup of distilled water
> 2 green-tea bags
> 3 tbsp. of granulated sugar

Bring the water to a rolling boil, pour it into a heat-proof bowl, and add the tea bags. Let them steep until the water is cool to the touch—about 15 minutes. Then stir in the sugar. Saturate a clean washcloth in the solution, and gently massage your skin using small circular motions. Rinse thoroughly with lukewarm water, and apply your favorite moisturizer. Repeat the process once a week to keep your skin clear, glowing, and younger looking.

Puffy-Face Fixer

Seasonal allergies, sunburn, and humidity conspire to make a puffy face as much a part of summertime as baseball and corn on the cob—only a lot less welcome, of course! If that sounds like you, here's good news: Ice cubes made from **GREEN TEA** and pureed blueberries can deflate your kisser, fast. Here's how:

Step 1. Pour 2 1/2 cups of boiling water over three green-tea bags and steep them for about 10 minutes. Remove the bags and stir in 3 tablespoons of organic raw honey.

Step 2. While the tea is cooling, puree 1/2 cup of fresh or frozen blueberries and 2 tablespoons of fresh-squeezed lemon juice in a blender until the mixture is mushy, but not liquefied.

Step 3. Mix the puree with the tea, pour the blend into an ice cube tray, and put it in the freezer.

Step 4. When the cubes are frozen, pop one out of the tray and rub it all over your face, concentrating on the puffiest areas, until the ice has melted. Blot your face lightly with a paper towel, but leave the slightly sticky residue on your skin for 20 to 30 minutes. Rinse it off with lukewarm water. *Note: Blueberries stain any fabric they touch, so do this procedure over a sink while you're wearing expendable clothing!*

HOW'S THAT?

Q *I've been hearing a lot about something called matcha. They're making drinks with it at my favorite coffee shop, and all I can figure out is that it's some kind of* **GREEN TEA.** *What's all the fuss about?*

A Matcha is, in fact, nothing more than green-tea leaves ground into a fine powder. It's being used everywhere from, as you've discovered, coffee shops to high-end cocktail lounges and restaurants. The antioxidant-rich powder is highly concentrated, so it delivers all of the skin- (and body-) nourishing benefits of regular green tea in a more potent form.

On Countertops

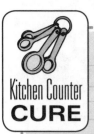

Kitchen Counter CURE

So-Smooth Smoothie

The antioxidants in **GREEN TEA** help prevent cell damage, thereby fending off wrinkles and keeping your skin soft and smooth. This drink is a simple way to enjoy all the benefits of this internal-beauty powerhouse.

¹/₂ cup of brewed green tea, chilled*

1 large peach, sliced

¹/₂ banana

1 tbsp. of organic raw honey

Puree the ingredients in a blender or food processor, and drink to your good looks and good health! *To speed up the process, make your tea by the quart, keep it in the fridge, and simply pour out as much as you need when it's time for a smoothie break. Use within two days.*

Meet Your Perfect Matcha

These finely ground **GREEN-TEA** leaves have become a key ingredient in many top-of-the-line beauty products. But it's easy, and a lot cheaper, to make your own. Here are some examples:

■ **Exfoliating, moisturizing mask.** Mix 3 teaspoons of matcha powder with 1¹/₂ teaspoons of distilled water and 1 teaspoon of honey to form a paste. (Add more matcha or water if necessary to get the right texture.) Smooth the paste onto your face, and leave it on for 15 to 30 minutes. Then gently massage it into your skin, and rinse with lukewarm water.

■ **Hydrating, cleansing mask.** Mix 3 teaspoons of matcha powder, 2 teaspoons of honey, and 5 teaspoons of plain yogurt, and spread the mixture over your face and neck. Leave it on for 15 minutes, and rinse with water.

■ **Softening, toning bath salts.** Combine equal parts of matcha powder and either sea salt or Epsom salts, and store the mixture in a tightly covered container at room temperature. At bath time, pour ¹/₄ cup of the blend under the spigot as you run warm water into the tub. Then settle in and soak for 20 minutes or so.

You can find matcha in the Asian-food sections of many supermarkets, as well as in health-food stores and online. Or, if you prefer, simply put regular green-tea leaves in your coffee grinder, and hold the "on" button down until you get a fine green powder.

SPOTLIGHT ON
NATURAL HAIR TREATMENTS

If you're still on the expensive hair-care bandwagon, it's high time to get off! Not only will going the homemade route save you money, it's also a kinder, gentler way to treat your treasured tresses. Here's just a sampling of easy hair treatments you can whip up with common kitchen countertop finds.

◆ Deep-condition damaged hair. Slice one **BANANA** into a medium-size bowl. Add 2 tablespoons of coconut milk and 1 tablespoon of coconut oil (use 2 tablespoons if your hair is extremely dry). Drizzle in 2 tablespoons of honey. Stir gently to mix, then spoon the contents into a blender and puree until the mixture is completely smooth, with no banana chunks. Massage the conditioner onto damp hair and cover with a shower cap. Leave on for 30 to 60 minutes, then rinse out, and shampoo as usual.

◆ Make a darkening hair rinse. Pour 2 cups of boiling water over two **BLACK-TEA** bags and steep, covered, in a pan for 15 minutes. Remove the tea bags, squeezing out the liquid. Reheat the tea to just the boiling point, take it off the stove, and add ¼ cup of dried sage leaves and 3 tablespoons of dried rosemary leaves. Steep the brew, covered, for 60 minutes, and strain the liquid into another container. Holding your head over a basin to catch the runoff, pour the tea through your freshly washed and rinsed hair. Repeat several times, working it through your hair, then dry and style your tresses as usual.

◆ Brighten blonde hair. Pour 2 cups of boiling water over two **CHAMOMILE TEA** bags and steep, covered, for 30 minutes. Then step into the shower and pour the tea over your just-washed hair, working it through. Repeat until you've used up all the tea, then shampoo and condition your hair as usual.

◆ Rev up the red highlights in your brown hair. After shampooing, rinse with strong black **COFFEE** that's been cooled to room temperature. Leave it on your hair for 15 minutes or so, and then rinse thoroughly with cool water.

Aspirin Balm for the Bikini Line

Ladies, after you shave, spritz the area with warm water in which you've dissolved two uncoated **ASPIRIN** tablets and a drop of glycerin. It's an easy way to keep ingrown hairs and razor bumps at bay.

Amazing Aspirin Exfoliant

The salicylic acid in **ASPIRIN** increases dead-cell exfoliation, which in turn helps minimize blotchy skin, fine lines, and wrinkles. To put this power to work for you, crush four uncoated aspirin tablets, and mix them with 1 teaspoon of fresh-squeezed lemon juice. Stir until the aspirin dissolves and forms a paste. Then smooth it evenly over your face, using cotton pads (and avoiding the eye area!). Leave it on for 10 minutes, then remove it using a cotton pad saturated in a solution of baking soda and warm water.

Note: You may feel a slight sting when you remove the mask, but don't worry—this is normal.

Clear Complexion Congestion

To unclog pores and soothe irritated, acne-prone skin, reach for **ASPIRIN**. It contains salicylic acid, which exfoliates and eases inflammation. Simply crush five uncoated aspirin tablets in a small bowl, adding 1 tablespoon each of honey and plain whole-milk yogurt. Mix well, then apply to your face and leave it on for 10 minutes. Remove the mask with a warm, wet washcloth, followed by a cool-water rinse, and gently pat your skin dry.

Back in the Day...

If Grandma Putt could see the price tags on some of those fancy dandruff shampoos, she'd hit the roof because this easy old-time treatment beats 'em all. Just mash five uncoated **ASPIRIN** tablets and put them in a bottle with 1 cup of apple cider vinegar and 1/3 cup of witch hazel. Cap the bottle and shake it to mix the ingredients. Shampoo as usual, then comb the solution through your hair. Wait 10 minutes, rinse with warm water, and wave those white-flake woes good-bye.

```
┌─────────────────────────────────┐
│                                 │
│         BEAUTY                  │
│          Bonus                  │
│  ─────────────────────────────  │
│       THE EYES HAVE IT           │
│  ─────────────────────────────  │
│                                 │
│  Eye makeup can be eye-         │
│  catching all right, but        │
│  trying to remove it with       │
│  commercial products can        │
│  irritate the tender tissue-thin│
│  skin around your peepers.      │
│  On the other hand, this        │
│  gentle combo will not only     │
│  clean off the colors you've    │
│  applied, but also soothe and   │
│  moisten your skin. Simply      │
│  mix 1 tablespoon each of       │
│  100 percent pure CASTOR        │
│  OIL, olive oil, and canola oil │
│  in a glass jar with a tight-   │
│  fitting lid. Then moisten a    │
│  tissue or cotton ball with the │
│  oil as needed (give the jar a  │
│  good shake first), and gently  │
│  wipe away your eye shadow,     │
│  eyeliner, or mascara.          │
│                                 │
└─────────────────────────────────┘
```

Soften Sandpaper Hands

Even the roughest, driest skin is no match for this moisturizing combo: Mix 1 teaspoon of 100 percent pure **CASTOR OIL** with 1 drop of either lemon oil or peppermint oil (available in health-food stores and many large supermarkets). Massage the mixture into your hands or feet at bedtime, put on cotton gloves or socks, and leave them on overnight. Smooth move!

Scoff at Scars

Applying a bit of 100 percent pure **CASTOR OIL** to both accidental and surgical wounds can greatly reduce scarring and may even prevent it altogether. Gently wipe the oil into your skin periodically throughout the day as the wound heals. (Be sure to let the oil dry thoroughly before it touches any fabric.) The secret "weapon" is castor oil's ability to increase your body's quantity of T lymphocytes (a.k.a. white blood cells), which studies have shown to play a vital role in skin healing.

Fade Age and Sun Spots

Are brown spots on your hands or face aging you before your time? You can lighten them up with the dynamic duo of vitamin E oil and **CASTOR OIL**. Simply apply vitamin E oil directly to the spots once a day, then at night, rub on some 100 percent pure castor oil. The unwelcome marks will begin to fade in just a few weeks.

De-Crease Your Face and Neck

CASTOR OIL can help minimize the appearance of fine lines with each passing year. At bedtime, just dab a little 100 percent pure castor oil into the creases in your neck and around your eyes and mouth. Unfortunately, it won't halt the parade of new lines, but it will help to slow down its pace.

Moisturize and Protect Thirsty Skin

CASTOR OIL adds moisture, but it also creates a protective barrier between your skin and the harsh environmental conditions of the sometimes not-so-great outdoors and indoors. Simply mix 1/2 cup of 100 percent pure castor oil with 2/3 cup of olive oil, and add 20 drops of your favorite essential oil. (Rose and geranium oils are both excellent for dry skin.) Use it as you would any other facial moisturizer.

Grow Lusher Lashes and Brows

Who wouldn't want to have thicker, fuller eyelashes? Just rub a little 100 percent pure **CASTOR OIL** over the base of your lashes before bed each night. It will prevent thinning and promote rapid growth of the hair. To thicken your eyebrows—whether they've become naturally sparse over time, or you've gone berserk with the tweezers and overplucked them— wipe a little castor oil over your brow line each night.

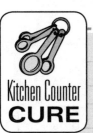

Kitchen Counter CURE

Tough-as-Nails Treatment

Here's an easy-to-make potion that will both strengthen and shine your nails.

2 tsp. of 100 percent pure CASTOR OIL
2 tsp. of salt
1 tsp. of wheat germ

Mix all of the ingredients together in a small bowl, then pour the mixture into a bottle with a tight-fitting cap. Shake well before using, and apply it to your nails and cuticles with a cotton ball.

Make Your Cuticles Cuter

CASTOR OIL and cocoa butter team up to keep your cuticles soft and neat. To make the conditioner, warm 4 tablespoons of cocoa butter over low heat until the butter liquefies. Stir in 4 tablespoons of 100 percent pure castor oil, and pour the mixture into a deep bowl. Let the potion cool a bit, then soak your fingers for 15 minutes. Rinse with warm water, and gently push back your cuticles. Store any leftover conditioner in a jar with a tight-fitting lid for up to three months at room temperature.

Fade Freckles in a Flash

Lots of folks think freckles are lovely, but if you're not one of them, this lotion can produce major freckle-fading feats:

Step 1. Rinse four medium-size dandelion leaves thoroughly, and tear them into small pieces.

Step 2. Mix the leaves with 5 tablespoons of 100 percent pure **CASTOR OIL** in a glass or enamel pan.

Step 3. Simmer the mixture, uncovered, over low heat for 10 minutes. Then turn off the heat, cover the pan, and let it steep for three hours.

Step 4. Strain the potion into a bottle with a tight-fitting lid.

Every evening, massage a few drops of the oil into the freckled area, and leave it on overnight. Come morning, rinse it off with lukewarm water. You should start to see dramatic results within just a week or so.

✍ Back in the Day...

There are more wart-removal remedies than you can shake a toad at, but this was one of my Grandma Putt's all-time favorites. Mix 2 parts 100 percent pure **CASTOR OIL** with 1 part baking soda to make a paste. Apply the paste to the wart, before bedtime, and cover it with a bandage. In the morning, remove the bandage, and rinse off any paste residue. Repeat until the wart is gone.

Cast Off the Frizzies

If hot, humid weather leaves your hair frizzed and frazzled, take heart—**CASTOR OIL** can calm down those flyaway strands. Just heat 1/4 to 1/2 cup (based on the length of your hair) of 100 percent pure castor oil in the microwave on the medium setting until warm, checking it frequently. Massage the warm oil onto the ends of your hair. Wait five minutes, then shampoo and condition your hair as usual.

Deep-Condition Your Tresses

If you have seriously dry, damaged hair, this **CASTOR OIL** mask will help improve the overall look of your locks, and add shine and smoothness, too. Start by gently heating 1 cup of plain yogurt in the microwave on low, until just warm. Add 3 tablespoons of 100 percent pure castor oil and stir well. Apply the mask to your hair from roots to ends, cover with a shower cap, and leave on for 30 minutes. Then shampoo and condition your hair as usual. Use this treatment two to three times a week for softer, healthier hair.

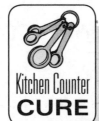

Kitchen Counter CURE

Ward Off Winter Weather

Cold, dry, windy weather can damage your skin fast—besides making it itch like crazy. This lotion acts like a suit of armor to protect your face and neck from Old Man Winter's ravages.

- 36 oz. of 100 percent pure CASTOR OIL
- 2 oz. of water
- 2–4 drops of frankincense oil*
- 2–4 drops of lavender oil*

Mix the castor oil and water in a plastic bottle that has a screw-on cap with a lift-up spout.** Add the frankincense and lavender oils, and shake to blend. If it's too thick or too thin, add a little more water or castor oil, as needed. To use the potion, shake the bottle, pour a small amount of the oil into your hands, and spread it over your face and neck—just be sure to avoid the eye area.

* Available in health-food stores, herbal-supply stores, and online.

** Available in the cosmetic or travel-supply section of drugstores and supermarkets.

In Cupboards

Epsom Detox Face Scrub

Your pretty face deserves an extra-thorough cleaning at night to remove your makeup, as well as all of the airborne gunk that your skin absorbs during the day. The good news is that you don't have to run out and buy a special intensive cleaner. Just mix ½ teaspoon of **EPSOM SALTS** with your regular cleansing cream. Massage it into your skin, and rinse with cool water. Follow up with your usual toner and moisturizer, and hit the road to dreamland.

Give Blackheads the Boot

Do you feel as though you're in a constant battle with blackheads? Well, victory is as close as your kitchen cupboard. Mix 1 teaspoon of **EPSOM SALTS** and 3 drops of iodine in ½ cup of boiling water. Let the mixture cool just enough so that you can stick your finger in it, then dab it onto each blackhead with a cotton ball, and let the solution dry. Repeat the procedure three or four times, reheating the solution if necessary. Gently remove the blackhead using a clean washcloth, and apply rubbing alcohol to the area.

Flawless Facial Mask

Soften your skin and draw out impurities with this quick and easy formula: Mix 1 tablespoon each of **EPSOM SALTS**, olive oil, and organic raw honey. (If you have oily skin, add a few drops of fresh lemon juice.) Smooth the mixture onto your face and neck, leave it on for 5 to 10 minutes, then rinse it off with warm water. Follow up with your usual moisturizer.

Back in the Day...

Long before fancy exfoliators came on the scene, my Grandma Putt and her lady friends used plain old **EPSOM SALTS** to remove dead skin cells and deep-down dirt from head to toe. It works as well now as it did then, and the process couldn't be simpler: Stand in the shower or bathtub, wet your skin, and then massage it with handfuls of the salts, starting with your feet and working up to your neck. When you're finished, rinse the stuff off and pat your skin dry. That's all there is to it!

Renew Your Feet

When sandal season is on the way, treat your winter-weary feet to this simple salt rub: Moisten a handful of **EPSOM SALTS** with a bit of olive oil. Then scrub your feet until the salts have dissolved and the oil has softened your skin. Rinse with lukewarm water.

Stop the Stench

No matter what the season, foot odor just plain stinks! To send the smell on its way, mix ½ cup of **EPSOM SALTS** in a foot basin filled with warm water, and soak your dogs for 10 minutes or so. Repeat daily.

Bath Salts Simplicity

Spa-worthy bath treats don't come any easier than this feel-good formula: Mix 1 cup each of baking soda, **EPSOM SALTS**, and sea salt or kosher salt, and store the blend in an airtight container. To use it, add about 2 tablespoons of the mixture to your bathwater. For an aromatic bath, add a few drops of your favorite essential oil as the tub fills.

BATHS À LA CARTE
There are many oils that can add aromatherapy power to an EPSOM SALTS bath, but here's a Baker's half dozen of excellent choices.

HERBAL OIL	WHAT IT DOES FOR YOU
Chamomile	Soothes and relaxes
Cinnamon	Energizes and stimulates
Eucalyptus	Clears internal airways
Geranium	Helps balance mind and body
Grapefruit	Lifts spirits
Lavender	Relaxes and rejuvenates
Peppermint	Cools and refreshes

Oily-Hair Repair

You don't have to put up with greasy locks. This simple solution will leave your hair soft, but not oily. Mix ¼ cup of **EPSOM SALTS** and ¼ cup of lemon juice in 1 quart of water, and let it sit for 24 hours. Just before using, mix well, then pour the solution onto your dry hair, wait 20 minutes, and shampoo. The excess oil will be gone, without leaving your scalp overly dry. *Note: This formula works equally well to remove hair spray buildup.*

Pump Up the Volume

This trick will add healthy fullness and bounce to your tresses. Here's what you need to do: In a pan, mix equal parts of **EPSOM SALTS** and a high-quality deep conditioner. Heat the mixture until it's warm, work it through your locks, and leave it on for 20 minutes or so. Then rinse with warm water.

Soothe Sore Lips

Chapped lips can be a year-round problem, whether you spend too much time in the cold winter wind or the hot summer sun. Return your kisser to kissable softness by mixing 2 tablespoons of **EPSOM SALTS** with 1 teaspoon of petroleum jelly. Gently massage the balm into your suffering lips, leave it on for five minutes, and then gently wipe it off with a tissue.

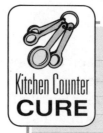

Kitchen Counter CURE

A Bouquet of Bath Crystals

Mix up a batch of this beautiful blend to soak your troubles away. While you're at it, multiply the recipe and make extra "servings" to give as birthday or Christmas presents.

½ cup of EPSOM SALTS

½ cup of fresh chamomile, lavender, or rosebuds

½ cup of sea salt

¼ cup of baking soda

15 drops of fragrance oil*

Food coloring (optional)

Blend the salts, flowers, and baking soda in a blender or food processor. Let the mixture sit for half an hour or so to dry a little, then add the oil and food coloring. Pour the blend into lidded glass jars. At bath time, add a heaping ½ cup of the mixture to the water.

* Use any kind you like to match or complement the flowers' fragrance.

Yield: About 1½ cups

It's Time to Get Glowing!

If your skin is chapped and flaking, with a dull, dry appearance, reach for some **EUCALYPTUS OIL**. Add a few drops to a gentle, unscented face cream, and use it as you would any other moisturizer. Your complexion will have its healthy glow back in no time at all!

Alleviate Acne

This spot treatment will help dry up breakouts fast, without irritating the rest of your skin. Simply mix 1 drop of **EUCALYPTUS OIL** with 3 drops of water. Then dip a cotton swab into the solution and dab it onto the blemish. Repeat dipping and dabbing for each spot. Let the solution air-dry on your skin, and go about your day.

Eucalyptus Hair Repair

Looking for a top-notch hair-care product? Look no further, because when it comes to healthy hair, **EUCALYPTUS OIL** is a triple-threat champ. It promotes hair growth, battles dandruff, and improves the elasticity of your locks (thereby leading to less breakage). Your job: Just add about 10 drops of the oil to a bottle of your regular shampoo, shake to mix, and wash your hair as usual.

HOW'S THAT?

Q *Jerry, I'm looking for relief from an itchy scalp. I've tried dandruff treatments, but I don't have dandruff, and they don't stop the itch. Help!*

A You can stop scratching with this solution: Mix 1½ ounces of white vinegar and 1 teaspoon of **EUCALYPTUS OIL** into 1 quart of water. While you're in the shower, pour this rinse over your hair, rub it in, and repeat until you've used up all of the solution. Then shampoo and condition as you usually do. Use this treatment every time you wash your hair, and it should end the itch once and for all.

BEAUTY
Bonus

LOOK BETTER FASTER

To keep your skin and hair healthy, eat fish two to three times a week, or take 1,000 milligrams of **FISH OIL** daily. The omega-3 fatty acids in the oil (and in fish) can help your skin retain water, which will keep it plump and smooth looking. In addition, thin, brittle hair may be an indicator of a fatty acid deficiency, so adding fish and fish oil to your diet will strengthen your tresses, too.

Fishy Scar Fader

FISH OIL and vitamin E oil team up to greatly reduce the appearance of scars, and sometimes even make them vanish entirely. The process is simple: First, squeeze the contents of a fish oil capsule and a vitamin E capsule into a bowl, and mix thoroughly. Gently rub all of the liquid into the scarred area, and let it air-dry completely. Repeat the procedure once a day, or as often as you can, until the proud skin (as the old-timers called it) diminishes. *Note: This same treatment works wonders for removing stretch marks caused by pregnancy or major weight gain or loss.*

Dive Deep for Dry-Skin Repair

Healthy, supple skin relies on essential fatty acids in your diet. A deficiency can leave your skin looking dried out and wrinkled. So pop a **FISH OIL** capsule once a day and/or eat one serving of foods containing omega-3 oils daily (salmon is an especially good source).

Thrash the Rash

If your skin has erupted in a red, bumpy rash on your forearms and thighs, it could be a telltale sign that you're lacking essential fatty acids—the kind found in **FISH OIL**, flaxseed oil, and evening primrose oil, all of which help keep skin lubricated, supple, and smooth. The solution? Take 1 teaspoon or 500 milligrams of fish oil three times a day. To help speed up the healing, you can also apply the oil directly to your rash. You should see your skin looking much healthier within a week or so. Just be sure to keep any clothing away from your oiled skin to avoid staining the fabric.

A Gem of a Jelly

Whether you've run out of a makeup essential and there's no time to shop, or you simply enjoy whipping up your own beauty products, here's a trio of DIY possibilities:

■ **Cream blusher.** Put 1 teaspoon or so of **PETROLEUM JELLY** in a bowl, and stir in a few scrapings of lipstick until it's well blended.

■ **Eye shadow.** Again, start with 1 teaspoon or so of petroleum jelly, but add a few drops of blue or green food coloring, and stir well.

■ **Lipstick.** Follow the same procedure described for eye shadow, but use red food coloring instead of blue or green. Better (and tastier) yet, use a pinch or two of cherry or strawberry Kool-Aid® powder instead of food coloring. Stir well to dissolve the powder.

Note: Adjust the amount of colorant to create a darker or lighter cosmetic.

Lip-Smacking Lip Gloss

What if you could have a moisturizing lip gloss that's your favorite shade and your favorite flavor? You can—and it's a snap to make yourself. In a bowl, thoroughly mix 1 tablespoon of **PETROLEUM JELLY**, 1/4 teaspoon of your favorite lipstick, and 2 to 4 drops of your favorite flavored extract. Scrape the mixture into a small, tight-lidded container. A clean plastic throat-lozenge container works well, too. Then tuck it into your pocket or purse, and use it to keep your lips smooth and kissable.

Back in the Day...

OUCH! The doorbell rang, and when you jumped up from the couch to answer it, you banged right into the coffee table! Well, don't chew yourself out for your clumsiness. Instead, treat your injury like Grandma would: Just measure out 5 parts **PETROLEUM JELLY** to 1 part ground hot pepper, then melt the jelly in a saucepan over low heat, and stir in the pepper. Let the gel cool, spoon it into a clean glass jar, and apply it to the bruised area once a day. (Just be sure to wear rubber or plastic gloves when applying the gel, because this stuff is hot!)

All-Over Scrub-a-Dub

Get ready for an exfoliating scrub that works wonders for sloughing off dead cells and softening the skin. Mix 2 parts brown sugar with 1 part **PETROLEUM JELLY** (add a little more petroleum jelly if the mixture is too thick). Scoop it out with your fingers, and massage it thoroughly onto your skin. Then rinse and follow up with your usual moisturizer.

Subdue Wayward Brows

Before you pluck, lube up your eyebrows with **PETROLEUM JELLY**. It'll make those stray hairs glide out smoothly and painlessly. And if your brows are unruly even after plucking, use petroleum jelly to instill a little discipline. Just put a dab of jelly on your fingertip or a new soft toothbrush, and sweep it across each brow from the inside to the outside. The result: a neat, trim look with no muss and no fuss.

Split-Ends Solution

Don't spend a fortune on hair potions that claim to cure split ends. Instead, get instant results with **PETROLEUM JELLY**. Just rub a little of the jelly between your palms, and wipe it onto your dry, cracked strands. If necessary, use it all over your hair to hold frizzy flyaway strands in place. When the jelly's job is done for the day (or evening), work some cornstarch into your hair to absorb the jelly, then wash it out with a clarifying shampoo. Follow up with your usual conditioner.

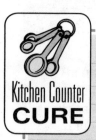

Kitchen Counter CURE

Mature-Skin Miracle Cream

This ultra-simple formula is perfect for extra-dry skin. To make it, mix a 13-ounce jar of **PETROLEUM JELLY**, a 15-ounce bottle of baby lotion (not oil), and a 16-ounce jar of vitamin E cream (not lotion) in a large bowl. (If you like, nuke the jelly in the microwave on medium for a few seconds to soften it up.) Mix well—the texture of the finished product should be somewhere between that of Cool Whip® and whipped butter. Store it in wide-mouth, lidded containers at room temperature, and use it as you would any other moisturizer.

BEAUTY
Bonus

SCENT-UOUS SOLID PERFUME

This aromatic formula has three advantages over commercial perfumes: First, the **PETROLEUM JELLY** makes it glide onto your pulse points more easily and stay there longer; second, you can customize the scent; and third, it costs a whole lot less than commercial versions! Here's all there is to it: Melt 1 cup of petroleum jelly and 1 ounce of beeswax in a double boiler over low heat. Remove the pan from the stove, and stir in 1 tablespoon of essential oil; let sit for a minute, then pour it into one or more dark-colored glass (not plastic) jars with tight-fitting lids. The perfume will firm up as it cools, and will keep at room temperature for up to two years. Just be sure to keep the perfume away from heat and sunlight, which can make it deteriorate quickly. *Note: Beeswax is available in health-food stores and online.*

A Dandy DIY De-Stinker

Do you really want to use a commercial, chemical-laden deodorant? No way! This simple concoction keeps you fresh smelling: Just mix 2 tablespoons each of baby powder, baking soda, and **PETROLEUM JELLY** in a pan. Heat the mixture on low until it's smooth and creamy. Then pour it into a jar that has a tight-fitting lid. Store at room temperature, and use it as you would any other antiperspirant.

A Tip to Dye For

And dye *with*. Keep hair dye formulas from flowing into your eyes by smearing a line of **PETROLEUM JELLY** above your eyebrows. For extra protection, especially if you are using a dark-colored hair dye, wipe a layer of jelly all around your hairline to prevent hard-to-remove skin stains. *Note: A line of jelly above the brows also works for keeping shampoo out of baby's (or Fido's) eyes.*

Save That Stunning Scent!

Dab a little **PETROLEUM JELLY** onto your pulse points, like your wrists and the sides of your neck, before you spray yourself with cologne or perfume. Your scintillating scent will last all day long, and well into the evening.

Bewitching Toners

Some store-bought toners contain acetone—the key ingredient in nail polish removers. Do you really want to use that stuff on your face? I don't think so! Instead, depending on your skin type, opt for one of these complexion-friendly formulas that get the job done, naturally:

For normal skin. Ingredients: ½ cup each of **WITCH HAZEL**, water, and peppermint tea (For instructions on making herbal tea, see "Spotlight on Healing with Herbs" on page 196).

For dry and mature skin. Ingredients: ½ cup each of witch hazel and water and 4 tablespoons each of aloe vera gel, glycerin, and rose water.

To make either type, mix the ingredients together in a bottle that has a tight-fitting cap. Store the container at room temperature, shaking it occasionally and before each use. Apply the toner to your face and neck with a cotton ball or pad. It will keep well for 8 to 10 months.

Back in the Day...

Although this skin firmer dates back to the 1600s, and was all the rage with Grandma Putt and her crowd, it's more popular today than ever before. And that's no wonder because it's cheap, is easy to make, and works like a dream to smooth and firm any type of skin. The simple procedure: Mix 3 tablespoons of alcohol-free **WITCH HAZEL** and 1 teaspoon of unfiltered apple cider vinegar in a bowl, then lightly beat in one egg white. Whip the mixture until it's foamy, and pop it into the refrigerator for five minutes or so. Apply the mixture to your warm, moist skin using a cotton pad. Leave it on for at least 30 minutes.

Dim the Shine

Commercial shine-control products dry out your skin, so make your own: Mix ⅓ cup of **WITCH HAZEL** with 1 cup of rose water and 1 cup of spring water, and store it in the refrigerator. (It'll keep for up to two weeks in a glass jar with a tight-fitting lid.) Then each morning and evening wipe the potion onto your face and neck using a cotton pad. *Note: You can buy rose water in health-food stores, herbal-supply stores, and online.*

SPOTLIGHT ON
COMPLEXION CURES

From bug bites to itchy rashes, skin ailments can be a health issue (see "Spotlight on Skin Problems" on page 60) or simply an unsightly inconvenience. Here are some kitchen cabinet finds that can help you look your best when your skin is conspiring against you:

◆ To ease inflammation after a bite or sting, dissolve two effervescent **ANTACID TABLETS** in a glass of water. Then moisten a soft cloth with the solution, and hold it on the bite site for 20 minutes.

◆ Moisturize seriously dry skin with **FISH OIL**. Rub a few drops of the oil into your skin until it is absorbed. For dry, cracked heels, use a generous amount of the oil as an overnight treatment. Pull on clean cotton socks and toddle off to bed.

◆ Treat heat rash or diaper rash with **MILK OF MAGNESIA**. Use a cotton pad to apply a generous layer of milk of magnesia over the affected skin. It will neutralize the acids that cause rashes and will also act as a natural disinfectant to prevent the problem from spreading.

◆ Soothe the sting of sunburn by gently covering your red-hot skin with a light layer of **MILK OF MAGNESIA**. Let it dry thoroughly before you dress or get ready for bed.

◆ Speed up the healing of dry, chapped lips with **PETROLEUM JELLY**. Dab it on lightly for daytime use if you don't like the greasy feel, but really glob it on at night to deep-condition your lips.

◆ Balance super-oily skin with **WITCH HAZEL**. The simple R_x: Pour witch hazel onto a cotton ball and sweep it across your face, paying particular attention to the oily areas. Let it air-dry on your skin before you put on any makeup. Repeat the procedure at night after washing your face.

Hop Off the Problem-Skin Merry-Go-Round

Countertop & Cupboard Appeal

It may seem logical to use commercial astringents when you're battling acne and similar skin problems. But these products dry out your skin, making it produce even more oil. So then you use more astringent, and start a vicious circle of no-win action. Fortunately, there is a gentle, natural alternative that will fight the bacteria without upping your oil production. Just mix 1 cup of **WITCH HAZEL**, 1/2 cup of strong chamomile tea, and 1/2 teaspoon of tea tree extract in a bottle with a tight-fitting cap, and store it at room temperature for up to nine months. Use it each morning and evening to keep your skin clear and soft. *Note: This potion also makes an excellent everyday toner for oily skin that's problem-free.*

Beat the Heat

When summer weather turns hot and humid, chill out by misting your skin with this cooling potion: Mix 2 teaspoons of **WITCH HAZEL**, 12 drops of lavender oil, and 10 drops of peppermint oil in an 8-ounce spray bottle, and fill the balance of the bottle with water. Keep it in the refrigerator, and reach for it anytime you feel too darn hot.

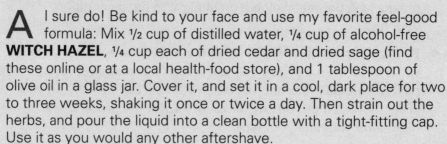

HOW'S THAT?

Q *Commercial aftershave lotions are chock-full of alcohol and all kinds of chemicals that irritate my face. Jerry, do you have a recipe for a gentler homemade aftershave for my sensitive skin?*

A I sure do! Be kind to your face and use my favorite feel-good formula: Mix 1/2 cup of distilled water, 1/4 cup of alcohol-free **WITCH HAZEL**, 1/4 cup each of dried cedar and dried sage (find these online or at a local health-food store), and 1 tablespoon of olive oil in a glass jar. Cover it, and set it in a cool, dark place for two to three weeks, shaking it once or twice a day. Then strain out the herbs, and pour the liquid into a clean bottle with a tight-fitting cap. Use it as you would any other aftershave.

Beauty

Smooth Like the Stars

Here's a not-so-confidential Hollywood secret—for decades, movie stars have used adhesive **TAPE** to temporarily lift their skin and smooth out wrinkles. In fact, Marlene Dietrich and Joan Crawford used tape, hidden under wigs, to pull their faces taut both on and off camera. But you don't have to go undercover to get the same effect. Just use tape strips at bedtime wherever you want to smooth out the wrinkles across your forehead and along your laugh lines. After a few weeks, you'll start to see results.

Tape and Trim

Tired of paying beauty-shop prices just to have your bangs trimmed? Then cut 'em yourself! When your hair is wet, run transparent **TAPE** across your forehead at eyebrow height, placing the top edge where you want the bottom of your bangs to be. Looking in a mirror, cut just above the tape. You'll have a professional salon look for zero bucks!

BEAUTY Bonus

EASY BROW TAMER

Do you have unruly eyebrows? Here's a simple way to get them under control: Each night at bedtime, press a piece of transparent **TAPE** across your brows. In the morning, gently pull it off, starting from the inner edge of your brow and pulling out toward your temple. Repeat each night until those little hairs know who's boss!

End Color Quandaries

When you can't decide what shade of fingernail polish to wear, cover a nail or two with transparent **TAPE**, and paint the polish over that. Keep experimenting until you've reached a final decision. Then remove the tape, and paint your nails.

Don't Share the Shades

Multishade eye shadow cases are a great convenience, but they tend to mix. Clean up those little compartments by blotting each surface with a piece of **TAPE**.

SPOTLIGHT ON
GIZMO & GADGET GLAM

While your kitchen countertops and cupboards may not be overflowing with potential beauty products, a quick search around the rest of the kitchen can turn up some pretty useful items, like these, for instance:

◆ Make your toothpaste last longer by squeezing the end of the tube with a large **BINDER CLIP.** This same trick works equally well for tubes of ointment, cream, hair gel, and even kitchen condiments that come in tubes, like minced garlic, pesto, and tomato paste.

◆ Do you break a nail every time you open an aspirin bottle? Save your nails (and your good humor) by keeping a **BOTTLE OPENER** right next to the aspirin—or any other bottle—that has a hard-to-pop top.

◆ A plastic **CUTLERY TRAY** is perfect for corralling lipsticks, eye pencils, makeup brushes, and other long, slender beauty items in your bathroom or vanity drawer.

◆ Use **ICE CUBE TRAYS** to freeze your favorite skin lotions. That way, you'll always have cool, soothing relief close at hand for sunburn, chapped skin, or insect bites.

◆ If you have long fingernails, or even not-so-long ones, it can be awkward and messy to use your fingers to scoop out beauty creams from jars. So keep your nails neat and use round **MEASURING SPOONS** instead. A ¼ teaspoon will hold the perfect amount for eye cream, while a 1-teaspoon measure is just about right for scooping face cream.

◆ Tuck a **MUFFIN TIN** into your bathroom or vanity drawer to hold the small stuff that tends to accumulate there, such as safety pins, trial-size bottles and tubes, and tiny jars of cosmetics. (If a muffin tin is too large to fit in your drawer, use an ice cube tray instead.)

Raise a Brush to Beer!

Want easy access to one of the most versatile hair-care products you could ever ask for? It's probably right in your kitchen. What is it? **BEER**! Here's a trio of ways to turn heads with a beautifying brewski:

- Boost your hair's volume and shine with this trick: In the shower, after shampooing, pour a bottle of beer over your head. (For best results, use a dark, rich brew that has a high yeast content, which means no "lite" brands!) The yeast and hops will swell your hair shafts and pump up the cuticles, while the beer's acidity will help remove any built-up product residue. Then rinse briefly with cool water. And don't worry—you won't smell like a brewery. The aroma will disappear as your hair dries.

- Beer also does a bang-up job as a setting lotion. Just pour some into a spray bottle and spritz your hair before styling it into the "do" of your choice.

- Hops (one of the main ingredients in beer) is a classic cure for dandruff. So to shake off the flakes, add a generous pour of beer to your regular shampoo, then lather up and rinse well.

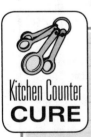

Kitchen Counter CURE

Dynamic Hair-Conditioning Duo

In the natural-beauty biz, **BEER** and honey are renowned as all-around individual champs. Here they team up in a conditioner that softens, shines, moisturizes, and strengthens your hair. To make it, pour a can or bottle of beer (preferably a dark, full-bodied brew) into a nonbreakable bowl, and let it go flat. In a separate container, mix 1 teaspoon of raw honey in 4 cups of warm water. After shampooing, pour the flat beer onto your hair, work it through the strands, and let it soak in for about two minutes. Rinse with cold water, and apply your usual conditioner. Then rinse again with the honey solution, and let your hair air-dry. Perform this routine once a month to keep your hair full, shiny, and beautifully manageable.

Zap Zits with Wine

RED WINE has anti-inflammatory and antiseptic properties, which are just the ticket for tackling tough breakouts. Simply pour some cheap wine on a cotton ball, and apply directly to each nasty bump. Let the wine air-dry.

Get Your Glow On

Here's a great way to get your skin glowing: Put a handful of dry oatmeal in a small bowl and add enough **RED WINE** to make a paste. Stir well, and apply to your clean skin as a mask. Sit back and relax for 15 minutes, then gently wipe off the mask with a warm, wet washcloth. Finish by splashing your face with cool water.

Wonderful Wine Face Treat

This **RED WINE** wonder mask will smooth and tighten your pores and leave your skin radiant. Start by brewing a cup of green tea and letting it cool to room temperature. Warm up 2 tablespoons of honey in the microwave for a few seconds (it should be runny but not hot). In a small bowl, mix 1 tablespoon of the green tea with the honey, adding 2 tablespoons of red wine and 1 tablespoon of plain yogurt. Stir until smooth. Spread the mask on your face with your fingers, staying away from your eyes, and relax for 15 minutes. Remove it with a warm, wet washcloth, rinse with cool water, and gently pat your skin dry.

BEAUTY Bonus

SILKY-SMOOTH SKIN TREATMENT

In the fight against aging skin, maintaining a smooth texture is half the battle. So enlist **RED WINE** in your quest to stop the clock. Combined with egg white and honey, it makes a rejuvenating mask that will have you feeling Sweet 16 again. Mix 1 egg white with 3 tablespoons of red wine and 1 tablespoon of organic raw honey until smooth. Spread the mask on your clean face, avoiding the eye area. Then sit or lie down and relax for 15 minutes. Remove by gently wiping with a warm, wet washcloth, then rinse with cool water and pat dry. Finish up with your usual moisturizer.

Shrink Your Pores

Tired of paying over-the-top prices for fancy astringents? Reach for the **VODKA** instead. Mix 3 parts distilled water with 1 part vodka, then apply to your face with a cotton ball and let air-dry. Use daily. If your skin becomes too dry, reduce the amount of vodka. If your skin is very oily, increase the vodka amount.

De-Gunk Your Hair

Styling products can leave your locks lackluster. So once a month, super-clean your hair with the help of **VODKA**. The recipe is simple: Pour your shampoo into your palm, then add about 1 teaspoon of vodka and swish it around with your finger to mix. Shampoo and condition as usual.

Discourage Dandruff

When you're searching for dandruff control, **VODKA** probably doesn't come to mind. But this weekly treatment works! Pour 1/2 cup of vodka into a glass jar with a tight-fitting lid. Add 2 teaspoons of crushed rosemary, put the lid on, and give the jar a shake. Set it in a spot where it won't get any sunlight, and let it "marinate" for three days. Then strain out the herb and massage the liquid into your dry scalp. Leave it on for one hour, and wash it out with a mild shampoo.

Back in the Day...

If you go through cans of hair spray like there's no tomorrow, take a hint from the past and use this old-as-the-hills recipe for locking your tresses in place: Slice 2 lemons and put them in a saucepan. Pour 2 cups of water over the lemons, cover the pot, and simmer on low heat for 30 minutes. Remove from the heat, take off the lid, and let the liquid cool for about 10 minutes. Then remove the lemon slices and stir in 1 tablespoon of **VODKA**. Pour the mixture into a spray bottle and use as you would any hair spray. Discard any unused spray after six months. *Note: This spray may lighten dark hair; to avoid a lightening effect, use sparingly and always cover your head when you are outdoors.*

SPOTLIGHT ON
DIY DEODORANTS

Yes, I know how easy it is to stroll down the deodorant aisle at your local superstore and grab the stick or roll-on brand that you've been using forever. But it wouldn't hurt to try something new, would it? Something that's all-natural, that tackles body odor just as well as— or even better than—conventional chemical-based antiperspirants? You may just find that your very own DIY concoction works better, and is less irritating, than your current brand. So go ahead, make your armpits happy by giving one (or more) of these a try!

◆ Fill a large, clean wide-mouth canning jar with grass clippings from a lawn that has not been treated with chemical pesticides or fertilizers. Cover the clippings with **VODKA** (any cheap brand will do), close the jar tightly, put it in a cool, dark place for 10 days, and shake it from time to time. After 10 days, strain out the grass clippings and pour the remaining liquid into a bottle (an old, clean roll-on deodorant bottle is perfect). If you don't have a roll-on bottle, any bottle with a tight-fitting cap will do. Then apply with your fingertips or a cotton pad.

◆ Make a spray deodorant by mixing ½ cup of witch hazel with 2 tablespoons of **VODKA**, 1 tablespoon of glycerin, and ½ teaspoon of the grass-vodka deodorant described above. Pour the solution into a handheld spray bottle and spritz your underarms.

◆ For a nicely scented DIY deodorant, add 5 to 10 drops of your favorite essential oil to either one of the above **VODKA** recipes; be sure to shake well to mix all of the ingredients before each use. Here are some of my favorite scents: bergamot, citrus, lavender, sandalwood, tea tree, and ylang-ylang. Experiment to find the fragrance that suits you best.

Note: If you're just not up to creating your own deodorant, give a deodorant stone a try. Its natural mineral salts fight odor, and you can also use it on your feet and any other, um, aromatic areas of your body.

CHAPTER 7

Foxy Fridge & Freezer Finds

When you reach into the fridge for a carton of milk or a few eggs, you probably don't realize that those items make more than just a tasty breakfast. They also are fine additions to your beauty routine. Don't believe me? Well, what if I told you that milk can make your skin glow and eggs can make your hair shine? That doesn't sound so far-fetched now, does it? But it's not only dairy products that can boost your beauty quotient. There are plenty of other goodies in your fridge and freezer that can help you look your very best. Read on for my tips and tricks on how to raid the fridge for a more beautiful you.

DAIRY PRODUCTS

Buttermilk for Beauty

Lactic acid is the key ingredient in many beauty products that exfoliate, soften, and brighten skin. **BUTTERMILK** is rich in lactic acid, so put it to work in this facial mask: Mix 1/4 cup of buttermilk with 1/4 cup of dry whole-milk powder (not nonfat) to form a paste. Spread it evenly over your face and neck, using a clean makeup brush. Let it dry for 20 minutes and rinse it off with cool water.

Buttermilk Moisture Boost

Treat your thirsty, dry skin to this nourishing drink: Mix 2 teaspoons of **BUTTERMILK** with a few drops each of almond oil and rose water (available in health-food stores and online). Using your fingertips, gently massage the mixture onto your clean face and neck and leave it on for 30 minutes or so. Rinse it off with warm water, and pat your skin dry.

Nifty Nail Nourisher

Need an easy, foolproof way to nourish and strengthen your fingernails? Try this: Beat 1 egg yolk, 1/4 cup of **BUTTERMILK**, and 1 tablespoon of honey in a small bowl. Soak your nails in the mixture for 10 minutes, and then rinse well with cool water. The buttermilk will soften dry cuticles, and the protein in the egg will make your nails as hard as, well, nails.

Out, Out, Dark Spots!

Here's a great way to lighten dark spots on your face: Grind dried orange peel (use a coffee grinder or mortar and pestle) and combine enough peels with 1/4 cup of **BUTTERMILK** to make a paste. Use your fingertips or a clean makeup brush to apply it to your face and let it dry completely. Then rinse the paste off with tepid water, and gently pat your skin dry. You should start to see the spots fading within 30 days.

Kitchen Counter

Dairy Delight Conditioner

This treat for dry, damaged hair comes straight from the fridge and leaves your hair shiny and smooth.

1 cup of plain yogurt
1/2 cup of BUTTERMILK
1 egg yolk
2 tbsp. of honey

Mix all of the ingredients together in a small shatterproof bowl. Bring the mixture into the shower with you, and apply it to your just-washed, wet hair, working it in all over your head. Step out of the shower and pull on a shower cap. Leave it on for 30 minutes or so, then rinse out the conditioner and dry and style your hair as usual.

Whip Up a Mini Face-Lift

Have you ever looked in the mirror and smoothed your face back to see how a new, rejuvenated you would look? Well, there's no need to go under the knife to get a fresh face—just grab an **EGG**! Separate the egg, and whisk the raw white with 1 tablespoon of honey. Wash your face, then use your fingertips to spread the mixture on, starting with your forehead, moving down your nose and across each cheek, and finishing just under your chin. You will soon feel the mask tighten. Leave it on for 20 minutes, then rinse it off with warm water and gently pat your skin dry.

Eggy Eye Relief

Do you look tired all of the time because of unsightly bags and dark circles under your eyes? Here's a trio of **EGG**-based quick fixes that'll leave you looking years younger:

BEAUTY
Bonus

EXFOLIATING BODY SCRUB

Why should your face get all the attention? You can have soft, caressable skin from head to toe, and here's one great way to get it: Start with the shells of five hard-boiled **EGGS**. Smash them into a fine powder with a mortar and pestle, and stir in 2 tablespoons of honey and 2 tablespoons of kosher salt to make a thick paste. Then step into the shower and get wet. Using a loofah or washcloth, rub the paste all over your body, paying particular attention to rough elbows, knees, and heels. Rinse off and pat dry. You'll feel silky smooth all over.

- Whisk one raw egg white, 1 tablespoon of finely shredded carrot, and 1 teaspoon of aloe vera juice until frothy. With a clean makeup brush, apply the mixture around and under your eyes. Allow it to dry for 30 minutes, then rinse it off with warm water and gently pat dry.

- Stir one raw egg white with 1 teaspoon of honey and 1 teaspoon of olive oil until thoroughly mixed. Lightly dab it around and under your eyes, wait 15 to 20 minutes, then rinse it off with warm water and gently pat dry.

- Apply one whisked raw egg white to your eye area with a clean makeup brush. Allow it to thoroughly dry on your skin, rinse it off with cool water, gently pat dry, and be on your way.

Unmask Beautiful Skin

Here's a treat for your face that will minimize fine lines and have you glowing: Stir together one raw **EGG** yolk, 2 teaspoons of very soft cooked rice (smash it into a pulp), 1 teaspoon of ground almonds (use a coffee grinder or mortar and pestle), and 10 drops of lemon juice. Mix well, then use your fingertips to apply the mask to your face. Sit back and relax for 20 to 30 minutes and allow the mask to dry completely. Then remove it with a warm, wet washcloth, rinse with cool water, and moisturize as usual.

DIY Pore-Cleansing Strips

Get rid of unsightly blackheads and reduce pore size with these homemade cleansing strips that work just as well as the pricey beauty-aisle brands. Start by thoroughly cleaning your face. Then rub the cut side of a lemon on the areas where you want to get rid of blackheads. Using your fingertips or a clean makeup brush, apply a layer of raw **EGG** white over the lemon juice and immediately cover each area with a strip of tissue paper. Leave it on for 20 minutes, or until the strips have dried completely. Then peel off the tissue paper, rinse your face with cool water, and gently pat your skin dry.

HOW'S THAT?

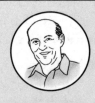

Q *A friend of mine swears that **EGG** shells can whiten teeth. I'm skeptical, but I guess it wouldn't hurt to give it a try, would it?*

A I *have* heard of this, and you're right—there's no harm in trying out this trick on yourself. Start by removing the shells from three hard-boiled eggs and drying the shells thoroughly. Then use a mortar and pestle or a coffee grinder to grind them into a fine powder. Store the powder in a jar with a tight-fitting lid. Whenever you clean your teeth, sprinkle about half a teaspoon of the eggshell powder on top of the toothpaste on your brush. The abrasive eggshell will help eliminate stains and get your choppers pearly white.

Back in the Day...

When it came to skin and hair care, my Grandma Putt and her friends had quite a few beauty secrets up their sleeves. Here's one that's especially good for oily skin that tends to break out: Stir 1 raw **EGG** into 1/2 cup of cooled, cooked oatmeal, mixing well. Add 1 tablespoon of lemon juice and blend thoroughly. Use your fingertips or a clean makeup brush to apply the paste to your face, and leave it on for 10 minutes. Then rinse it off with warm water, and gently pat your skin dry.

Eggy Stretch Mark Eraser

Lessen the look of ugly stretch marks with this soothing massage oil. In a small bowl, mix one raw **EGG** white with a few drops of almond oil. With your fingertips, massage it into the marks for three to five minutes, then leave the mixture on your skin for another 10 minutes before you rinse it off with warm water and pat your skin dry. Use this treatment several times a week.

Lemon and Egg Acne Aid

Here's an easy way to reduce the look of unsightly acne scars and other skin discolorations. Mix together one raw **EGG** and the juice of one lemon. Using your fingertips, apply it to any scar, pimple, and/or dark spot on your face. Let the mixture dry completely, rinse it off with warm water, and gently pat your skin dry. Repeat once a week, and watch those marks fade.

Super-Simple Eyelash Enhancer

If you long for lush lashes, this simple serum will do the trick. In a small bowl, mix together one raw **EGG** yolk, 2 teaspoons of glycerin (available online), and 1 teaspoon of olive oil. Mix well, then dip an unused, clean mascara wand into the serum and gently sweep the wand from the base to the tips of your eyelashes. Repeat two to three times. Discard the remaining mixture. Leave it on your lashes for 15 minutes, then rinse it off with cool water. For best results, use each evening after removing your makeup. *Note: Thoroughly clean your mascara brush with hot, soapy water after each use, and use it only for this serum. Or use disposable mascara wands, which you can buy at beauty-supply stores.*

Hydrating Hair Mask

De-stress your tresses with this luxurious treatment that will put the shine and bounce back into your hair. Start by smashing half of a ripe avocado and half of a ripe banana together in a medium-size bowl. Add one beaten raw **EGG** and 2 teaspoons of olive oil and mix well. Apply the mask to your dry hair, cover with a shower cap, and go read a good book for a half hour. When the time is up, wash out the mask with a mild shampoo, followed by your usual hair conditioner.

Restorative Tonic for Tresses

Give your hair some tender loving care with this tea tonic, guaranteed to make your mane the talk of the town! Brew a cup of green tea and measure out 2 tablespoons into a small bowl. Add one raw **EGG** yolk and beat with a fork until frothy. Pour the mixture over your head, working it into your dry hair with your fingertips. Then sit down and enjoy your hot tea while the tonic does it magic. After 30 minutes or so, wash it out with your regular shampoo, followed by your usual conditioner.

Dandy Dandruff Detonator

EGGS can help combat problems like dandruff and dry scalp. Beat two raw egg whites in a small bowl and add 4 tablespoons of coconut oil, stirring until smooth. Apply the mixture to your wet hair and scalp, and brush it through to distribute evenly. Leave it in your hair for an hour, then rinse it out with lukewarm water. Follow with your usual shampoo and conditioner.

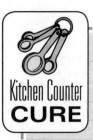

Kitchen Counter **CURE**

Shine-On Conditioner

This all-natural conditioner will add shine and soften your hair, and the recipe is simple: Beat two **EGG** yolks until they're frothy, and then beat in 1 cup of water and 1 teaspoon of baby oil or olive oil. Work the mixture through your wet hair as you would any other conditioner, wait for a minute or two, and rinse thoroughly with cool water.

Make Mine Milk

If your blotchy, uneven skin tone is tempting you to drop big bucks on a pricey commercial potion, stop right there. Before you open your wallet, try one—or both—of these **MILK** treatments:

- In a small bowl, mix 2 tablespoons of milk, 1 tablespoon of honey, and 1 tablespoon of lemon juice, stirring well. Using your fingertips or a makeup brush, apply the mixture to your just-washed face. Leave it on for 15 minutes, or until it is completely dry, then rinse it off with cool water and gently pat your skin dry. Use twice a week and watch those blotches fade.

- Before bed, soak a cotton ball in milk, and dab the dark skin areas. Allow the milk to dry, then hit the sack. Wash your face in the morning.

Back in the Day...

Just about every day we seem to hear of some scientific proof confirming what we've known all along. That sure is true when it comes to a great deal of my Grandma Putt's rules to live by. Here's another one that she always knew: Stress (or getting all hot and bothered, as she put it) is bad for your health, and detracts from your good looks, too. So do your body and soul a favor, and whip up this simple soother: Mix 4 cups of dry **MILK**, 2 cups of cornstarch, and a few drops of your favorite scented oil in a blender. Store the mixture in an airtight container at room temperature. Whenever you feel the need, add ½ cup to a tub of hot bathwater and relax.

Moo Juice Rejuvenator

Turn back the clock with a **MILK** and honey combo that will make your skin radiant and youthful. In a small bowl, mix 2 tablespoons of dry milk, 2 tablespoons of warm water, and 1 tablespoon of honey and stir until a paste forms. Using your fingertips, apply the paste to your face in small circles, starting at your forehead, working down over your nose and across your cheeks, and ending just under your chin. Then sit back and relax for a half hour or so, until the mask is completely dry. Rinse it off with warm water, and gently pat your skin dry.

BEAUTY Bonus

SPRAY-ON CONDITIONER

Put the magic of **MILK** to work restoring dry, damaged hair. Simply replace your usual conditioner with whole milk at least twice a week. Fill a handheld spray bottle with enough milk to cover your entire head of hair and bring it into the shower. After washing your hair as usual, squeeze out the excess water, then aim and spray. Comb your milk-soaked hair to evenly cover the strands, and wait 10 minutes before rinsing well with warm water. If your hair is extremely dry, add a tablespoon of olive oil to the milk in the sprayer and shake it well before using.

Super-Simple Scrub

Use a **MILK** scrub on your face to get rid of dead skin cells and make your skin glow. Start by dissolving 1 teaspoon of table salt in a cup of very hot water. Add instant nonfat dry milk, 1/2 cup at a time, until you have a thick paste. When it is cooled to room temperature, scoop up the paste with your fingers and scrub your face with it. Rinse it off with lukewarm water, and gently pat your skin dry.

Soothing Skin Smoother

To help smooth out fine lines and get your face glowing, mash half a banana and add a few spoonfuls of whole **MILK** to make a paste. Using your fingertips, apply the paste to your clean, damp skin and leave it on for 15 minutes. Rinse it off with warm water, gently pat your skin dry, and follow with your usual moisturizer.

Easy Acne Treatment

Get breakouts under control with **MILK**. The lactic acid in milk helps to brighten up your complexion and is a gentle exfoliant. Just mix a few tablespoons of whole milk with enough flour to create a thin paste. Apply it to your spots at bedtime, being sure it's completely dry before you climb into bed. In the morning, rinse your face with cool water and gently pat dry.

A Milky Moisture Pack

This hair pack is just what your dull, dry hair needs to rev up the moisture and sheen. Break an egg into 1 cup of whole **MILK**, and beat with a fork until well combined. Get into the shower and wet your hair. Squeeze out as much water as you can, then pour the mixture over your damp tresses and massage it all over your head. Leave the pack on for 20 minutes, then shampoo and condition as usual.

Cool the Burn

Ease the pain of sunburn with **MILK**. Pour a cup or so of whole milk (or even half-and-half) into a bowl. Dip a soft, clean cloth into the milk, and gently lay the wet compress on your sizzling skin. Hold it there for 15 minutes or so, then rinse the milk off with cool water and let your skin air-dry. Repeat throughout the day.

Nurture Your Nails

Are you embarrassed by your ragged nails? Here's a simple solution: Soak your fingernails in a mixture of 1/4 cup of warm whole **MILK** and one beaten egg yolk for about 10 minutes. Then rinse with cool water and dry your nails thoroughly. This nourishing mixture will help to smooth cuticles and strengthen nails so they're less likely to crack or split.

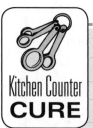

Kitchen Counter CURE

Mocha Milk Mask

Here's a facial treat that is so yummy you'll be tempted to take a sip as you mix it up, but try to save some for your skin!

- **3 tbsp. of whole MILK**
- **1 tbsp. of cocoa powder**
- **1 tbsp. of instant coffee**

In a small bowl, mix all of the ingredients together, adding a few more drops of milk if the mask is too thick to spread. Using your fingertips or a clean makeup brush, apply the mixture evenly to your face. Leave it on for 15 minutes, then rinse it off with warm water, gently pat your skin dry, and follow up with your usual facial moisturizer.

SPOTLIGHT ON
SKIN SMOOTHERS

No matter how well you take care of your skin, there are still times when you need to make that extra effort to achieve soft and smooth results. Perhaps dry, indoor heat (or air-conditioning!) has wreaked havoc on your epidermis, or maybe you've spent a bit too much time out in the sun, and now your skin needs extra TLC. Or you may just want quick relief for dry elbows and knees. Whatever type of skin you're in, try these tips to get your "smooth" on.

◆ To soften rough elbows and knees, add enough dry oatmeal to 4 tablespoons of **BUTTERMILK** to make a paste. Apply to all the rough places and leave on for 10 minutes before rinsing and patting dry.

◆ To reduce the appearance of large facial pores, beat one **EGG**, and mix it with about 1 tablespoon of honey. Spread the mixture onto your face, and leave it on for 20 minutes or so. Then rinse it off to reveal skin that's softer, firmer, and smoother than before.

◆ Rumor has it that Cleopatra took **MILK** baths to keep her skin silky smooth. It can work for you, too. Simply add 1 or 2 gallons of whole milk to a bathtub of warm water, then slip in and soak for about 20 minutes. Rinse well so you don't smell like a dairy, and apply your usual body moisturizer while your skin is still slightly damp to lock in essential moisture.

◆ Reveal smooth, younger-looking skin by applying a thick layer of plain whole-milk **YOGURT** to your face. Leave it on for 20 minutes, and rinse it off with lukewarm water. Repeat the process at least once a week—more often if you have the time.

◆ Mix 2 parts plain whole-milk **YOGURT** with 1 part honey, and spread the mixture over your face. Then lean back and relax for 15 minutes or so. Rinse the combo off with warm water, and enjoy the results: calmer spirits and smoother, softer skin!

A Little Culture Goes a Long Way...

Put **YOGURT's** live active cultures to good use in this super-simple facial mask. Using your fingertips, apply a thick layer of plain whole-milk yogurt to your clean face and neck, lie down, and relax for 20 minutes. Then rinse it off with warm water, and gently pat your skin dry.

Spot-On Anti-Spot Treatment

YOGURT that contains live active cultures is just what you need to battle blemishes. With your fingertips, rub plain low-fat yogurt directly into any blemish-prone areas. Allow it to thoroughly dry on your skin, then rinse it off with lukewarm water and gently pat your skin dry.

Instant Eye Lift

Reduce the look of sags, bags, and dark under-eye circles while you sleep! Gently tap a thin layer of plain whole-milk **YOGURT** around each eye. Leave it on for 15 minutes, then gently blot with a tissue, and toddle off to bed. Do this nightly, and you'll soon start to see an improvement.

Fabulous Foot Scrub

Smooth your dry feet with **YOGURT**. Stir 1/2 cup of ground walnuts into 1/2 cup of plain whole-milk yogurt. Use it to exfoliate dry patches and calluses on your feet. Rinse with warm water and dry your toes completely before you put on footwear.

HOW'S THAT?

Q *I've got some dark spots on the backs of my hands and a few on my face. I really don't like the chemical concoctions that are available as skin lighteners. Do you have a gentler, more natural alternative?*

A I sure do! Mix 2 tablespoons of plain whole-milk **YOGURT** with a few drops of lemon juice and leave it on the affected skin for about 30 minutes before rinsing off. Yogurt contains mild bleaching properties that can help even out skin tone.

Sweet Skin Saver

Here's a rejuvenating cocoa mask that will leave your skin glowing: In a small bowl, combine 2 tablespoons of plain whole-milk **YOGURT**, 1 tablespoon of cocoa powder, 1 tablespoon of ground oats (grind uncooked rolled oats in a coffee grinder or food processor), and 1 teaspoon of honey. Gently massage the mixture onto your still-moist, freshly washed face. Leave it on for 15 minutes, then rinse with warm water, gently pat your skin dry, and follow up with your usual facial moisturizer. Repeat once a week for maximum benefits.

Complexion Perfection

You should never spend top dollar for skin treatments! Good ol' **YOGURT** contains lactic acid, a prime component of many chemical peels that are offered in doctors' offices. By gently exfoliating the top layers of the skin, yogurt can clear up blemishes and discolorations and may help reduce fine lines and wrinkles. Here's the how-to: In a small bowl, mix 1 cup of plain whole-milk yogurt, 1 tablespoon of honey, and 2 to 3 drops of almond or olive oil. Stir well. Using your fingertips or a clean makeup brush, apply the mask to your freshly washed and dried face. Leave it on for 30 minutes, then rinse it off with warm water and gently pat your skin dry.

BEAUTY
Bonus

SOOTHING SUNBURN SOLUTION

You *know* each application of sunscreen only protects your skin for an hour or so, but let's face it, sometimes you just plain forget to keep slathering it on. So what's the best way to treat the resulting sizzled, sunburned skin? Why, with **YOGURT**, of course! The zinc in yogurt helps cool the burn, and this calming concoction really does the trick: Mix a few drops of chamomile oil into $\frac{1}{2}$ cup of plain whole-milk yogurt, and gently apply it to your singed skin. Let the mixture dry completely, then rinse it off with cool water and let your skin air-dry. Repeat several times each day until the sting is out and your skin is looking and feeling back to normal. And next time, don't forget to keep applying the sunscreen!

Fantastic Frizz Fighter

Are you tired of fighting frizzy hair? Don't despair—**YOGURT** can tame your tresses and make them more manageable. Just mix together 3 tablespoons of plain whole-milk yogurt, 2 tablespoons of coconut oil, and 4 teaspoons of aloe vera gel. (Depending on the length of your hair, you may need to double or even triple this recipe.) Divide your dry hair into sections, and apply the paste evenly on each section from root to tip. Then put on a shower cap and relax for 30 minutes. When the time is up, wash your hair with a mild shampoo, followed by your usual conditioner.

Kick Up the Color

Are your locks losing their luster? Is that expensive color fading fast? Here's how plain whole-milk **YOGURT** can make your hair tones richer and more radiant. How you use it depends on your natural hair color.

- **For brunettes.** Mix ½ cup of yogurt, ½ cup of cocoa powder, 1 teaspoon of apple cider vinegar, and 1 teaspoon of honey to form a smooth paste. Apply the mixture to your freshly shampooed hair, and leave it on for two to three minutes. Then rinse and style as usual.

- **For redheads.** In a blender or food processor, mix 3 tablespoons of yogurt, 2 tablespoons of honey, and three medium-size chopped carrots (or ½ cup of cranberries if you want copper undertones) to get a coarse paste. After shampooing, work the mixture through your wet hair. Leave it on for one to two minutes, and then rinse it out. Follow up with your usual styling routine.

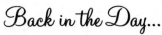

Back in the Day...

Don't let dandruff ruin your hairdo. Try this old-as-the-hills flake fighter for healthy hair: In a small bowl, mix 1 cup of plain whole-milk **YOGURT** with 2 teaspoons of ground black pepper. Wash and towel-dry your hair, then apply the yogurt-pepper mixture to your scalp, massaging it in thoroughly. Wait 15 minutes, then rinse it with warm water. Repeat daily, and your dandruff should disappear within a week. Use the treatment once a week to keep the flakes at bay.

BEAUTY
Bonus

TRESS R$_x$

Styling products can build up in your hair, making it dull, lifeless, and limp. To make it shiny and bouncy again, simply massage ½ cup of plain whole-milk **YOGURT** into your damp hair, cover with a shower cap, and leave it on for 30 minutes. Rinse it off first with warm water, then with cool water. Follow up with your usual shampoo and conditioner.

Defeat Hair Damage

From cold winter winds to hot, sunny summer days, the weather can take its toll on your tresses. So pamper your hair with this nourishing, hydrating treatment, and liven up those limp locks. Use a whisk to whip ½ cup of plain whole-milk **YOGURT** with 2 beaten eggs and 2 tablespoons of almond oil. Apply the treatment to your freshly washed, damp hair and leave it on for 30 minutes. Rinse it with lukewarm water and style.

Ultimate Hair Healer

You can spend a small fortune on deep-conditioning treatments for dry, damaged hair, but don't do it! This rich repair serum does the job at a fraction of the cost of those high-priced hair products. In a medium-size bowl, using a hand mixer, beat ½ cup of plain whole-milk **YOGURT**, ½ cup of full-fat mayonnaise, and one raw egg white. Slather the conditioner onto your head, and thoroughly coat all of your hair strands, concentrating on the ends. Put on a shower cap, and tuck tissues or cotton balls around the edges to catch any drips. Leave it on for 30 minutes or so. Rinse thoroughly with lukewarm water. (Don't use hot water, or you'll wind up with a head full of scrambled eggs!) You can follow up with a mild shampoo, or just dry and style your hair as usual.

Get Your Shine On

Give your hair a healthy gleam with this shine-enhancing treatment. In a small bowl, beat one raw egg white until it's foamy, then stir in 6 tablespoons of plain whole-milk **YOGURT**. Apply the mixture to your freshly washed, towel-dried hair from roots to tips and leave it on for 15 minutes. Then rinse it out with lukewarm water.

Easy Wrinkle Eraser

Enzymes in **APPLES** help your skin retain moisture and have a soothing, cooling effect. They also help to reduce inflammation and the appearance of fine lines and wrinkles. So what are you waiting for? Grab an apple, core it, peel it, finely grate it, and apply the mush to your face. Leave it on for 15 minutes, then rinse it off with warm water and gently pat your skin dry.

The Apple of Your Eye

Place a very thin slice of **APPLE** under each eye to reduce dark circles and puffiness. Leave them in place for 20 minutes, then remove the slices and rinse your eye area with lukewarm water. Gently pat dry, and follow up with your usual eye moisturizer.

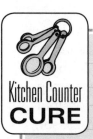

Kitchen Counter CURE

Nifty Night Cream

As we age, our skin begins to lose its youthful elasticity. Coax it back with this luxurious night cream.

1 APPLE
1 cup of olive oil
1 cup of rose water*

Wash and dry the apple, but don't peel it. Remove the stem, core the apple, then cut it in half and remove the seeds. Cut into small pieces and place them in a blender or food processor. Slowly add the olive oil until a paste forms. Put water in the bottom of a double boiler and add the apple-oil mixture in the top part; heat it until it's just lukewarm. (If you don't have a double boiler, substitute a saucepan and a heat-proof bowl.) Don't let the apple cook—if it does, the key ingredient (malic acid) will dissipate. Set the mixture aside until it cools to room temperature, then add the rose water and stir until the ingredients are thoroughly combined. Store the cream in the fridge, where it will keep for up to six days. Use it nightly before bed. *Available in health-food stores and online.*

Anti-Acne Apple Treatment

Let the power of **APPLE** enzymes clear up breakouts fast. Finely grate half of a cored, peeled apple, and mix thoroughly with 4 teaspoons of honey. Using your fingertips, lightly tap the treatment onto the affected areas. Leave it on your skin for 15 minutes, then rinse it off with luke-warm water and gently pat your skin dry. Repeat every night.

Appealing Apple Cleanser

The natural acids in **APPLES** help to remove excess oil from the skin and prevent breakouts, leaving your face with a healthy glow. This cleanser makes the most of apple's potent powers: Finely grate one-quarter of a cored, peeled apple and mix it thoroughly with 2 tablespoons of whole milk and 1 teaspoon of honey. Using your fingertips, apply the cleanser to your face and neck, massaging in circles. Rinse it off with warm water, and gently pat your skin dry.

All-Purpose Applesauce

This no-frills sauce won't win any culinary taste awards, but it's just the ticket for facial and hair treatments. Peel and core two medium-size **APPLES**, put them in a small baking dish, and pour about 1/8 cup of water over them. Bake them in a 350°F oven for 15 minutes, or until they're slightly mushy. Puree the apples in a blender or food processor, and use the sauce to wash your hair or in any facial mask that calls for applesauce. Store leftovers in the refrigerator and use within a week.

Back in the Day...

Get ready for compliments on your shiny, healthy hair after you use this old-as-the-hills deep-clean treatment. Simply scoop up a handful of All-Purpose **APPLESAUCE** (see above), and massage it deeply into your dry hair and scalp. Leave it on for 10 minutes, then rinse thoroughly. Your hair will be so smooth you won't have to follow up with conditioner. Just style as usual and be on your way.

Feed Your Skin

If you're looking for a skin-firming facial mask, this easy formula is the answer to your prayers: Mix 1 tablespoon of All-Purpose **APPLESAUCE** (at left) with 1 tablespoon of wheat germ. With your fingertips or a clean makeup brush, apply the mixture to your face, starting at your forehead, working down your nose and across your cheeks, and ending just under your chin. Leave it on for 15 minutes, then rinse it off with warm water, gently pat your skin dry, and follow up with your usual facial moisturizer.

Apple Magic Mask

You can't beat this **APPLE**-infused treatment—it soothes and nourishes your skin while providing gentle exfoliating action. Finely grate one-quarter of a peeled, cored apple and mix it with 1 tablespoon of uncooked rolled oats, 1 teaspoon of heavy cream, and 1 teaspoon of honey. Using your fingertips, apply the mask to your face, massaging it into your skin. Leave it on for 10 minutes, then rinse it off with warm water, gently pat your skin dry, and follow up with your usual facial moisturizer.

BEAUTY
Bonus

BACK-IN-BALANCE SKIN SOOTHER

For skin that really needs some TLC, this **APPLE** mask has it all, from gentle fruit acids that tone to oatmeal that exfoliates and buttermilk that calms. Best of all, it uses half an apple, so you can enjoy the other half while your mask works its wonders. Start by coring and paring one apple. Then cut it in half, and set aside one half to eat later. Chop the remaining half into small chunks and put them into a food processor or blender. Add one 1.5-ounce packet of colloidal oatmeal, 1 tablespoon of buttermilk, and 1 tablespoon of oat bran to the apple chunks, and puree until the ingredients reach a thick, paste-like consistency. Using your fingertips or a clean makeup brush, apply the mask to your face, starting at your forehead, going down your nose and across your cheeks, and ending just under your chin. Leave it on for 10 minutes, then rinse it off with warm water and gently pat your skin dry. Store any leftover mixture in an airtight container in the refrigerator for up to three days.

De-Puff Your Peepers

This tip is so simple, you won't believe it actually works—but it does! The next time you look in the mirror and puffy, dark-circled eyes are staring back at you, head right into the kitchen and slice up a ripe **AVOCADO**. Then sit back, place one avocado slice over each eye, and relax for 20 minutes. Remove the slices, splash your eyes with cool water, and gently pat dry. You should see almost-instant results.

A Treat for Your Feet

This tasty tootsie treat soothes dry, cracked skin and leaves your feet smooth as silk. Using a fork, smash one pitted, peeled ripe **AVOCADO** until it's creamy. Sit down on the floor with a towel under your feet and massage the avocado well into both feet, paying particular attention to your heels. Leave it on for about 15 minutes, then rinse it off with warm water and pat your skin dry.

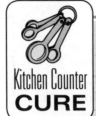

Kitchen Counter CURE

Halt-the-Oil Skin Mask

If you're looking for a mask that will sop up facial oil, but not leave your skin feeling like sandpaper, this balanced blend is for you.

½ ripe AVOCADO, halved, pitted, and peeled
1 raw egg white
1 teaspoon of lemon juice

In a blender, combine all of the ingredients until smooth. Using your fingertips, apply the mask evenly to your face, avoiding the eye area. Leave it on for 20 minutes, then rinse it off with warm water and gently pat your skin dry.

Aaahhh ... Avocado Skin Treatment

This gentle mask works wonders on mature, dry skin, but you can add some lemon juice to it if your skin is oily, so everyone wins! Peel and smash half of a ripe **AVOCADO** in a small bowl. Stir in 2 tablespoons of honey and 1 tablespoon of sugar. Add 1 teaspoon of lemon juice if you have oily skin. Rinse your face with warm water to open up your pores. Using your fingertips, apply the avocado mixture to your face and neck, massaging it into your skin in small circles, and avoiding the eye area. Leave it on for 15 minutes, then rinse it off with warm water and gently pat your skin dry.

Awesome Avocado Mask

Make the most of the moisturizing oils in **AVOCADOS** by adding honey, a natural antibacterial, and soothing yogurt to gently clean and soften your skin while tightening pores. In a small bowl, use a fork to smash half of a pitted, peeled ripe avocado until smooth. Stir in 1 tablespoon of honey and 1 tablespoon of plain yogurt. Combine well. Using your fingertips, apply the mask evenly to your face. Leave it on for 20 minutes, then rinse it off with warm water and gently pat your skin dry.

Tap Your Inner Beauty...

With the inside of an **AVOCADO** peel! Whenever you peel an avocado for a recipe, use the inside of the skin on *your* skin as a facial moisturizer. Rub the inside of the peel onto your clean face and use your fingertips to work it in. Leave it on for 20 minutes, then rinse it off with warm water.

Healing Hair Mask

This rich mixture helps hair retain moisture, leaving you with shiny, manageable locks. Put half of a pitted and peeled ripe **AVOCADO** in a small bowl and smash it with a fork until smooth. Add one raw egg yolk and $1/2$ teaspoon of olive oil, and use a whisk to thoroughly combine. Divide your dry hair into sections, holding with hair clips. Massage the avocado mask into each section from scalp to tips, concentrating on the ends. Leave it on for 30 minutes, then rinse with warm water and style.

HOW'S THAT?

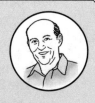

Q *Jerry, my hands are a mess from all the gardening I do, and they need help fast! Any suggestions for a natural hand lotion?*

A The answer, my friend, is **AVOCADO**. In a small bowl, use a fork to smash half of a pitted, peeled avocado. Mix in 4 tablespoons of uncooked rolled oats, one raw egg white, and 1 tablespoon of lemon juice. Massage the mixture into your hands, leave it on for 15 minutes, then rinse and dry. Your hands will be soft and smooth in no time.

Foxy Fridge & Freezer Finds

SPOTLIGHT ON
FRUITY FACE FRESHENERS

Sure, you can buy lots of fancy lotions and potions that promise to make your skin youthful and glowing. But why spend big bucks when Mother Nature does the same job, at a fraction of the cost? Here's just a sampling of fabulous fruity face treatments that will have you looking your best:

◆ Refresh your face with this lightly fragrant scrub that tones and brightens skin. Just grind several dried **APRICOT** pits in a food processor or coffee grinder until you have a coarse powder. Stir in enough rose water (available in health-food stores and online) to make a thick paste, and using your fingertips, apply it to your face, avoiding the eye area. Gently massage the scrub into your face in circles to remove dull, dead skin and get your glow back. Then rinse it off with warm water, and gently pat your skin dry.

◆ Soothe and freshen with an **AVOCADO** facial cleanser. In a small bowl, combine one beaten egg yolk, ½ cup of whole milk, and half of a peeled avocado. Beat the mixture with a fork until it is thin and creamy. Use cotton balls to apply it to your face, using gentle, circular motions. Rinse it off with warm water, and gently pat your skin dry.

◆ Minimize tiny lines and wrinkles around your eyes and mouth. Just cut green seedless **GRAPES** in half, and squeeze the juice right onto the little creases. (This treatment is especially good for dry, sensitive skin.)

◆ Whip up a triple-treat face cream that will remove makeup and clean and soften your skin. In a small bowl, mix the juice of one **LIME** with ½ cup of mayonnaise (the real kind, made with eggs and oil, not the lower-fat version) and 1 tablespoon of melted butter (not margarine). Spoon the cream into a glass jar with a tight-fitting lid, and store it in the refrigerator. Use your fingertips to scoop out the cleanser and massage it into your face in small circles. Rinse well with lukewarm water, and gently pat your skin dry.

Best Blackberry Mask

What's the best way to use a handful of **BLACKBERRIES**? Turn them into this nourishing face mask! Start with six ripe blackberries and mash them in a small bowl. Stir in 1 teaspoon of honey and mix well. Using your fingertips, apply the mixture to your face and neck, then relax until the mask is completely dry. Remove it with a warm, wet washcloth, then rinse your face and neck with cool water and gently pat your skin dry.

Brightening Blackberry Cleanser

Freshen up and nourish your skin with this berry good cleanser. Mash three ripe **BLACKBERRIES** in a small bowl, and mix in 2 tablespoons of plain yogurt and 1 teaspoon of rose water (available in health-food stores and online). Gently massage the mixture onto your face for 30 seconds, avoiding the eye area. Rinse it off with cool water, gently pat your skin dry, and follow up with your usual facial moisturizer.

Rejuvenating Facial

Use this facial treatment once or twice a week for smooth, hydrated skin. In a blender, puree five ripe **BLACKBERRIES**, 3 tablespoons of plain whole-milk yogurt, 1/4 teaspoon of lemon juice, and a pinch of ground nutmeg. Use your fingertips to apply the mixture evenly to your face and neck, avoiding the eye area. Leave it on for 20 minutes, then rinse it off with lukewarm water and gently pat your skin dry.

Back in the Day...

Long before commercial acne treatments came on the scene, Grandma Putt swore by the power of **BLACKBERRIES** to clear up breakouts. In a small bowl, mash a handful of fresh blackberries to a pulp. Stir in 3 drops of lime juice and a dash of turmeric powder, and mix well. Wash your face, then use your fingertips to apply the treatment to all of the affected areas, avoiding your eyes. Leave it on for 20 minutes, then rinse it off with lukewarm water and pat your skin dry.

BEAUTY
Bonus

COOL COMPLEXION CLEARER

Here's a skin-clearing and firming treatment that is truly cool. Smash ¼ cup of **BLUEBERRIES** in a small bowl until they're pulpy. Add 1 tablespoon each of honey and olive oil and stir well to make a paste. Put the bowl in the freezer for 10 minutes. Using your fingertips or a clean makeup brush, apply the chilled mask evenly to your face, avoiding the eye area. Leave it on for 20 minutes, then rinse it off with lukewarm water.

Super Scrub

Your skin will sparkle with this berry-rich exfoliating scrub. Gently smash a handful of **BLUEBERRIES** in a medium-size bowl. Add 1 tablespoon of ground almonds (use a coffee grinder or mortar and pestle) and 1 tablespoon of plain whole-milk yogurt, and stir well to make a paste. Using your fingertips, slowly massage the scrub into your face in small circles, starting at your forehead and ending just under your chin. Use a warm, wet washcloth to remove the scrub, then rinse your face with cool water and gently pat your skin dry.

Fool Father Time

Turn back the clock with this **BLUEBERRY** anti-aging mask. In a small bowl, smash ¼ cup of blueberries until pulpy. Add 1 tablespoon of ground oats (grind uncooked rolled oats in a coffee grinder or food processor) and 1 teaspoon of lime juice. Mix well to form a paste. Using your fingertips, apply the mask to your face and leave it on until completely dry. Rinse it off with lukewarm water, and gently pat your skin dry.

Three-Berry Hand and Foot Therapy

The fruity acids in berries help to slough off dead skin and restore skin's youthful appearance. So put this therapeutic mix to work on your rough hands and calloused feet: In a blender, puree ¾ cup each of **BLUEBERRIES**, raspberries, and strawberries, along with ½ cup of kefir (drinkable yogurt). Apply generously to your hands and feet, massaging it into your skin for a minute or two. Leave the treatment on for 15 minutes, then rinse it off with warm water and pat your skin dry. Follow up with a rich body moisturizer.

Rah, Rah, Raspberries!

The antioxidants in **RASPBERRIES** do your body good, inside and out. So when you've had your fill of eating these ruby-red berries, it's time to use them to soothe and smooth your skin. Give this anti-aging mask a try: Mash up a handful of raspberries in a small bowl and stir in 1 teaspoon of honey, mixing well. Using your fingertips, apply the mask evenly to your clean face, avoiding the eye area. Leave it on for 15 minutes, then rinse it off with lukewarm water and gently pat your skin dry.

Oil-Removing Mask

If you have oily skin, this treatment will sop up the oil and tighten pores without overly drying your skin. In a blender, puree 1 cup of plain low-fat yogurt and ½ cup of **RASPBERRIES** until smooth. Using your fingertips or a clean makeup brush, apply the mixture to your freshly washed face and leave it on for 15 minutes. Use a warm, wet washcloth to remove it, then rinse your face with cool water and gently pat your skin dry.

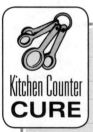

Kitchen Counter CURE

Seedy Scrub

Put the power of **RASPBERRIES** to work all over your body with this seedy, exfoliating bath scrub.

1 cup of raspberries, rinsed and dried

4 cups of granulated sugar

½ cup of extra virgin olive oil

½ teaspoon of grapefruit oil

½ teaspoon of lavender oil

Put a kitchen strainer over a bowl and put five or six berries into the strainer. Use the back of a large dessert spoon to smash the berries, leaving behind the seedy pulp. Continue until you have used all of the berries. Put the seedy pulp in a blender along with the sugar, olive oil, and essential oils, and blend well. Pour the scrub into a shatterproof container and bring it into the shower. Rub your skin all over with the scrub (if it's too sticky for you, wet your skin first), then rinse well.

Attack Acne

STRAWBERRIES are rich in salicylic acid, considered effective in treating acne. This mask helps clear up breakouts without overly drying your skin. Mash five strawberries in a small bowl and stir in 1 tablespoon of honey and the juice from one-quarter of a lemon. Mix well. Using your fingertips, apply the paste evenly to your face, avoiding the eye area. Wait 10 minutes, then rinse with warm water and gently pat your skin dry.

Strawberry Smoothie

Moisturize and rejuvenate your skin with this **STRAWBERRY** smoother. In a blender, puree ½ cup of strawberries and 1 tablespoon of full-fat sour cream. Using your fingertips, apply the mask to your face and relax for 20 minutes. Rinse with lukewarm water, and gently pat your skin dry.

Blotch Buster

Is your skin blotchy? Are your pores pronounced? This **STRAWBERRY** and banana combo will brighten your skin, leaving you with a healthy glow. In a blender, puree ¼ cup of strawberries, 1 ripe banana, ¼ cup of plain yogurt, and 1 tablespoon of honey. Using your fingertips or a clean makeup brush, spread the mixture evenly on your freshly washed face. Leave it on for 20 minutes, then wash it off using a warm, wet washcloth, rinse your face with cool water, and gently pat your skin dry.

HOW'S THAT?

Q **STRAWBERRIES** *can fade freckles? My cousin told me, but I have my doubts. I love to eat strawberries, so why waste them on my skin?*

A First of all, yes, I've heard of this trick, and a lot of folks say it really does work. Second, you only need half of a strawberry, so don't be so stingy! Just slice a large fresh berry in half, pop one half in your mouth, and rub the cut side of the other half over your freckles. Let it air-dry on your skin. Repeat every day or two until your speckles disappear, or at least become less noticeable.

Sweet Cheeky Treat

Soften and tone your cheeks (and the rest of your face) with this exfoliating **CHERRY** scrub. Puree six pitted cherries, 1 teaspoon of brown sugar, and 1 teaspoon of ground almonds (use a coffee grinder or mortar and pestle). Then add ¼ cup of honey and a few teaspoons of plain yogurt and mix well. Using your fingertips or a clean makeup brush, apply the toner to your freshly washed face, avoiding the eye area. Leave it on for about 10 minutes, then rinse it off with lukewarm water and gently pat your skin dry.

See Spots Run!

If your face has dark spots from sun exposure, hyperpigmentation, or acne, conquer them with **CHERRIES**. In a medium bowl, smash six pitted cherries until pulpy. Add 1 teaspoon of honey and 1 teaspoon of turmeric and mix well. Smooth the mixture evenly over your face, avoiding the eye area, and leave it on for 15 minutes. Rinse it off with lukewarm water, and gently pat your skin dry.

Age-Defying Face Mask

Get younger-looking skin with this fruity formula. In a small bowl, mash together six pitted **CHERRIES** and four strawberries. Wash your face, but don't dry it. Using your fingertips or a clean makeup brush, apply the mixture evenly to your face and neck. Leave the mask on for 10 minutes, then remove it with a warm, wet washcloth. Rinse your face with cool water, and gently pat your skin dry.

Speedy Sloughing Treatment

This exfoliating mask will deep-clean your pores and reveal fresh, healthy skin. Mix 1 tablespoon of instant oatmeal with 2 tablespoons of **CHERRY** juice (smash cherries through a kitchen strainer with the back of a spoon to release the juice) until you have a thick paste. Apply the paste to your face, avoiding the eye area, and massage it into your skin for one minute. Then leave it on for 10 minutes before removing it with a warm, wet washcloth. Rinse your face with cool water, and gently pat your skin dry.

Satisfy Thirsty Skin

Give a good, long drink to your dull, dry skin with this pulpy paste. Smash 10 pitted **CHERRIES** in a bowl, then put the pulp into a blender along with one peeled, sliced ripe peach and 1 teaspoon of extra virgin olive oil, and mix until well blended. Apply the paste to your face and neck. Leave it on for 10 minutes, then rinse it off with lukewarm water and pat your skin dry. Follow with your usual moisturizer.

Best Blotting Mask

Folks with oily skin can count on **CHERRIES** to come to their aid, too. Whisk one raw egg white until it forms peaks. Stir in 10 pitted, smashed cherries, 2 tablespoons of cornmeal, and 1 tablespoon of honey. Using your fingertips, apply the mask to your face, avoiding the eye area. Leave it on for 20 minutes, then remove it with a warm, wet washcloth. Rinse your face with cool water, and gently pat your skin dry.

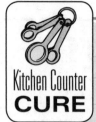

Kitchen Counter CURE

Cherry Color Corrector

Want to add shine and enhance the color of your brown or auburn hair? **CHERRIES** help balance pH levels, which are key for hair growth. Black tea boosts the color of drab, dull tresses.

- **2 cups of water**
- **8 black-tea bags**
- **1 cup of 100 percent cherry juice**

Start with clean, dry hair. Bring the water to a boil and steep the tea bags for 10 minutes. Remove the bags and let the tea cool, then stir in the cherry juice. Step into the shower, and pour the mixture over your head, working it into the roots with your fingers. Leave it in for 45 minutes, then rinse with clear, warm water—no shampoo.

Glow with Grapes

It's hard to believe that inside a tiny **GRAPE** there are some powerful antioxidants that fight skin aging and brighten the complexion. This super scrub will have you glowing. Put 10 red or purple grapes (the deeper the fruit color, the more antioxidants the fruit contains) in a blender or food processor. Add 1 tablespoon of cornmeal and 1 tablespoon of vitamin E oil, and blend until a paste forms. Using your fingertips, apply the paste to your face, avoiding the eye area, and massage it into your skin in small circles. Rinse it off with warm water, and gently pat your skin dry.

Minimize Pores

GRAPES can make your skin tighter and brighter and shrink enlarged pores. First, wash and dry your face, then put four grapes in a kitchen strainer over a bowl and smash them with the back of a spoon to release their juice. Add 1 teaspoon of honey to the juice and mix well. Apply the treatment to your face and leave it on for 20 minutes. Rinse it off with warm water, and gently pat your skin dry.

Turn Back the Clock

Well, not literally. But **GRAPES** can help keep aging skin soft and smooth, and that's half the battle. Mash three grapes with 3 tablespoons of aloe vera gel. Smooth the mix onto your face and leave it on for 20 minutes. Rinse it off with lukewarm water, and gently pat your skin dry.

Back in the Day...

My Grandma Putt knew a thing or two about taking care of skin. And when it came to dealing with acne, or any skin irritation, she reached into her refrigerator for some **GRAPES.** Just peel the skin from any color grape, and press the inner side of the peel onto the infected area. Relax for 20 minutes, keeping the affected area flat so the peels don't slide off. Then remove them and rinse with cool water. Gently pat your skin dry.

The Kiwi Cure

As we age, dark spots and discolorations seem to appear out of thin air. But you can bring back a more even skin tone with this **KIWI** treatment. Cut one kiwi in half and scoop out the fruity pulp. Mix it in a small bowl with 1 teaspoon of lemon juice and 1 teaspoon of uncooked rolled oats. Stir to make a paste. Apply the mixture to your face and leave it on for 10 minutes. Rinse it off with lukewarm water, and gently pat your skin dry.

Soothe and Smooth

Slow down the hands of time with this rich, creamy **KIWI** fix. In a small bowl, smash the pulp of one peeled kiwi with half of a ripe avocado. Stir in 1 teaspoon of honey, and mix well until smooth. Using your fingertips or a clean makeup brush, apply the paste to your face and neck. Wait 15 minutes, then rinse it off with lukewarm water and gently pat dry.

Quick Oil Absorber

Do you have oily, breakout-prone skin? Then let the fruity acids and enzymes in **KIWI** give your complexion a healthy do-over. Before you go to bed, cut a kiwi in half and rub the cut half over your face. Let it air-dry, then toddle off to bed. In the morning, rinse your face with cool water and pat your skin dry.

HOW'S THAT?

Q *From time to time, my local grocery store has a sale on bags of KIWIS. I love the fruit, but there's only so much a person can eat before it starts to go bad. How else can I enjoy this wonderful fruit?*

A You're in luck, as you can see by the kiwi tips on this page. And here's one more to help you make the most of all that fruit and get your skin glowing: Peel and smash one kiwi in a small bowl. Add 1 tablespoon of yogurt and mix well. Apply the mixture evenly to your face and leave it on for 15 minutes. Then rinse it off with lukewarm water, and gently pat your skin dry.

When Life Gives You Lemons ...

Make a skin toner! In a small bowl, mix 2 tablespoons of **LEMON** juice with 2 tablespoons of honey. Using your fingertips or a clean makeup brush, apply the mixture to your face and neck. Leave it on for 10 minutes, then remove with a warm, wet washcloth. Rinse your face and neck with cool water, and pat your skin dry.

Blemish-Fighting Face Mask

Banish breakouts with this **LEMON** mask: In a small bowl, mix 3 tablespoons of lemon juice, 3 tablespoons of honey, and 2 tablespoons of ground cinnamon. Using your fingertips or a clean makeup brush, apply the mask evenly to your face. Leave it on until it dries completely, then rinse it off with lukewarm water and gently pat your skin dry.

BEAUTY
Bonus

SKIN SOOO SOFT

Soften and tone your skin in one smooth move. Beat a large egg white until it forms peaks, and then fold in the juice of half a **LEMON**. Using your fingertips or a clean make-up brush, apply it to your face and neck. Leave it on for 20 minutes, and rinse with cool water. Gently pat dry, then use a cotton pad to spread witch hazel over your skin and let it air-dry.

Lemony Blackhead Lifter

Combat blackheads with the power of **LEMON**. At bedtime, rub some lemon juice onto your skin. Let it air-dry, then hit the sack. In the morning, rinse your face with cool water, and gently pat your skin dry.

Super-Sour Body Scrub

Use this brisk, tangy scrub in your morning shower to wake up your senses and get your day off to a sunny start. In a shatterproof bowl, mix 1/2 cup of **LEMON** juice with 1/4 cup of sugar. Step into the shower, and use the rub all over your body, massaging until the sugar granules dissolve. Rinse off with warm water, and pat dry.

Everyday Face Wash

Lighten up uneven skin tone with this gentle daily cleanser. First thing every morning, mix 2 tablespoons of whole milk with 1 tablespoon of **LEMON** juice, and use your fingertips or a clean makeup brush to apply it to your face. Leave it on for one to two minutes, then rinse it off with lukewarm water and gently pat your skin dry.

Fountain of Youth Night Lotion

For soft, supple, younger-looking skin, nothing beats this overnight treatment. In a small bowl, mix 2 tablespoons of **LEMON** juice with 2 tablespoons of glycerin (available online) and 1 tablespoon of rose water (available in health-food stores and online). Using your fingertips, apply the lotion to your skin, massaging in small circles across your forehead, down your nose, across your cheeks, over your chin, and down your neck. Use it every night before bedtime and wake up to a more youthful you.

Nice Nails Made Easy

If your fingernails or toenails are dingy or discolored after years of using nail polish, give them a new lease on life with **LEMON**. Make them stronger and whiter by soaking them in lemon juice for 10 minutes, once a week. (Just make sure your fingers and toes are free of cuts or scrapes, or you'll get a stinging surprise!) Then brush them with a half-and-half solution of white vinegar and warm water, rinse well with warm water, and pat your skin dry, being sure to completely dry the area between your toes.

Back in the Day...

Treat your cracked, dry feet to Grandma Putt's favorite moisturizing routine. Just combine 1 tablespoon of **LEMON** juice with one ripe, smashed banana, 2 tablespoons of honey, and 2 tablespoons of soft margarine. Stir the ingredients until creamy, then massage the mixture onto your clean, dry feet. Pull on a pair of cotton socks, and hit the sack. Come morning, your feet will feel as soft as a baby's.

Terrific Tootsie Treat

Pep up tired, funky feet with this invigorating scrub. In a small bowl, mix 1 cup of sea salt, the zest from one **LEMON**, ½ cup of sweet almond oil (available online), and 8 drops of peppermint oil. Pour the concoction into a jar with a tight-fitting lid and store it in the refrigerator, where it will keep for two weeks. To use, spoon out a handful and massage your wet feet with the scrub. Rinse it off with warm water and thoroughly dry between your toes.

Oil-Busting Toner

Clear up oily, breakout-prone skin with this terrific toner. Start by brewing one strong cup of mint tea. Measure out ¼ cup and set it aside in a small bowl. When the tea in the bowl has cooled to room temperature, add ¼ cup of **LEMON** juice and ¼ cup of rose water (available in health-food stores and online) and stir well. Pour the mixture into a bottle with a tight-fitting cap and put it in the refrigerator. Every evening, after you've washed your face, apply the chilled toner with a cotton ball (shake the bottle first).

Ditch the Dandruff

All it takes is a little **LEMON** juice to put an end to dandruff. Apply 1 tablespoon of it to your dry hair, massaging it well into your scalp, then shampoo as usual, and rinse with clear water. Rinse again, this time using a mixture of 2 tablespoons of lemon juice and 2 cups of water. Repeat every other day until the white flakes flee for good.

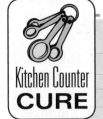

Kitchen Counter CURE

Lemony Fresh Hair Gel

Tame wild tresses and control frizz with this super-simple citrus hair gel.

- **1 cup of water**
- **1 packet of Knox® unflavored gelatin**
- **2 tablespoons of LEMON juice**

Warm the water and gelatin over low heat in a saucepan until the gelatin is completely dissolved. Remove from the heat and stir in the lemon juice. Let the mixture cool until set, then spoon it into a jar with a tight-fitting lid and store it in the refrigerator for up to two weeks. Use as you would any commercial hair gel.

Lighten Up with Limes

If dark spots and uneven skin tone are dragging you down, lighten up with **LIME**. Cut a lime into quarters and use one quarter at a time to squeeze out the juice onto a cotton ball. Apply the juice directly to your skin and leave it on for 30 minutes. Rinse it off with cool water, and gently pat dry.

Another Bright Idea...

Make your skin lighter and brighter with this quick trick: Cut a **LIME** into quarters and peel each section. Rub the inside of the peel over any dark spots and discolorations on your face and/or the back of your hands. Let your skin air-dry, then apply sunscreen before you head out the door.

Rx for Blemishes

Harness the power of the citric acid in **LIMES** and the antibacterial properties of honey to wage war against acne. In a small bowl, mix 3 tablespoons of lime juice with 2 tablespoons of honey. Using your fingertips and working in small circles, massage the paste onto your blemished skin. Leave it on for two minutes, then use a warm, wet washcloth to remove it. Rinse your face with cool water, and gently pat dry. Perform this routine three times a week until your skin is clear.

HOW'S THAT?

Q *Jerry, every year my cousin sends me a carton of LIMES grown in his Florida backyard. Apart from using them in homemade face treatments (not to mention margaritas), how else can I put them to good use?*

A Oh, how I wish I had your problem! Limes are handy for all kinds of health and beauty uses (see page 85 for limey health tips). Here's a lime infusion that will refresh tired eyes: Mix 1 tablespoon of lime juice into 5 tablespoons of ice water. Soak two cotton balls in the cold lime water and squeeze out the excess liquid. Close your eyes and place the wet cotton balls on your eyelids for about 10 minutes. Remove the cotton and gently pat your skin dry.

Supple Skin Supplier

Make your dry skin smooth and supple again with this **LIME** facial. Break one egg yolk into a small bowl, and add 1 tablespoon of lime juice and 1 teaspoon of extra virgin olive oil. Whisk until blended. Using your fingertips or a clean makeup brush, apply the mask evenly to your face and neck. Allow it to dry completely, then rinse it off with lukewarm water and gently pat your skin dry.

Body Beautifier

This **LIME** and milk overnight body moisturizer can't be beat. Just before you go to bed, bring 1 cup of milk to a boil, remove it from the heat, and stir in 1 teaspoon of glycerin (available online) and the fresh-squeezed juice of one lime. Let the mixture cool to room temperature, then massage it into your face, hands, and feet and hop under the covers. Store any extra moisturizer, tightly covered, in the refrigerator, and use it within a week.

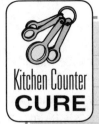

Kitchen Counter CURE

Blonde Booster

If you want to make your blonde hair lighter, don't rush off to the beauty salon. Raid the fridge and mix up this citrusy concoction, instead.

Juice of 2 LIMES
Juice of 1 lemon
2 tbsp. of mild shampoo

Wait for a clear, sunny day. Mix the juices and the shampoo in a container, wrap a towel around your shoulders, and carefully pour the solution onto your hair and massage it in. Then head outside and sit in the sun for 15 to 20 minutes. Come back inside and rinse your hair thoroughly before applying a conditioner. Keep repeating daily until your blah blonde color becomes brilliant.

Dandruff Defeater

Say "so long!" to your itchy scalp with this no-more-flakes fix: Cut a **LIME** in half, and rub the cut side all along your scalp, squeezing out the lime juice and working it into your skin. Let it sit for two minutes, then wash your hair with a mild shampoo and condition as usual. Use this treatment every time you wash your hair, and your flakes will soon be history, leaving you with a healthy scalp.

Blackhead Buster

MANGOES can help remove black-heads. Use this paste every night and you'll soon be on your way to clearer skin. Cut a ripe mango in slices around the center pit and discard the pit. Peel one slice and mash enough to fill 1 teaspoon. Put the mashed fruit in a small bowl, and wrap the remaining fruit slices in plastic wrap and put them in the fridge for use later. Then add 1/2 teaspoon of milk and 1/2 teaspoon of honey to the mashed mango and stir until well mixed. Apply the paste to your face, rubbing in small circles from forehead to chin. Leave it on for two minutes, then remove with a warm, wet washcloth. Rinse your face with cool water, and gently pat your skin dry.

BEAUTY
Bonus

A SERIOUSLY SIMPLE SCRUB

Don't toss those **MANGO** skins out! After you've used the fruit, use the skins as a rejuvenating body scrub. Just step into the shower and get wet. Rub the cut sides of fresh skins all over your body, starting at your neck and moving downward. Leave it on for 10 minutes so your skin absorbs the fruit enzymes, then rinse off with warm water and pat dry.

Marvelous Mango Mask

Get your complexion glowing with this **MANGO** facial, and you'll be setting the stage for the makings of an excellent body scrub (see below). Cut one ripe mango in slices around the center pit and discard the pit. Mash enough fruit to fill 2 tablespoons. Set aside the skins and remaining slices. Put the mashed fruit on a plate. Using a fork, work in 1 teaspoon of honey and mash until smooth. Apply the mask to your face, working in small circles from forehead to chin. Leave it on while you prepare the Moisturizing Mango Body Scrub (below).

Moisturizing Mango Body Scrub

Use this super-smoothing body scrub in your next bath or shower, and your skin will feel like silk. Put the remaining peeled **MANGO** slices from "Marvelous Mango Mask" (above) into a blender with 1/2 cup of sugar, 2 tablespoons of whole milk, and 1 tablespoon of honey. Blend thoroughly, bring the mixture into the shower, and rub the scrub all over your body. Rinse with warm water, then cool water.

Time-Saving Facial Mask

This easy mask takes advantage of the active fruit enzymes in **MANGO** to exfoliate and refresh your skin. Peel and slice a ripe mango, and put the peeled slices in a blender. Add enough plain yogurt to cover, and blend well, adding more yogurt if needed, to make a smooth paste. Apply the paste evenly to your face and neck. Leave it on for 15 minutes, then rinse it off with lukewarm water and gently pat your skin dry.

Dark-Spot Eraser

MANGO skins can reduce the look of dark spots and blotches on your face and hands. Place several fresh mango skins on a cookie sheet and put them out in the sun until they are thoroughly dried. Or, place the sheet in the oven at its lowest setting and cook until the skins are completely dried, checking frequently so they don't burn. Then grind the dried skins in a coffee grinder. Store the grounds in a tightly sealed container. To use, mix 1 tablespoon of ground mango with 1 tablespoon of plain yogurt. Stir well, and apply to any dark spots and blemishes. Leave the treatment on for 30 minutes, then wipe it off with a tissue.

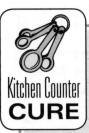

Kitchen Counter CURE

Mango Mud Mask

This nourishing facial mask is good for all skin types. The honey and cream act as moisturizers, and also help to slough off dull, dead skin, leaving you looking luminous.

- **¹/₄ of a MANGO, peeled and chopped**
- **¹/₄ cup of heavy cream (Use milk if you have oily skin.)**
- **1 tbsp. of honey**
- **1 tbsp. of finely ground oats (Grind uncooked rolled oats in a coffee grinder or food processor.)**

Put the mango into a food processor and puree until you have a paste. Add the cream or milk and the honey, and puree, adding more dairy if needed to keep it smooth. Add the finely ground oats and blend until combined (it's okay if it's a bit lumpy). Apply the mask evenly to your clean face and neck, and leave it on for 15 minutes. Wash it off with a warm, wet washcloth, rinse your skin with cool water, and dry.

Very A-Peeling Orange Scrub

To keep your skin looking its best, you need to exfoliate regularly to slough off dull, dead skin cells. And nothing could be better than to use **ORANGE** peels as the primary ingredient in any scrub, whether for your face or your body. They're easy to prepare: Every time you peel an orange, place the peels on a cookie sheet and put it out in the sun until the peels are dry. Or, put the sheet in the oven at its lowest temperature and check every half hour until the peels are dry and curling. Grind the dry peels in a food processor or coffee grinder, until you have either a coarse powder (for body scrubs) or a fine powder (for facial scrubs). Store in a tightly sealed container.

Restore Radiance

Get your face glowing with this **ORANGE** and cream mask. Stir 1 tablespoon of orange peel powder (see "Very A-Peeling Orange Scrub," above) into 2 tablespoons of heavy cream. Using a clean makeup brush, apply the mask to your face, avoiding the eye area. Leave it on for 10 minutes, then tissue off. Rinse your face with lukewarm water, and gently pat your skin dry.

Calm Distressed Skin

If your face is prone to breakouts, give your skin a break with an **ORANGE** peel mask. Mix 2 tablespoons of orange peel powder (see "Very A-Peeling Orange Scrub," above) with 3 tablespoons of plain low-fat yogurt. Apply the mask to your face, massaging it into your skin in small circles. Leave it on for 15 minutes, then rinse it off with lukewarm water and gently pat your skin dry.

BEAUTY
Bonus

QUICK AND EASY BODY SCRUB

You can still take advantage of a skin-saving **ORANGE** scrub even when you haven't had the time to dry a bunch of orange peels. Just grab an orange, peel it, and wrap the fresh rind in a large piece of gauze or cheesecloth. Then hop into the shower, and rub the scrubber all over your body. The acid and vitamin C in the orange peel will firm and tone your skin just as well as any other orange-based scrub!

Excellent Exfoliant

Bring back that youthful glow with this exfoliating face mask. In a small bowl, mix 2 teaspoons of **ORANGE** peel powder (see "Very A-Peeling Orange Scrub," at left) with 2 teaspoons of plain whole-milk yogurt and 1 teaspoon of honey. Apply the mask to your just-cleaned face. Leave it on for 25 minutes, then rinse it off with lukewarm water. Rinse your face with cool water, and gently pat your skin dry.

Outstanding Orange Toner

Firm up your face and shrink oversized pores with an **ORANGE** peel toner. Start with fresh peels from two oranges. Put them into a heat-proof bowl and pour 1 cup of boiling water over them. Cover the bowl with another bowl or a pot lid, and let the mixture steep overnight at room temperature. The next day, pour off the liquid into a bottle and store it in the refrigerator. To use, pour some toner on a cotton ball and sweep it across your face. Allow it to air-dry. Make a fresh batch every two weeks.

OJ Is OK

Here's a cool tip that will brighten up dull, lackluster skin and control oiliness: Extract the juice from two **ORANGES** and pour it into an ice cube tray. Freeze the juice overnight, and the next day, pop out a cube and gently rub it all over your face. Leave the juice on for 10 minutes, then rinse it off with cool water and gently pat your skin dry.

Back in the Day...

Get your glow on with this old-fashioned citrusy body scrub that ladies have been using for decades to keep their skin luminous. Extract the juice from one **ORANGE** into a small shatterproof bowl. Stir in 1/2 cup of brown sugar and 1 tablespoon of extra virgin olive oil or vitamin E oil. Mix well. Then step into the shower and slather your body with the scrub, focusing on rough elbows, knees, and heels. Massage it in well, then rinse off and pat your skin dry.

Good-Enough-to-Eat Face Cream

This **ORANGE** blend softens and helps detoxify your skin. Plus, it's so safe, you can eat the leftovers! Take two sections from a peeled navel orange and chop them up. Put the pieces in a food processor or blender and add 2 ounces of softened full-fat cream cheese, 1 teaspoon of honey, and ½ teaspoon of lemon juice. Blend until the mixture has a soft, spreadable texture, and use a spatula to scrape it into a bowl. Using your fingertips, apply a thin layer of the spread to your face and neck, and leave it on for 15 minutes or so, or until it's dried. Remove it with a warm, wet washcloth, then rinse your face and neck with cool water to close your pores, and gently pat your skin dry. If there's any mixture left in the bowl, spread it on a cracker, toast, or bagel, and enjoy!

BEAUTY
Bonus

RADIANCE RESTORER

Bring back the brilliance to dull, drab hair with this **ORANGE** conditioner. Extract the juice from one orange and mix it in a shatterproof bowl with ½ cup of water and 1 teaspoon of honey. Step into the shower and shampoo your hair. Pour the orange water over your head, and massage it into your hair from roots to tips. Leave it on for 10 minutes before rinsing it out with warm water. Dry and style your hair as usual, and admire your soft, shiny tresses.

Detox Your Locks

The gunky buildup of hair products can leave your tresses in distress. Clear it all out and get your hair back to good health with this potent **ORANGE** and lemon aid: Extract the juice from one orange and one lemon, putting it through a sieve to catch the pulp. Pour the juices into a small bowl. Add 1 tablespoon of extra virgin olive oil and 1 tablespoon of honey and mix well. Wrap a towel around your shoulders to catch any drips, and massage the mixture into your dry hair from roots to tips. Leave it on your hair for one hour, then shampoo and condition as usual. Use this surge-of-citrus cleansing treatment once a month to keep your mane looking its best.

Simply Seedy Face Mask

After you eat a **PAPAYA**, don't toss the seeds—use them in this enzyme-rich facial mask. You'll need 3 tablespoons of papaya seeds, 1 tablespoon of ripe papaya fruit, 1 tablespoon of honey, and 1 teaspoon of coconut or almond oil. Put all of the ingredients into a blender or food processor and blend until they reach the consistency of rough sand. Apply the mask evenly to your face (avoiding the eye area), neck, and upper chest. Leave it on for 10 minutes, then rinse it off with warm water and gently pat dry. *Note: Papaya is rich in enzymes and alpha hydroxy acids, which create a slight burning sensation. If it starts to irritate, remove the mask immediately.*

Pleasing Papaya Facial

Perk up your complexion and rejuvenate your skin with this **PAPAYA** treatment. In a small bowl, mash enough ripe papaya to make 2 tablespoons. Stir in 1 teaspoon of honey and mix well. Apply the mask to your clean face, avoiding the eye area. Leave it on for 15 minutes (or less if it starts to irritate your skin), then rinse it off with lukewarm water and gently pat your skin dry.

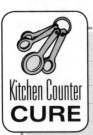

Kitchen Counter CURE

Easy Exfoliating Mask

Improve your skin tone with the power of papain. This enzyme in **PAPAYA** removes dead skin cells and tightens pores, leaving your skin smooth and clear. Papain levels are particularly high in unripe papaya, so if you have sensitive skin, only use very ripe papaya in this and other facial recipes.

¼ cup of peeled, seeded, diced papaya
¼ cup of 100 percent pure pumpkin (*not* pumpkin pie mix)
½ tsp. of honey
½ tsp. of plain yogurt
1 egg white (for oily skin) or 1 egg yolk (for dry skin)

Put all of the ingredients into a blender or food processor and puree until smooth. If the mixture is too runny, add more diced papaya. Apply the mask to your clean face, avoiding the eye area. Leave it on for 15 minutes (or less if it starts to irritate your skin), then rinse your face with lukewarm water, followed by cool water. Gently pat your skin dry.

Skin-ny Papaya Scrub

This easy body scrub leaves skin so soft, you won't need to use body lotion afterward. The next time you peel a **PAPAYA**, take the fresh skins right into the shower. Get your face and body wet, and rub the cut sides of the peels all over. Wait for 10 minutes, then shower off with warm water.

Rise and Shine Scrub

Start your day with this invigorating body scrub. In a small bowl, mash enough ripe **PAPAYA** to make 3 tablespoons. Stir in the juice of one lemon, 2 tablespoons of brown sugar, and 2 drops of your favorite scented essential oil. Then step into the shower and get your face and body wet. Rub the scrub all over, and leave it on for 10 minutes (or less if it starts to irritate your skin) before showering it off with warm water.

Love-Your-Skin Remedy

Do you battle dry, flaky, rough skin? Well, it's time to bring in the big gun …**PAPAYA**. Smash a peeled, seeded papaya in a medium-size bowl, and apply a thin layer to your face, neck, and anywhere else you have dry skin. Wait 10 minutes (or less if it starts to irritate your skin), then rinse it off with lukewarm water, followed by cool water. Gently pat your skin dry.

Back in the Day…

Now, I know what you're thinking: There's no way Grandma Putt would have known what to do with a **PAPAYA**. And you're right; tropical fruits were nowhere to be found in grocery stores of yore. But times do change, and I'm sure she'd approve of all the wonderful uses we've found for these delightful fruits, like this facial mask that lightens dark spots. Put 1 cup of ripe, chopped papaya into a blender or food processor. Add 1 teaspoon of honey, 1 teaspoon of plain yogurt, and 1 teaspoon of vitamin E oil. Blend to make a smooth paste. Massage the paste onto your damp skin, from forehead to chin, in small circles. Leave it on for 10 minutes (or less if it starts to irritate your skin). Then rinse your face with lukewarm water, followed by cool water, and dry.

Just Peachy Skin Firmer

Firm and tighten saggy skin with **PEACH** peels. Just before you hit the sack, massage your face gently with the inside of a fresh peach peel for a few minutes, then go to bed. You'll wake up to firmer, fresher skin in the morning, thanks to the astringent action of the peach juice.

Vein-Eraser Treatment

This gentle **PEACH** face mask is particularly good for minimizing the appearance of small broken capillaries and spider veins. Cut one very ripe peach in half, and remove the stone and skin. In a small bowl, smash the peeled fruit with the back of a spoon, then stir in 2 tablespoons of plain whole-milk yogurt. Using your fingers or a clean makeup brush, apply the mask to your clean face. Lie down and rest for 20 minutes, then rinse your face with lukewarm water and gently pat your skin dry.

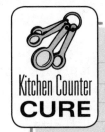

Kitchen Counter CURE

Hand Healer

This intensive treatment works magic on over-worked and aging hands. Apply it just before bedtime and in the morning you'll have softer, healthier-looking hands.

2 tablespoons of almond oil
2 teaspoons of fresh PEACH juice, with pulp removed
1/2 teaspoon of honey

In a small bowl, mix all of the ingredients thoroughly. Then dip your fingers into the moisturizer and rub it all over your hands. Pull on a pair of white cotton gloves and slip into bed. In the morning, remove the gloves, rinse your hands with lukewarm water, and gently pat your skin dry.

Peachy Pore Reducer

Do you have oily skin and enlarged pores? Then give this treatment a try. With regular use, it will shrink your pores and leave your skin smooth but not oily. Peel and remove the stone from one ripe **PEACH** and put the fruit in a blender. Add one raw egg white and blend until smooth. Using your fingertips or a clean makeup brush, apply the mixture to your clean face, avoiding the eye area, and leave it on for 30 minutes. Remove it with a warm, wet washcloth, and gently pat your skin dry.

A Peach of a Toner

This formula is perfect for dry, flaky skin. Peel two **PEACHES**, remove the stones, and use a spoon to smash the fruit in a medium-size bowl. Add 1 teaspoon of heavy cream and enough extra virgin olive oil to make a smooth paste. Apply the mixture to your face and wait 10 minutes. Rinse it off with lukewarm water, and gently pat your face dry.

Triple-Treat Face Mask

Can one facial treatment nourish, hydrate, and smooth your skin? Yes! Peel one ripe **PEACH** and remove the stone. In a small bowl, smash the fruit with a spoon until it's pulpy. Stir in 1 tablespoon of honey and add enough uncooked rolled oats to make a thick paste. Apply it evenly to your face and leave it on for 15 minutes. Remove it with a warm, wet washcloth, rinse your face with cool water, and gently pat your skin dry.

Complexion Correction

Everyone wants silky, smooth, more youthful skin. Here's how to get it: Peel and remove the stone from one very ripe **PEACH**. Put the fruit in a small bowl, and use a spoon to smash it. Add one raw egg white, and combine it with the fruit until a creamy mixture forms. Apply the mask to your face and neck and relax for a half hour. Rinse the mask off with lukewarm water, and pat your skin dry.

Back in the Day...

Grandma Putt picked her prized **PEACHES** to bake delicious pies. But there were always a couple extra peaches that sat around and got real soft. But even then, they were put to good use as the main ingredient for this facial cleanser: Peel one peach and remove the stone. Cube the fruit and put it into a small saucepan. Mince fresh leaves from one sprig of peppermint and add them to the pot, along with the juice from one lemon. Heat the mixture on low heat, stirring occasionally, until it is very mushy. Remove from the heat and use the back of a spoon to smash it into a smooth paste. Let it cool until it's warm, then use your fingertips to massage the cleanser into your skin in small circles. Rinse it off with warm water, and pat your face dry. Spoon any remaining mixture into a jar with a tight-fitting lid and store it in the refrigerator for up to three days.

Pore-Perfecting Pear Scrub

The natural enzymes in **PEARS** help eliminate complexion-dulling dead skin cells. Peel one very ripe pear, and place it in a small bowl. Smash the fruit with enough uncooked rolled oats and water to make a paste. Massage the paste into your skin, from forehead to chin. Remove it with a warm, wet washcloth, and rinse your face with cool water.

Refreshing Face Mask

Renew your complexion with this soothing **PEAR** treatment. In a small bowl, mix slices of one very ripe pear with 2 tablespoons of heavy cream and 1 tablespoon of honey. Apply the mixture to your face. Leave it on for 15 minutes, then rinse it off with lukewarm water.

Pears for Hair

If every day is a bad-hair day for you, this **PEAR** treatment will leave you with bouncy, shiny locks. In a small bowl, smash a peeled, very ripe pear and mix it with 2 tablespoons each of apple cider vinegar and water. Place a towel around your shoulders to catch any drips, and pour the mixture over your dry head. Work it into your hair from roots to tips, then wait 15 minutes before rinsing it out with warm water. Follow up with your usual conditioner.

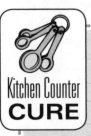

Kitchen Counter CURE

Fruity Face Saver

Here's a fresh fruit formula that will soften your face, invigorate your senses—and smell like a yummy fruit salad.

6 strawberries
1/2 of an apple, peeled and with seeds removed
1/2 of a PEAR, peeled and with seeds removed
4 tbsp. of orange juice
Honey

Puree the fruits with the orange juice in a blender or food processor. Apply a thin layer of honey to your face, then smooth on the fruit mixture. Relax for 40 minutes, then rinse with lukewarm water.

BEAUTY
Bonus

PIÑA COLADA FACIAL

Here's a cocktail you can not only drink, but also apply to your face for fabulous results. Put four fresh, peeled **PINEAPPLE** slices into a blender or food processor along with 2 tablespoons of coconut milk. Puree until smooth. Using your fingertips or a clean makeup brush, apply the mask to your clean face and neck, avoiding the eye area. Leave it on for five minutes, then remove it with a warm, wet washcloth. Rinse your face with cool water, and gently pat your skin dry.

Tropical Treat

Nothing beats alpha hydroxy acids for refining skin tone, erasing fine lines, and giving you a more youthful appearance. That's why they're the main ingredient in many expensive beauty creams and lotions. But you can save your pennies and concoct your own facial treatment that rivals the pricey ones by using fresh **PINEAPPLE**. It's the enzyme bromelain in the fruit that does the trick. In a blender, puree 1 cup of fresh pineapple chunks and half of a fresh papaya (peeled and seeded). Pour the mixture into a bowl and stir in 2 tablespoons of honey. Using your fingertips or a clean makeup brush, apply it to your clean face and neck, avoiding the eye area. Leave it on for five minutes, then rinse it off with lukewarm water, followed by cool water. Gently pat your skin dry. *Note: The enzymes in pineapple can irritate sensitive skin. If you feel any discomfort, remove the mask ASAP.*

Perfect Your Pores

The enzymes found in **PINEAPPLE** act as rejuvenating agents to exfoliate and unclog pores. Put them to work for your distressed skin with this pore-shrinking facial treatment. Slice a fresh pineapple into rings. Remove the outer skin and place four rings in a blender (cut them to fit, if needed). Add 3 tablespoons of extra virgin olive oil and 1 tablespoon of honey, and puree until smooth. Using your fingertips or a clean makeup brush, apply the mixture to your clean face, avoiding the eye area. Lie down and relax for 10 to 15 minutes, then rinse your face with lukewarm water and gently pat your skin dry.

Simple Skin Support

Hydration is the key to healthy-looking skin. While you should certainly drink plenty of water throughout the day to keep skin plump and fresh, what you put on the outside is important, too. So give this simple treatment a try. Pour 3 tablespoons of fresh **PINEAPPLE** juice in a small bowl and add one raw egg yolk and a splash of whole milk. Mix well. Using your fingertips or a clean makeup brush, apply the mixture to your face, avoiding the eye area. Leave it on for five minutes, then rinse it off with lukewarm water and gently pat your skin dry.

Basic Body Scrub

The same enzymes that make **PINEAPPLE** work wonders on your face are also beneficial to the rest of your skin. And this is about as basic a technique as you can get: Cut a fresh pineapple into four large wedges and remove the rough peel. Bring them into the shower with you. Wet your skin, then rub the wedges all over your body, including your face (avoid the eye area). Leave the juice on for two or three minutes, then rinse it off thoroughly with warm water, and pat your skin dry.

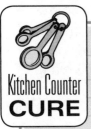

Kitchen Counter CURE

Pampering Pineapple Scrub

When your skin could use some serious TLC, whip up a batch of **PINEAPPLE** scrub and show the world a revived, fresh face.

1 cup of fresh pineapple chunks
1 tbsp. of fresh pineapple juice
1 tbsp. of honey
1 tbsp. of uncooked rolled oats

In a medium bowl, crush the pineapple chunks until they're pulpy. Add the remaining ingredients and mix well. Wet your face with warm water to open up the pores, then massage the scrub into your skin in small circles, from forehead to chin. Be sure to keep the scrub away from your eyes. Leave it on for five minutes, then use a warm, wet washcloth to gently wipe it away. Rinse your face with cool water, and pat your skin dry.

Fruit Salad for Neat Feet

Treat your tootsies to this mixed-fruit scrub that will leave your feet soft and smooth. Before you begin, grab a towel and a roll of plastic wrap (or two plastic grocery bags) and set them aside. Then slice, peel, and finely chop a fresh **PINEAPPLE** to make ½ cup, and put it in a medium bowl. Finely chop half of a peeled lemon, half of an unpeeled apple, and one-quarter of a peeled grapefruit and add to the bowl. Stir in 2 teaspoons of anise extract and 1 teaspoon of kosher or sea salt. Mix well. Sit down in a chair and put a towel under your feet. Scoop up the scrub and rub it all over your feet, paying attention to rough heels. Wrap your feet in plastic wrap or tie a plastic grocery bag over each foot. Sit back and relax for 30 minutes while the fruit enzymes go to work. Remove the wrapping or bags, rinse your feet with lukewarm water, and pat dry, making sure the spaces between your toes are completely dry.

Cuticle Cure

Besides being an eyesore, dry cuticles can crack and become infected. Make them soft and supple again with **PINEAPPLE**. In a small bowl, blend 2 tablespoons of fresh pineapple juice with 1 raw egg yolk, and mix well. Using a fingertip, apply the mixture to your cuticles, gently massaging all around the nail bed. Leave it on for five minutes, then use a cotton swab to gently push back your softened cuticles. Rinse your fingers with lukewarm water and slather on your favorite hand cream.

Back in the Day...

John Dole started his first **PINEAPPLE** plantation in Hawaii in 1900. Since then, Americans have been enjoying the fruit in salads, ice creams, and desserts. Grandma Putt loved pineapple, and once she discovered this facial mask recipe that tightens and tones, she shared it with all of her friends. In a blender, puree two large, fresh pineapple chunks with one raw egg white and 1 teaspoon of honey. Apply the mask to your face, avoiding the eye area. Leave it on for five minutes, then wash it off with lukewarm water. Rinse your face with cool water, and gently pat your skin dry.

A Cool Retreat

Summer heat can take a toll on your skin. So give your face a mini-vacation with this cool **WATERMELON** facial. Just peel and remove the seeds from a slice of watermelon, and mash it in a glass or ceramic bowl until it's about the consistency of thin applesauce. Put it in the fridge to get it nice and cool. Wash your face so it's squeaky clean. Spread the melon over your face, lie down, and put a piece of gauze or cheesecloth over the fruit (otherwise, it may slide off). Relax for 30 minutes, then rinse it off with lukewarm water and gently pat your skin dry.

Watermelon Wake-Up

This **WATERMELON** toner tightens up pores with its astringent action. Combine ¼ cup of watermelon juice with 2 tablespoons of honey. Apply it to your face with a cotton ball, concentrating on your trouble spots. Leave it on for two minutes, then rinse with lukewarm water and gently pat your skin dry.

Best Burn Soother

Treat your sizzling summer skin to this chilly remedy. In a medium-size bowl, mix equal portions of smashed **WATERMELON** and cucumber pulp (puree peeled cucumber slices in a blender to get the pulp). Using your fingertips, gently apply the pack to your face or other sunburned skin. Cover with a piece of gauze or cheesecloth to keep it in place. Leave the pack on for 20 minutes, then rinse it off with cool water and let your skin air-dry.

BEAUTY
Bonus

A BIG WIN FOR SKIN

This winning combo leaves your skin soft and glowing: In a small bowl, mix 3 tablespoons of smashed **WATERMELON** with 3 tablespoons of plain yogurt. Using your fingertips or a clean makeup brush, apply the mask to your face and neck, and leave it on for 10 minutes. Rinse it off with lukewarm water, and gently pat your skin dry. The lactic acid and enzymes in the yogurt will help to gently exfoliate and purify, while the watermelon hydrates and heals. Now that's a one-two punch worth taking!

Wonderful Watermelon Skin Savers

When it comes to rescuing troubled skin, **WATERMELON** is the winner. Whether you're fighting the ravages of time, trying to hydrate dry skin, or struggling with uneven skin tone, this trio of facials will get the job done:

- **For aging skin.** Mix 3 tablespoons of smashed watermelon with 3 tablespoons of mashed ripe avocado. Apply the combination evenly to your face and neck. Leave it on for 20 minutes before rinsing with lukewarm water. Gently pat your skin dry.

- **For dry skin.** Combine 3 tablespoons of smashed watermelon with 3 tablespoons of honey. Using your fingertips, apply the mixture evenly to your face and neck. Leave it on for 15 to 20 minutes, then rinse it off with lukewarm water and gently pat your skin dry.

- **For blotchy, uneven skin.** Mix 3 tablespoons of smashed watermelon with 1 tablespoon of freshly crushed mint leaves. Pour into an ice cube tray and freeze. Rub an ice cube on your face to tighten up pores and soothe troubled skin. Leave the residue on for 10 minutes, then rinse it off with cool water and gently pat your skin dry.

HOW'S THAT?

Q *My feet are a mess. Now that summer's here, I'm too embarrassed to have them be seen. Do you have any easy ways I can get them in good enough shape that I can wear sandals and not be ashamed?*

A Give this **WATERMELON** foot treatment a try—it just may get you back into flip-flops fast. Press ½ cup of cut-up watermelon through a strainer set over a bowl to extract the juice, and set it aside. Use a coffee grinder or mortar and pestle to roughly crush enough almonds to fill 2 tablespoons. Mix the crushed almonds with the watermelon juice, then stir in ¼ cup of plain whole-milk yogurt. Massage the rub into your feet, really working it into your rough skin. Leave it on for 10 minutes, then tissue it off. Rinse with lukewarm water and thoroughly dry your feet, especially between your toes. Repeat this routine daily, and you should see noticeable results within a week.

Healthy Hydrator

If you have extremely dry skin, this **CABBAGE** and milk combo will serve your thirsty epidermis a healing drink. Pour 2 cups of whole milk in a saucepan. Add 2 cups of chopped cabbage and bring to a boil over medium-low heat, stirring frequently so the milk doesn't scorch. Take the mixture off the heat and let it cool to room temperature. Then pour it into a blender and puree until it's a thick paste. Using your fingertips or a clean makeup brush, apply the mask evenly to your face and neck. Leave it on for 30 minutes. Rinse it off with lukewarm water, and gently pat your skin dry.

Spruce Up with Juice

The vitamins in fresh **CABBAGE** juice can improve the tone and texture of your skin. And it's easy to whip up a batch. You'll need 3 cups of chopped green cabbage and 1 3/4 cups of water. Boil the water in a teakettle. Put the chopped cabbage in a blender and pour the boiling water over it. Blend at low speed, stopping when the water is green, with chunks of cabbage still visible. Switch to high speed and blend for another 10 seconds. Pour the liquid through a strainer and into a clean jar with a tight-fitting lid. Store in the refrigerator for up to two weeks. To use this complexion corrector, pour some juice on a cotton ball, wipe it over your just-washed face, and let your skin air-dry.

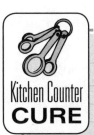

Kitchen Counter CURE

Hair-Growth Stimulator

Just like other green vegetables, **CABBAGE** is loaded with vitamin A, which can stimulate hair growth. So if your locks are losing their luster, try this treatment twice a week to help bring back your crowning glory: Blend 1/2 cup of boiled cabbage and 1/8 cup of fresh lemon juice in a blender on high until a thick paste forms. Using your fingertips, massage the paste onto your scalp, working from roots to tips. Leave it in your hair for 30 minutes, then shampoo and condition as usual.

Yes, Carrots Can ...

Fight wrinkles, improve skin's elasticity, and repair and tone skin texture. Not bad for rabbit food, eh? Put power-packed **CARROTS** to work for you by slicing three large ones and boiling them until they're soft. Mash them in a medium-size bowl and add 3 tablespoons of honey. Massage the mixture onto your face from forehead to chin, using a circular motion, and leave it on for 20 minutes. Rinse it off with lukewarm water, and gently pat your skin dry. *Note: Before you use carrot juice or pulp on your face, test it on an inconspicuous spot to make sure it doesn't turn your skin slightly— but temporarily!—orange.*

Back in the Day...

When Grandma Putt and her friends wanted to pamper their faces, they made their own skin cleansers and softeners using ingredients fresh from their gardens and kitchens. This was one of their favorites—and it still works as well now as it did decades ago. Mix 1/4 cup of grated **CARROTS** with 1 1/2 teaspoons of full-fat mayonnaise. Using your fingertips or a clean makeup brush, apply the mixture evenly to your face and neck. Leave it on for 15 minutes, rinse it off with lukewarm water, and gently pat your skin dry.

Easy On, Easy Off Mask

Nothing beats this **CARROT** peel-off mask for getting your skin really deep-down clean. Follow this simple routine:

1. Mix 1/2 cup of fresh carrot juice, 1/2 teaspoon of lemon juice, and 1 teaspoon of unflavored gelatin in a microwave-safe bowl.

2. Heat in the microwave for 30 seconds, or until the gelatin dissolves. Stir well, and refrigerate for 30 minutes to let the mixture thicken to a spreadable consistency. Don't let it get as firm as a gelatin salad!

3. Soak a washcloth in very warm water, and hold the cloth to your face for 15 minutes. Smooth the gelatin mixture over your freshly steamed skin. When the mask has dried, carefully peel it off.

4. Rinse your face with warm water, then rinse with cold water. Gently pat your skin dry, and apply your usual moisturizer.

Carroty Complexion Clearer

Don't let acne get the best of you. Even occasional breakouts can cause distress, so banish blemishes with this fix. Boil three **CARROTS** until they're soft, and mash them in a medium-size bowl. Mix $1/2$ cup of the pulp with just enough dry milk to form a smooth paste. Using your fingertips or a clean makeup brush, apply it to your face and leave it on for 20 minutes. Wash it off with lukewarm water, and pat your skin dry.

For a More Manageable Mane ...

Treat your head to **CARROTS**. Grate one medium-size carrot into a shatterproof bowl and bring it with you into the shower. Wet your hair and squeeze out the water. Cover the drain with a piece of screen or old panty hose, then massage the carrot gratings into your hair from roots to tips. Wait 15 minutes, and rinse them out with warm water, no shampoo. Follow up with your usual conditioner.

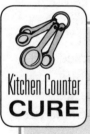

Kitchen Counter CURE

Ultimate Hair Conditioner

This luxurious treatment reduces dandruff, minimizes hair loss, helps preserve the natural elasticity of your hair—and makes it shine, shine, shine!

> **1 large CARROT, sliced**
> **1 medium-size banana, sliced**
> **$1/3$ cup of honey, warmed**
> **$1/4$ cup of olive oil**
> **Water**

Boil the carrot slices in water until they're soft. Strain off the water, and puree the carrots and the banana in a blender or food processor until they're smooth, with no lumps. Pour the mixture into a bowl, stir in the honey and olive oil, and mix well. Massage the conditioner into your hair, coating it completely from roots to tips. Cover your hair with a shower cap, and go about your business for at least 45 minutes, or up to eight hours for an extra-intensive treatment. Rinse your hair thoroughly with warm water, then shampoo and condition as usual.

Fresh Vegetables

BEAUTY
Bonus

DOUBLEHEADER FOR HAIR

Don't even bother with commercial two-in-one products that shampoo and condition your hair in one step. Instead, make your own by pureeing a peeled, diced **CUCUMBER** and a peeled, sliced lemon in a blender or food processor. Use a sieve to strain out the seeds, and bring the puree with you into the shower. Wash your hair with the dynamic duo, and rinse it out. The lemon cleans your tresses like nobody's business, while the cuke acts as a terrific conditioning agent.

Cool as a Cucumber Eye Pack

Tired, puffy eyes add years to your face, and no one I know wants to look any older than they already are! If you agree, put your peepers back in their place with this cool **CUCUMBER** pack. Wash and cut a fresh cucumber in half. Set aside one half, and finely grate the other half, cut side down, on a kitchen grater until you have $1/2$ cup. Spread the grated cuke down the middle of an 8-by-11-inch piece of cheesecloth. Fold up the short ends, then overlap with the long ends, like a burrito. Place the pack in the fridge for 20 minutes or so to cool. Then sit back or lie down and place the pack over your tired eyes for a half hour. When the time is up, you'll look relaxed and refreshed and oh-so-youthful, too! *Note: Toss the pack and make a fresh one whenever you want to use this treatment.*

Calming Cuke Toner

This refreshing toner is very mild and works well for all skin types. It's the perfect antidote for a puffy face. Chop half of a **CUCUMBER**, with the peel on, and put it in a blender or food processor. Add 3 tablespoons of witch hazel and 2 tablespoons of distilled water and blend until smooth. Pour the mixture through a fine-mesh sieve to remove the solids. Pour the remaining liquid into a clean bottle with a tight-fitting lid and store it in the refrigerator, where it will keep for up to two weeks. To use, pour the toner onto a cotton ball, wipe it across your clean face, and let it air-dry. It's the perfect treatment for a hot summer day!

Cukes Cut Chlorine

Do you spend a lot of time in the pool? Then this **CUCUMBER** conditioner is for you. It works wonders on hair damaged by chlorinated water. Place one-quarter of a peeled cucumber, one egg, and 1 tablespoon of olive oil in a blender and puree until smooth. Pour the mixture into a shatterproof container, and bring it with you into the shower. Wash your hair as usual, squeeze out as much water as you can, then spread the cuke conditioner evenly through your hair, from roots to tips, and leave it on for 10 minutes. Rinse it out with warm water and dry and style your hair as usual. Use once a week during the summer months, or year-round if you swim all year.

Soothing Cucumber Mask

This **CUCUMBER** and avocado mask will get your skin glowing. It can be used immediately, or refrigerated for up to 30 minutes. Place $1/2$ cup of chopped, peeled cucumber in a blender. Add $1/2$ cup of chopped, peeled avocado, one raw egg white, and 2 teaspoons of dry milk. Blend until the ingredients reach a smooth, paste-like consistency. With your fingertips, massage the mask onto your face and neck using circular motions. Relax for 30 minutes, or until the mask is completely dry. Remove it with lukewarm water, then rinse your face with cool water and gently pat your skin dry.

Back in the Day...

Smooth and tone your skin with this **CUCUMBER** puree facial that's been a well-kept beauty secret for ages. Peel one cucumber, cut it into slices, and puree on high speed in a blender until it has a pulpy consistency. Using your fingertips, apply the paste to your skin, massaging it in small circles from your forehead to your chin. Rinse it off with lukewarm water, and gently pat your skin dry.

SPOTLIGHT ON
AGING SKIN SOLUTIONS

Time marches on, but your face doesn't have to reveal its true age! Put the power of fresh vegetables to work on shrinking pores, minimizing fine lines, and leaving your skin with a youthful, healthy glow. Raid the produce drawer in your fridge for these turn-back-the-clock beauty boosters:

◆ An anti-aging **ASPARAGUS** mask will help slough off dull, dead skin. Steam two stalks of asparagus until they just start to soften, then slice them and put the slices in a blender. Add the juice of half a lemon and puree until a paste forms. Apply the paste to your face, avoiding the eye area. Leave it on for 10 minutes, then use a warm, wet washcloth to remove it. Rinse your face with cool water, and gently pat your skin dry.

◆ Minimize dark circles and decrease puffy eyes with a **BROCCOLI** mask. Put 2 tablespoons of grated raw broccoli in a blender. Add 2 tablespoons of instant coffee (caffeinated) and 1 tablespoon of water. Blend until a paste forms, adding more water if needed. Gently pat the paste under and around your eyes, being careful not to get any in your eyes. Leave it on for 20 minutes, then remove with cotton pads soaked in cool water.

◆ This **CABBAGE** mask will help tighten sagging skin. In a blender, puree 1/4 cup of chopped cabbage, 2 tablespoons of rice flour, and one raw egg white. Apply the mask evenly to your face and neck and leave it on for 20 minutes. Rinse it off with lukewarm water, then rinse with cool water and gently pat your skin dry.

◆ Tighten your pores with a **CUCUMBER** toner. Chop half of an unpeeled cucumber and put it in a blender or food processor. Add 2 tablespoons of honey, 1 tablespoon of apple cider vinegar, and 1 tablespoon of fresh-squeezed lemon juice. Blend well. Apply the toner to your face, avoiding the area around your eyes. Leave it on for 10 minutes, then rinse it off with lukewarm water, followed by cool water. Gently pat your skin dry.

CHAPTER 8

Pretty Pointers from the Pantry

If you think that baking supplies are only good for baking, you're in for a treat. Cornmeal, for instance, does double duty as a skin moisturizer and an exfoliant. And mustard isn't just for garnishing hot dogs—it plays the starring role in feel-good masks and scrubs. In fact, there are dozens of products on your pantry shelves that you've probably never considered using outside of the kitchen. So turn on your light-up beauty mirror and change your mind about that—and look your best while you're at it!

BAKING SUPPLIES

Better Body Scrub

If you're ready for a body scrub that's free of harsh chemicals and cloying perfumes—and doesn't cost an arm and a leg—then grab a box of **BAKING SODA**! It's the perfect base for an all-over scrub. Just mix 3 parts baking soda, 1 part ground oatmeal (grind uncooked rolled oats in a food processor), and 1 part water. Step into the shower, and rub the paste in circles from your neck to your toes to exfoliate and soften your skin. Rinse with warm water.

BEAUTY
Bonus

BAKING SODA BLEMISH BLASTER

Dry up blemishes fast without irritating your skin. In a small bowl, combine 1 tablespoon of **BAKING SODA** with ½ tablespoon of honey. Using your fingertips, apply the paste directly onto each spot, or for a major breakout, apply it evenly over your entire face. Leave it on for about 15 minutes, then rinse it off with lukewarm water, followed by cool water, and pat your skin dry.

Now That's a Bright Idea!

Lighten up dark age spots and brighten uneven skin tone with **BAKING SODA**. In a small bowl, mix 2 tablespoons of baking soda with 1 tablespoon of lemon juice and a few drops of extra virgin olive oil to make a paste. Wash your face and pat it dry. Using your fingertips, apply the paste to your face from forehead to chin. Leave it on for 10 minutes, then rinse it off with lukewarm water and gently pat your skin dry.

Soothing Spa Pedi

Treat your feet to the ultimate spa experience, right at home. Start with a soothing footbath of 3 parts **BAKING SODA** to 1 part warm water. Add a few drops of your favorite essential oil, and soak your feet for 20 minutes. Then exfoliate rough heels with a paste of baking soda and water. Rinse off with warm water, apply a rich moisturizing lotion to your legs and feet, and wrap a warm towel around them. Rest for 15 minutes before removing the wraps. You'll have salon-smooth legs and feet, without the salon price tag!

Blissful Bath Mix

There's no better way to unwind from a stressful day than with a nice relaxing bath, so add ½ cup of **BAKING SODA** to running water as you fill the tub, then sink in and say "aaahhh." The baking soda will neutralize acids on your skin and help wash away oil and perspiration, leaving your skin soft, smooth, and soothed.

Can the Tan

Many people use self-tanners instead of sunning themselves, and that's a smart way to reduce your risk of developing skin cancer. But self-tanners don't always live up to their hype, and you can end up with orange skin, or ugly dark streaks instead of a gorgeous tan. If this happens to you, don't hide inside until the faux glow fades. Instead, mix up this easy exfoliator to help fade away the blotchy mess, fast. Mix 3 parts **BAKING SODA** with 1 part warm water, and use it in the shower to scrub your skin. Its gentle action will make quick work of reversing that unflattering hue.

Perfecting Nail Prep

Get your nails clean and ready for a manicure with **BAKING SODA**. Start by dipping a nailbrush into a handful of baking soda, and gently scrub under and over your nails. In a small bowl, make a paste of 3 parts baking soda to 1 part warm water. Scoop it up and rub it all over your fingers and hands to exfoliate rough spots. Rinse with warm water, and thoroughly dry your hands and nails before applying polish.

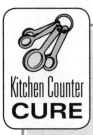

Kitchen Counter
CURE

Callus Corrective

Got tough calluses on your feet? Start clearing them away with this bedtime treatment that softens and exfoliates, thanks to the powers of **BAKING SODA**.

Baking soda
Water
Lavender oil
Brown sugar

A half hour before you go to bed, mix 2 tablespoons of baking soda in a basin of warm water. Stir in a few drops of the oil. In a small bowl, mix 3 parts baking soda, 1 part brown sugar, and 1 part warm water, and set aside. Soak your feet in the basin for 20 minutes. While they're still wet, use the scrub all over your feet, paying attention to the calloused areas. Rinse with warm water, thoroughly dry your feet, and apply moisturizer. Then pull on cotton socks and toddle off to bed. In the morning, your calluses will be noticeably softer.

Corny Skin Savers

Whether your skin is sensitive, dry, oily, or a combination of all three, a **CORNMEAL** concoction will leave your face looking and feeling its very best. Start with a washed, damp face, then whip up one of these:

- **Sensitive-skin soother.** Brew 1 cup of chamomile tea and let it cool to room temperature. Stir in $1/4$ cup of cornmeal and 1 teaspoon of dry milk, and mix well. Apply the paste evenly to your face and neck. Leave it on for 15 minutes, then rinse it off with lukewarm water followed by cool water, and gently pat your skin dry.

- **Super scrub.** In a small bowl, combine 2 tablespoons each of cornmeal, uncooked rolled oats, and wheat germ. To use, measure out 1 tablespoon of the mixture and add enough water to make a paste. Apply it to your face, massaging in small circles. Rinse it off with lukewarm water, followed by cool water, and gently pat your skin dry. Pour the remaining mixture into a container with a tight-fitting lid, and store it in the refrigerator for up to one month.

- **Oil buster.** In a small bowl, combine 2 tablespoons each of plain yogurt and cornmeal, add 1 teaspoon of lemon juice, and blend well. Apply the paste to your face and leave it on for five minutes. Rinse it off with lukewarm water, followed by cool water, and dry.

Back in the Day...

Folks have been suffering from athlete's foot since the dawn of time, which is why there are so many pricey antifungal lotions on the market, but before dipping into your wallet, you may want to give this old-time treatment a try. Find a pan large enough to hold both of your feet, and pour **CORNMEAL** into the pan to a depth of 1 inch. Add enough warm (not hot!) water to reach a depth of 2 inches. Do not mix; just let the pan sit for about an hour until the contents look like mush. Then pull up a chair, sit down, and slide your feet into the pan, adding a bit more warm water if needed so that the mush surrounds your feet. Soak for 15 minutes or so, then pull your feet out, rinse them with warm water, and thoroughly dry your toes before putting on any footwear.

Nourishing Facial Mask

Here's a sweet solution for dry skin: In a small bowl, mix 2 tablespoons of **CORNMEAL**, 2 tablespoons of plain yogurt, and 1 tablespoon of honey to form a creamy paste. Apply it to your face and leave the mask in place for 15 minutes. Rinse it off with lukewarm water, and pat dry.

Anti-Aging Exfoliant

Diminish the look of fine lines with this fragrant mask. In a bowl, mix 1/2 cup of **CORNMEAL**, 1/2 cup of plain yogurt, and 5 drops each of lavender, patchouli, and grapefruit oils. Stir well, then cover the bowl with plastic wrap and put it in the refrigerator for two hours. To use, scoop up the scrub with your hands, and gently massage it over your clean, damp face and neck. Remove it with a warm, wet washcloth, rinse, and pat dry.

Fab Foot Freshener

Keep your feet pretty with this **CORNMEAL** scrub. In a bowl, combine 3 tablespoons of cornmeal with 2 tablespoons of fresh mashed avocado and stir well. Sit down with a towel under your bare feet. Scoop up the mixture and work it into your tootsies, focusing on calluses and rough, dry areas. Rinse well with warm water and thoroughly dry your feet. Repeat twice a week.

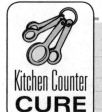

Kitchen Counter CURE

Cornmeal Soap

This super-simple soap recipe whips up in a flash with no special equipment. You'll end up with a small bar of soap that's perfect for scrubbing your hands and feet. Include the essential oil if you want a fragrant cleanser.

- **½ cup of CORNMEAL**
- **½ cup of grated mild bar soap (such as Ivory®)**
- **1 ½ tablespoons of cooking oil**
- **1 tablespoon of water**
- **1–2 drops of your favorite essential oil (optional)**

Pulse the cornmeal and soap in a food processor until grainy. Remove the mixture from the processor and place it in a bowl along with the cooking oil and water; add the essential oil if you decide to use it. Mix with your hands until the ingredients are well blended. Form the mixture into a ball and allow it to harden at room temperature.

Firming Face Mask

Give your face a mini-lift with this **CORNSTARCH** mask. In a small bowl, whisk 1/4 cup of cornstarch with one raw egg white and 2 tablespoons of whole milk until well blended. Apply the mask to your face, avoiding the eye area, and leave it on for 20 minutes. Rinse it off with lukewarm water, followed by cool water, and gently pat your skin dry.

Mascara Magic

Give your eyes more oomph with this simple trick that thickens mascara and adds volume to your lashes. Start by knocking a full wand of your mascara against a small, clean plate so that mascara drops off. Repeat until you have a small blob. Add just a pinch of **CORNSTARCH** and mix it in with a toothpick. Apply the new and improved makeup with a clean mascara wand and admire your new bright-eyed look.

BEAUTY
Bonus

DIY DRY SHAMPOO

Soak up excess hair oil or add a beauty boost to your lifeless locks with **CORNSTARCH**. Just dust some along your part, leave it on for about two minutes, then comb or brush it out. You can create a scented version by mixing a few drops of essential oil into 1/4 cup of cornstarch and applying it along your part with a clean makeup brush.

Bold Bronzer

Artfully applied bronzer along your cheeks and temples adds a dramatic touch, and gives the illusion of a slimmer profile. Before you spend your money in the makeup aisle, give this DIY bronzer a try: On a small plate, combine 1 1/2 tablespoons of cinnamon with 1 tablespoon of **CORNSTARCH**. Mix well with a fork, then apply it with a clean blush brush.

Make Mine Matte

If you love the look of matte lipstick but have a drawer full of glosses, don't toss 'em! Instead dust your lips with a bit of **CORNSTARCH**, rubbing it in so there is no white trace. Then apply your glossy lipstick on top for a smooth matte finish.

Bargain Body Butter

At about three dollars a can, nothing beats unflavored **VEGETABLE SHORTENING** as an economical body butter. It's made from soybean oil and, unlike most commercial body lotions, contains no water, so it can really deep-condition skin. After your next shower, dab it on your elbows, knees, and heels, and rub it in well. Then put just a tiny dab on your lips to soften your kisser.

Speedy Smoother

Fancy hand creams don't hold a candle to good ol' **VEGETABLE SHORTENING**. So stop buying them, and do this instead: Scoop out a dollop of the shortening and rub it into your hands. Voilà! Smooth, soft skin in an instant, and without the fancy price tag.

Nifty Nighttime Moisturizer

Give your skin a youthful glow with this super-easy bedtime treatment. Simply smooth a palmful of **VEGETABLE SHORTENING** onto your face before bed, as you would any other night cream. Then hit the sack, and wake up to a glowing complexion.

First-Rate Foot Repair

Feet that are really dry and calloused all but cry out for this super-softening routine: Just before you go to bed, rub some **VEGETABLE SHORTENING** into your skin. Then put on a pair of old cotton socks. Besides protecting your sheets, the covering will force the shortening to penetrate deeper into your skin. Come morning, simply wipe any residual "grease" off with a tissue, and be on your way.

Back in the Day...

My Grandma Putt rarely wore eye makeup or any other kind of cosmetics. But when she did brush on mascara for a very special occasion, like a wedding or christening, she took it off with **VEGETABLE SHORTENING**. She just dabbed a little onto her eyelids, then gently wiped it over her lashes with a cotton pad. Give it a try; my guess is that you'll never go back to commercial makeup removers again!

SPOTLIGHT ON
SKIN SAVERS

Baking supplies come in handy not only when you're whipping up delectable desserts, but also when you need to treat minor burns, prevent chafed skin, block body odor, or ... the list goes on and on. Here are just a few examples of easy ways to save your skin with baking ingredients you already have on hand:

◆ **Burn salve.** In a large bowl, mix 1 tablespoon of **BAKING SODA** and 1 tablespoon of **CORNSTARCH** in 8 cups of warm water. Soak a washcloth in the solution and gently place it on the burn for 30 minutes. Then let your skin air-dry.

◆ **Anti-chafing powder.** Running a marathon or just hiking around town? Prevent chafing with a quick dusting of **CORNSTARCH** behind your knees, between your thighs, under your arms, and anywhere else you need it. Cornstarch also helps clothes slip on and off more easily when you're hot and sweaty.

◆ **DIY deodorant.** Simply wipe rubbing alcohol across your underarms, then brush on some **CORNSTARCH**. For a more involved concoction, mix equal amounts of baking soda, coconut oil, and cornstarch (add a few drops of essential oil if you'd like a scented version), and pour it into an empty deodorant stick if you have one, or a paper cup. The mixture congeals quickly and won't melt, and it lasts about three months at room temperature. Simply peel the cup down as you use up the deodorant.

◆ **Odor chaser.** Stop the stink of smelly shoes by sprinkling some **CORNSTARCH** into them before you put them on.

◆ **Bottom soother.** Before you put a fresh diaper on a baby, wipe a light coat of **VEGETABLE SHORTENING** onto his bottom. It'll form a moisture barrier and help prevent diaper rash. By the way, this works equally well for those folks who wear adult incontinence briefs or diapers.

Barley Beautifier

If you're longing for fresher, brighter skin, **BARLEY** is the answer to your prayers. In a small bowl, combine 1 tablespoon of barley powder (use a blender or food processor to crush barley into a fine powder), 1 tablespoon of lemon or lime juice, and 1 tablespoon of milk. Mix until you have a thick paste, adjusting ingredient amounts as needed. Using a clean makeup brush, apply the paste to your face, avoiding your eyes and lips. Leave it on for 10 minutes, then rinse it off with lukewarm water, and gently pat your skin dry.

Easy Everyday Cleanser

Homemade facial cleansers don't get any easier than this one. Start by crushing **BARLEY** in your blender or food processor until you have a fine powder. Mix 1 teaspoon of the powder with a splash of milk or water in the palm of your hand, and use it to wash your face. Rinse with cool water, and gently pat your skin dry. Store any leftover powder in a jar with a tight-fitting lid for up to one month.

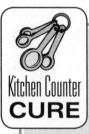

Kitchen Counter CURE

Barley Body Scrub

Bring lackluster, dry, and aging skin back to life with this refreshing **BARLEY** and cranberry body scrub. The barley helps exfoliate dead skin cells while the antioxidants in the cranberries provide anti-aging benefits.

- 1/2 cup of frozen whole cranberries
- 1/4 cup of barley powder*
- 1/4 cup of coconut oil or extra virgin olive oil
- 1/4 cup of sugar

Place the ingredients in a blender and puree for 20 seconds. Spoon the scrub into a shatterproof container and bring it into the shower. Wet your body, then apply the scrub, paying particular attention to rough, dry areas such as knees and elbows. Rinse off and pat your skin dry.
* Use a blender or food processor to crush barley into a fine powder.

Bran Banishes Blemishes

Acne and blackheads don't stand a chance against this remarkable remover: Just mix 2 tablespoons of **BRAN** with enough water to make a paste. (Add a teaspoon or so of H_2O at a time, until you get a spreadable consistency.) Smooth it onto your freshly washed face, avoiding the eye area, and leave it on for 20 minutes or so. Rinse it off with warm water, splash your skin with cool water to close your pores, and gently pat your face dry. Finish by applying your usual toner and moisturizer. Repeat this procedure once a week to keep your skin clear and fresh.

Beautiful Bran Body Scrub

Your skin couldn't ask for a healthier scrub than this one. Here's the easy formula: Mix 1/2 cup of **BRAN** and 1/2 cup of finely ground almonds in a heat-proof bowl, and gradually stir in 1 cup of hot green tea until you have a thick, spreadable paste. Let it cool to room temperature, then add 10 drops of lavender oil, and mix well. Bring it into the shower with you and massage the mixture onto your dry body, working in small circles from your face down to your toes, paying particular attention to any rough, dry areas. Then rinse with lukewarm water, and pat your skin dry.

BEAUTY
Bonus

BENEFICIAL BRAN BATH

Give your dry, sensitive skin some extra TLC with this soothing soak. Start by putting 3/4 cup of wheat **BRAN** and 1/2 cup of oat bran in a medium pot with 2 cups of cold water. Bring the mixture to a boil, then cover the pot, lower the heat, and simmer for 30 minutes. Pour the mixture through a fine sieve and set the liquid aside. Place the bran solids in a small cloth sack or panty hose toe, tie it closed, and thoroughly squeeze out any excess liquid into the liquid you set aside. Save the sack for later. Add 5 tablespoons of heavy cream and 4 tablespoons of honey to the liquid and mix well. Run a warm bath and add the liquid and the bran sack to the bathwater. While bathing, squeeze the sack gently from time to time to ensure that all the beneficial components of the bran are fully extracted.

Fresh Face Cleanser

Give your skin a fresh, clean glow by washing it with **OATMEAL**. Just grind about ¼ cup of uncooked rolled oats in a coffee grinder or food processor until they're the consistency of coarse flour. In a small bowl, mix the oats with enough heavy cream to make a paste. (If you have oily skin, substitute skim milk.) Let the mixture thicken for a minute or two, then apply the paste to your face and neck, massaging in small circles. Rinse it off with warm water, then cool water, and pat your skin dry.

Bowl of Oats Scrubber

When you want a gentle way to soften up rough heels, knees, and elbows, reach for **OATMEAL**. In a bowl, mix together 1 part baking soda, 1 part uncooked rolled oats, and 3 parts water. Use a washcloth to apply the scrub to your body in a circular motion, paying attention to areas that are rough, dry, or cracked. Rinse with warm water, and pat dry.

Basic Blackhead Buster

This simple solution will banish blackheads fast. Make a paste of 3 teaspoons of uncooked rolled **OATS** and 1 teaspoon of water, and rub it into the affected areas. Leave it on for 10 minutes, rinse with warm water, and pat dry.

HOW'S THAT?

Q *Hey, Jerry, my hair is dry, so I don't wash it every day, but I do want it to stay clean between washings. I've tried some of the dry shampoos my wife has, but, between you and me, they're a bit too fragrant for my taste. Do you have a natural solution that will clean my hair and not make me smell like a girl?*

A Relax, buddy, I've got you covered. Just grab a handful of dry **OATMEAL** and work it through your hair with your fingers. Let it sit for a minute or two, then brush it all out. The cereal will remove the oil, leaving your hair clean, but not smelling like a lollipop or floral bouquet!

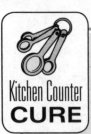

Kitchen Counter CURE

Oh, So Softening Scrub

If you're battling dry skin, an exfoliant is your best friend. This **OATMEAL** scrub will slough off those dead skin cells, leaving you soft and smooth.

2 cups of finely ground uncooked rolled oats*

1 cup of baking soda

3/4 cup of whole milk

1/2 cup of kosher salt or sea salt

1/4 cup of honey

1/4 cup of olive oil

1 tbsp. of vitamin E oil

20 drops of your favorite essential oil

Mix the first five ingredients together in a bowl, then stir in the oils. Pour the mixture into a wide-mouth jar with a tight-fitting lid. It will keep for a week at room temperature and for three weeks in the refrigerator. To use it, scoop a handful of the scrub out of the jar, massage it into your skin, and rinse it off in the shower or tub. Just be sure to cover the drain with a piece of fabric to snag the oatmeal particles.

* Use a coffee grinder or food processor.

Yield: About 4 cups

Combo Complexion Care

When your face has both dry and oily zones, using a different product for each area can be a time-consuming nuisance, especially if you make your own beauty products. The solution? This once-a-month **OATMEAL** cleansing mask that's good for *all* types of skin. Grind up 1 cup of uncooked rolled oats in a blender. Add one raw egg white, 1/2 cup of skim milk, and 3 drops of almond oil, and blend to form a smooth paste. Spread it over your face and neck (avoiding the eye area), and leave it there for 30 minutes or so. Rinse it off with lukewarm water.

Magical Meal Mask

Reveal glowing, radiant skin with this **OATMEAL** facial mask. Mix 2 tablespoons of ground uncooked rolled oats (use a coffee grinder or food processor) with 3 tablespoons of sour cream. Wait a bit for the oats to expand, then add a few drops of lemon juice. Using your fingertips, apply the mask to your face, massaging in a circular motion from forehead to chin. Leave it on for 20 minutes, then remove it with a warm, wet washcloth, rinse with cool water, and pat dry.

Rice Is Nice...

For toning your skin and keeping it smooth and bright. So whip up a batch of this **RICE** water toner to have on hand. Start with 1 cup of rice (not the instant kind) and 6 cups of water. Cook the rice until soft. Pour the contents of the pot into a colander that is set over a large bowl to separate the cooked rice from the remaining water. Store the cooked rice in the refrigerator to eat later, and let the rice water in the bowl cool to room temperature. Pour it into a jar or bottle that has a tight-fitting lid, and keep it in the refrigerator for up to one week. To use the toner, simply pour some onto a cotton ball, swoop it over your clean face, and let it air-dry.

Brightening Face Mask

Battle the aging effects of dark spots with this **RICE** flour mask that lightens and brightens your complexion. In a small bowl, mix 1 heaping tablespoon of rice flour and 1 teaspoon of half-and-half. Mix well, and continue to add the half-and-half one teaspoon at a time until you have a very smooth, slightly thick paste. Using a clean makeup brush, apply the paste evenly to your face (avoiding the eye area), your neck, and your upper chest. Leave it on for 20 to 30 minutes, or until it's dry. Remove the mask with a warm, wet washcloth, then rinse with cool water and gently pat your skin dry.

BEAUTY
Bonus

THYME-FOR-RICE TONER

Here's a DIY toner that's good for all skin types and gentle enough to use every time you wash your face: Using the back of a spoon or a mortar and pestle, crush enough uncooked **RICE** to equal 2 teaspoons and put it in a heat-proof bowl. Add two chopped sprigs of fresh thyme (or substitute ½ tablespoon of dried thyme), and pour ½ cup of boiling water over them. Stir in the juice from half of a lemon. Let the mixture steep for 15 minutes, then strain out the solids. Pour the liquid into a bottle with a tight-fitting cap, store it in the refrigerator, and pull it out to use as you would any other toner.

SPOTLIGHT ON
BEAUTY BATHS

We all know that a nice long soak can do wonders for frazzled nerves or distressed skin. But a bath can also enhance your beauty. Try one or more of these, and you'll feel relaxed and radiant. Just one note: Before you start your bath, cover the drain with a piece of fabric or a plastic drain cover to snag any grains and prevent clogging.

◆ **Beautifying bran bath.** Put ½ cup of oat **BRAN** in a medium pot with 2 cups of cold water. Bring the mixture to a boil, then cover the pot, lower the heat, and simmer for 30 minutes. Pour the mixture through a fine sieve and set the liquid aside. Place the bran solids in a small cloth sack or panty hose toe, tie it closed, and thoroughly squeeze out any excess liquid into the reserved liquid. Set the sack aside. Add 1 cup of white cosmetic clay (available online) and 4 tablespoons of honey to the liquid and mix well. Run a warm bath and add the liquid and the bran sack to the bathwater. While bathing, squeeze the sack gently from time to time to ensure that all the beneficial components of the bran are fully extracted.

◆ **Oats, milk, and honey blend.** Put ½ cup of uncooked rolled **OATS**, ¼ cup of dry whole-milk powder, and 2 tablespoons of honey in an all-cotton muslin or cheesecloth bag. Tie it shut with a cord, and hang it under the spigot as you fill the tub. The running water will disperse the super-softening trio throughout your bath.

◆ **Skin-soothing soak.** Warm up 2 tablespoons of honey in the microwave until it's runny. Pour the honey under warm running bathwater, then add 1 cup of uncooked rolled **OATS**, 4 tablespoons of dry milk, 3 tablespoons of aloe vera gel, and 3 tablespoons of dried mint to the rising water while stirring to mix it all.

◆ **Relaxing rice bath.** Pour ¾ cup of **RICE** bran powder (available in Asian markets and online) under warm running water as you fill the tub. Add several drops of lavender oil or your favorite fragrant oil.

When your bath is done, pamper yourself a bit more by wrapping up in a heated towel. Then lie down and think happy thoughts.

Take a Break from Breakouts

This **HORSERADISH** lotion will help dry up pimples and, when used regularly, will keep 'em from coming back. Finely grate a piece of fresh horseradish until you have 1/4 cup. Put it in a clean jar with a tight-fitting lid, and add 1/2 cup of buttermilk and 2 tablespoons of glycerin (available online). Put the lid on and shake the jar to thoroughly mix the contents. Store the jar in the refrigerator overnight. In the morning, strain out the solids and save the lotion in another clean jar or bottle. Twice a day, apply it to your blemishes with a cotton ball and let it air-dry. Use the lotion nightly as a toner on your freshly washed face. Keep it in the refrigerator and use within two weeks.

A Fine Face Brightener

Bring back the glow with this super-easy facial mask. Place 2 tablespoons of prepared **HORSERADISH** in a small bowl. Add 3 tablespoons of sour cream and 1 tablespoon of ground oats (grind uncooked rolled oats in a coffee grinder or food processor) and stir to mix well. Apply the mask to your face, massaging it in small circles from your forehead to your chin. Leave it on for 10 minutes, then remove it with a warm, wet washcloth. Rinse with cool water, and gently pat your skin dry.

Back in the Day...

Drive dandruff to defeat with this tried-and-true remedy from Grandma's time. Mix equal parts of prepared **HORSERADISH** and apple cider vinegar in a shatterproof container and bring it into the shower. Get your hair damp, and pour the mixture over the top of your head (keep your eyes closed to avoid any irritation) and massage it well into your scalp. Wait two to three minutes, then rinse it out thoroughly and follow up with your usual shampoo and conditioner. Use two to three times a week until the flakes flee.

Marvelous Mayo Facial

Whether your skin is oily, dry, or somewhere in between, **MAYONNAISE** can help it look its best. Place 1/3 cup of mayonnaise (the full-fat kind) in a small bowl. If your skin is oily or acne prone, add 3 tablespoons of fresh-squeezed lemon juice and stir well. For dry skin, add 3 tablespoons of an exfoliating agent, such as Epsom salts or baking soda, and stir well. If your skin is sensitive or normal, don't add anything to the mayonnaise. Using your fingertips, massage the mixture onto your clean, dry face, avoiding the eye area. Leave it on for 20 minutes, then remove with a warm, wet washcloth. Rinse with cool water, and pat your skin dry.

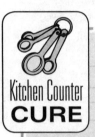

Kitchen Counter CURE

Homemade Cold Cream

Here's a DIY formula that will not only remove makeup, but also clean and soften your skin at the same time.

½ cup of full-fat MAYONNAISE

2 tbsp. of melted butter

Juice of 1 lemon or lime

Combine all of the ingredients in a small bowl, then spoon the mixture into a glass jar with a tight-fitting lid. Store the jar in the refrigerator and let the cream firm up. To use, scoop out a palmful and massage it onto your face in small circles from forehead to chin. Tissue it off, then rinse with cool water and gently pat your skin dry.

A Mayo Mask-erade

Here's a super-simple facial mask that soothes, softens, and is suitable for all skin types. Just mix 5 drops of chamomile oil into 1/3 cup of full-fat **MAYONNAISE**. Smooth the mixture over your face and neck, and leave it on for 20 minutes. Rinse if off with lukewarm water and gently pat your skin dry.

Miraculous Moisturizing Mayo

Full-fat **MAYONNAISE** provides deep-down moisture to thirsty skin. In a small bowl, mix 1/3 cup of mayonnaise and 3 tablespoons of baby oil. Stir well. Using your fingertips, smooth the mixture onto your face, neck, and any other part(s) of your body that could use some softening. Leave it on for 20 minutes, then rinse with lukewarm water and pat your skin dry.

A Mayo Mani

Make that, a mayo pre-mani. Get your nails ready for a manicure by dipping your clean fingers into a small bowl of full-fat **MAYONNAISE**. Let them linger for five minutes, then massage the mayo around your nails and cuticles. Leave it on for another five minutes, then rinse it off with lukewarm water and pat your skin dry.

Mayo for Your Mane

Plain old **MAYONNAISE** makes a great hair conditioner. Start by shampooing your hair as you normally do. Then towel it dry, and massage full-fat mayo (not the low-fat kind and not the miracle salad dressing!) into your hair from roots to tips. Cover your head with a shower cap and go about your business for a half hour or so. When the time's up, shampoo the mixture out and condition your hair as usual.

Ultra-Moisturizing Mayo Hair Mask

This luscious treatment not only deeply moisturizes dull locks, but also adds strength and shine to your tresses. Mix $1/2$ cup each of full-fat **MAYONNAISE** and honey in a small bowl. Stir until thoroughly blended. Scoop the mixture out with your fingers and coat your dry hair from roots to tips, making sure every strand is covered. Leave the mask on for one hour, then shampoo it out and follow up with your usual conditioner.

HOW'S THAT?

Q *Jerry, I hope you can help me win an argument with my wife. I recently came in from a day of yard work with a sunburned neck. She wanted to slather it with MAYONNAISE, and I told her, "No way!" She insists it can ease sunburn pain. Is she nuts, or what?*

A Sorry, pal, but your wife is right. Cold mayo straight from the fridge can take the sting out of sunburn, and fast. But be prepared next time, and remember to wear sunscreen (and leave the mayo for your tuna sandwich)!

Not Just for Hot Dogs...

I'm talking about **MUSTARD**, of course! It not only enhances the flavor of your food, but enhances your beauty, too. Try this mustard mask and see for yourself: Spread a thin layer of classic yellow mustard on your face, avoiding the eye area. Wait 10 minutes, then rinse it off with lukewarm water and gently pat your skin dry. Your face will be smooth and glowing. *Note: If you have sensitive skin, test first by putting some mustard on the inside of your wrist. Wait 15 minutes; no rash? No problem—you can proceed.*

Mighty Mustard Scrub

Get rid of blackheads and dead skin cells with this powerful facial scrub. In a small bowl, mix 1 tablespoon of honey, 1 tablespoon of lemon juice, and 1 tablespoon of **MUSTARD** seeds (available in grocery stores and online). Stir well. Using your fingertips, apply the scrub to your face in small circles from forehead to chin, focusing on oily areas. Leave it on for three minutes, then remove it with a warm, wet washcloth. Rinse with cool water, and pat your skin dry.

Supple Skin Scrub

Your skin will become soft and smooth with this **MUSTARD** scrub. Mix 1 tablespoon of mustard seeds with 2 tablespoons of rose oil and stir well. Using your fingertips, apply the scrub to your face in small circles from forehead to chin. Leave it on for five minutes, then rinse.

BEAUTY
Bonus

SUMMER SANDAL SOAK

No, I don't mean soak your sandals! Instead, treat your feet to this relaxing **MUSTARD** mixture so your toes are ready to bare all. Measure 3 tablespoons of yellow mustard into a pan of warm water. Stir well to dissolve the mustard, then slip your feet into the spicy water and soak 'em for 15 minutes or so. To tackle rough heels, grab a handful of mustard seeds and start scrubbing. Rinse with clear water and thoroughly dry your feet, paying particular attention to the spaces between your toes. Now slide your feet into some sandals and show off those smooth tootsies!

SPOTLIGHT ON
SPICY BEAUTY SOLUTIONS

Maybe you never acquired a taste for horseradish, hot-pepper sauce, or pungent mustards, so those bottles and jars are just collecting dust in your pantry. Or perhaps you're a huge fan of the hot stuff, but you often end up with not quite enough at the bottom of the jar to do much with, recipe-wise. Well, whichever camp you're in, here's a handful of great ways to use up those last few drops or spoonfuls of these spicy condiments:

◆ Add shine and bounce to dull tresses with this dynamic duo: Combine 3 tablespoons of prepared **HORSERADISH** with ⅓ cup of full-fat mayonnaise in a small bowl and mix well. Then step into the shower and pour the mixture over your damp hair. Work it in from roots to tips, then put on a shower cap. After 30 minutes, shampoo and condition as usual.

◆ Plump up thin lips by combining ¼ teaspoon of **HOT-PEPPER SAUCE** and a pea-size dollop of petroleum jelly. Mix thoroughly, then use your finger or a lip brush to apply to your kisser.

◆ Give limp hair a new lease on life with this hair strengthener: Generously sprinkle **HOT-PEPPER SAUCE** over your damp head, massaging it into your scalp and along your hair from roots to tips. Leave it on for two minutes, then shampoo and condition as usual.

◆ Exfoliate and hydrate your face by combining 1 tablespoon of **MUSTARD** seeds with 2 tablespoons of aloe vera gel in a small bowl. Using your fingertips, apply the scrub to your face in small circles from forehead to chin. Then rinse it off with lukewarm water and gently pat your skin dry.

◆ Treat delicate, aging skin to a creamy wash. Combine 1 tablespoon of yellow **MUSTARD** with 2 tablespoons of heavy cream in a small bowl. Using your fingertips, apply the wash to your face in small circles from forehead to chin. Leave it on for three minutes, then rinse it off with lukewarm water and gently pat your skin dry.

Amazing Almond Scrub

Get your glow on with this invigorating **ALMOND** face scrub. Warm up 1 tablespoon of dark organic honey just until it becomes runny by putting it in a small glass bowl immersed in hot water (or microwave it for a few seconds). Stir in 2 tablespoons of finely ground almonds (use a coffee grinder or food processor) and 1/2 teaspoon of fresh-squeezed lemon juice. Stir well. Using your fingertips, apply the scrub to your face in a circular motion from forehead to chin, avoiding the eye area. Leave it on for five minutes, then rinse it off with lukewarm water and dry.

Beneficial Body Scrub

A combination of avocado and **ALMONDS** leaves your skin smooth, supple, and hydrated. Smash a ripe avocado into a small shatterproof bowl. Grind enough almonds to equal 2 tablespoons, and combine them with 1 cup of uncooked rolled oats in another shatterproof bowl. Bring the bowls into the shower. Get wet, then turn off the water and scoop up the avocado and massage it all over your skin. Pour the almond-oatmeal mixture onto a wet washcloth, and rub it right over the avocado. Leave the scrub on for 10 minutes, then shower it off with warm water.

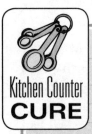

Kitchen Counter CURE

Fresh-from-the-Kitchen Cleanser

Here's a facial cleanser that's perfect for all skin types. Plus, you can put it together in a flash and keep it on hand for daily use. Put 1 cup each of **ALMONDS**, uncooked rolled oats, and dried orange peel in a blender or food processor, and chop the ingredients until they form a fine powder. Scoop some into the palm of your hand, add a few drops of water, and rub it onto your face. Rinse with warm water, gently pat your skin dry, and follow up with your favorite toner and moisturizer. Store the remaining mixture in an airtight container at room temperature.

Creamy Walnut Cleanser

Your face will feel super clean and fresh with this creamy, nutty, citrusy cleanser. And it takes just a few minutes to put it all together. Start by grinding enough shelled **WALNUTS** in a coffee grinder or food processor to equal 2 tablespoons. In a small bowl, mix the ground nuts with 2 tablespoons of heavy cream and 1 teaspoon of fresh-squeezed lime juice. Using your fingertips, gently massage the cleanser into your wet face in a circular motion from your forehead to your chin. Wash it off with lukewarm water, then rinse with cool water and gently pat your skin dry. Follow up with your usual moisturizer.

Walnut Wonder Scrub

Ditch dry skin while soothing it at the same time with this scrub that works equally well for normal and combination complexions. Use this treatment two to three times a week to keep your face looking smooth and vibrant. Mix 1/4 cup of plain yogurt and 1/4 cup of ground shelled **WALNUTS** (use a coffee grinder or food processor). Using your fingertips, apply the scrub to your clean face in a circular motion from your forehead to your chin. Wash it off with lukewarm water, then rinse with cool water and gently pat your skin dry. Follow up with a toner and your usual moisturizer.

BEAUTY
Hint

WALNUT POWER PACK

Reap the beauty benefits of **WALNUTS** by preparing this powerful face pack that not only moisturizes, but also makes fine lines and wrinkles seem to disappear. Place four shelled walnuts, 2 tablespoons of heavy cream, 2 teaspoons of uncooked rolled oats, 1 teaspoon of honey, and 1 teaspoon of olive oil in a blender and blend until you have a smooth paste. Using a clean makeup brush, apply the pack to your face and neck, and allow it to dry completely. Then wash it off with a warm, wet washcloth, rinse with cool water, and gently pat your skin dry.

SPOTLIGHT ON
INNER BEAUTY

The same vitamins, minerals, and other compounds that make nuts so good for your health (see page 123 to learn about the health benefits of nuts) also make them a powerful addition to your beauty-care arsenal. So while you're busy whipping up the facials and scrubs in this section, you can also snack on their main nut ingredient. In fact, one serving of nuts every day (a small handful) can help keep your nails, skin, and hair healthy and younger looking. If you need any more enticement to add nuts to your daily diet, just take a gander at this list of their beautifying nutrients, from A to Z:

◆ **Alpha-linolenic acid. WALNUTS** are packed with this omega-3 fatty acid, which, among other feats, moisturizes your hair, nourishes and softens your skin, relieves skin disorders such as acne and eczema, and helps fight aging.

◆ **B-complex vitamins.** These include riboflavin, niacin, thiamine, pantothenic acid, vitamin B_6, and folates, and are essential for optimum health and well-being, along with healthy skin and hair. The B team includes **ALMONDS** and pecans.

◆ **Selenium.** This mighty mineral helps hair grow thick and shiny. Among all foods, **BRAZIL NUTS** rank as one of the most potent sources of selenium.

◆ **Vitamin E.** It aids in tissue repair, thereby slowing down your skin's aging process. Your prime dietary helpers: **ALMONDS**, cashews, peanuts, and **WALNUTS**.

◆ **Zinc.** The big Z keeps your hair shiny, helps prevent hair loss, aids in healing acne and scabs on your skin, and guards against white spots on your fingernails and toenails. **ALMONDS**, cashews, pecans, and **WALNUTS** are all rich in zinc.

Remember, all nuts are "energy dense," which means they have a high concentration of calories per bite, so don't overindulge! Just keep your portions small (no more than 1 ounce per day), and avoid salted, processed versions.

Captivating Coconut Scrub

COCONUT OIL is a creamy solid at room temperature that turns liquid when heated, so it's the perfect base for this body scrub. Melt 1/2 cup of coconut oil over very low heat, then pour it over 1 cup of brown sugar or coarse salt, and mix thoroughly. Stir in 5 drops of pure vanilla extract or an essential oil. Step into the shower and massage the mixture into your skin from neck to toes, rinse it off with warm water, and pat dry.

Quick Coconut Conditioner

Hold a jar of **COCONUT OIL** under warm water, then apply a generous amount to your just-washed hair, working it through the strands. Cover your head with a shower cap, then wait 10 minutes. No need to shampoo or condition—just rinse, dry, and be on your way!

Super Lip Saver

Chase away chapped lips with ultra-hydrating **COCONUT OIL**. Spoon solid coconut oil into a clean contact lens holder or other small container. Keep it in your purse or pocket, and use your finger to dab the creamy treatment on your lips throughout the day.

Back in the Day...

After World War II, **COCONUT OIL** was sold in England as "margarine" and in the United States as "coconut butter." It wasn't until the 1960s that the coconut oil we find today started appearing on American store shelves. My Grandma Putt used that old-time "coconut butter" to moisturize her cuticles, and so can you. Rub a small amount of solid coconut oil onto each of your cuticles, allowing it to be absorbed to strengthen your nails and hydrate the delicate cuticle skin.

Clean-Sweep Coconut Wipes

Stubborn makeup comes off with ease when you use these **COCONUT OIL** face wipes. Lay a dozen round cotton pads on a baking sheet with sides. Put 1/4 cup of solid coconut oil in a microwave-safe container and heat it on low, watching carefully, until melted. Pour the melted oil over the cotton pads, and let them soak overnight. In the morning, store the pads in a plastic ziplock bag. Just one wipe will take the day's dirt and makeup off your face, and they're portable, so you can take them on the road.

Soothing Body Butter

Soften your skin with **COCONUT OIL** and honey. It's a treat worthy of an ultra-fancy spa—for a fraction of the price. Here's the simple process:

1. Gather the goods. You'll need 2 tablespoons of solid coconut oil, 1 tablespoon of honey, 2 drops of pure vanilla extract or peppermint oil, a small bowl, and enough soft cotton bath towels to cover your body.

2. Mix all of the ingredients together in the bowl.

3. Spread the towels out in your bathtub, and wet them with hot water.

4. Rub the butter all over your body, settle into the tub, and wrap yourself in the hot towels. Then lie back and relax until the towels have cooled to room temperature.

5. Rinse yourself off, pat dry, and smooth plain coconut oil onto your skin to seal in the moisture.

HOW'S THAT?

Q *I'm tired of spending an arm and a leg on shaving cream. And I keep thinking there's got to be a good, cheap alternative that's not full of all those unpronounceable chemicals in the store-bought stuff. Am I right?*

A Yep, you're right, and the answer is as close as your pantry. Simply smooth some solid **COCONUT OIL** onto your about-to-be-shaved skin, whether it's your face, legs, or underarms. It will give you a clean, close shave and leave your skin healthily hydrated.

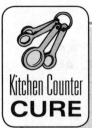

Kitchen Counter CURE

3 Cheers for Olive Oil!

Whether your skin is normal, dry, or oily, one of these weekly **OLIVE OIL** treatments will have you loving the skin you're in:

- **Normal skin.** In a blender, puree 1/2 cup of plain yogurt with 2 tablespoons of extra virgin olive oil. Apply the mixture to your face and neck. Leave it on for 15 minutes, then remove it with a warm, wet washcloth and gently pat your skin dry.

- **Dry skin.** In a small bowl, combine 1 tablespoon of extra virgin olive oil, one raw egg yolk, and 1 tablespoon of flour. Add more oil if needed to make the paste thin enough to spread on your face. Apply it to your face and leave it on for 20 minutes. Remove it with a warm, wet washcloth, then gently dry.

- **Oily skin.** In a small bowl, combine 1 cup of uncooked rolled oats, 1/2 cup of plain yogurt, 1 tablespoon of extra virgin olive oil, and 1 tablespoon of kosher or sea salt. Stir well. Apply the paste to your face, massaging in small circles from forehead to chin. Leave it on for 15 minutes, then remove it with a warm, wet washcloth. Rinse your face with cool water, and gently dry.

Magical Moisturizer

If you're looking for an easy, no-frills moisturizer that will leave you glowing, let **OLIVE OIL** work its magic on your skin. Apply the oil to your face, massaging in small circles from forehead to chin. Wait 10 minutes, then rinse with warm water and gently pat dry.

Simple Wrinkle Remover

As we all know, a life well lived involves good days and bad. And over time, the accompanying smiles and frowns begin to leave their mark. Erase those lines with twice-weekly use of this **OLIVE OIL** formula: Start by washing and drying your face. Wait 10 minutes, then spread a thin layer of milk of magnesia on your face with a cotton pad, avoiding the eye area. Let it dry completely, then apply a second layer of milk of magnesia, which will dissolve the first one. After you wipe it all off with a warm, wet washcloth, heat 1/4 cup of extra virgin olive oil in a small pan over low heat until it's just lukewarm. Apply it to your face with a cotton pad and leave it on for five minutes. Remove the oil with a few swipes of refrigerated witch hazel on a cotton ball, and let your skin air-dry.

Oils & Vinegars

Outstanding Olive Oil Facial

Here's a facial treatment that's quick and easy to make and will leave your skin with a wonderful glow. In a small bowl, combine one raw egg yolk and 2 tablespoons of extra virgin **OLIVE OIL**. If you have oily skin, stir in 1 teaspoon of lemon juice. Using your fingertips or a clean makeup brush, apply the mask to your clean face and leave it on for 10 minutes. Rinse with lukewarm water, then cool water, and gently pat your skin dry.

Oil-Reducing Mask

It may sound crazy to treat oily skin with more oil, but this mask will really help cleanse impurities from your skin and tighten your pores. In a small bowl, mix 1 tablespoon of white cosmetic clay (available online) with 1 tablespoon of extra virgin **OLIVE OIL**. Using your fingertips or a clean makeup brush, apply the mask to your clean face and leave it on for 20 to 30 minutes, or until the mask is dry. Remove it with a warm, wet washcloth, then rinse your face with cool water, and gently pat your skin dry. Follow up with a toner and your usual anti-aging moisturizer.

Chapped Lip Fix

Soothe and heal dry, cracked, chapped lips with this **OLIVE OIL** treatment. In a small bowl, combine 1 teaspoon of extra virgin olive oil with $1/2$ teaspoon of sugar and $1/8$ teaspoon of lemon juice. Use your fingertip to massage the scrub across your lips to exfoliate the dead skin. Rinse with lukewarm water, and gently pat your lips dry. Then apply a very thin layer of plain extra virgin olive oil to your lips to keep them soft and smooth.

BEAUTY
Bonus

TAME FLYAWAY STRANDS

If you regularly blow-dry your hair, here's a way to give your dry tresses some of the moisture and shine they've lost from all of that heat processing. Simply rub a few drops of extra virgin **OLIVE OIL** between your palms, and apply it to your flyaway hair ends.

Put on a Sunny Face

SUNFLOWER OIL is a key ingredient in many commercial beauty products for two reasons: It's rich in the moisturizing power of fatty acids and vitamins A, D, and E. Plus, it has a light texture that makes it easy for your skin to absorb. This mask is especially beneficial for dry or aging skin: Mix 2 tablespoons of sunflower oil with half a mashed banana, and apply to your freshly washed face. Leave it on for 20 minutes, then rinse it off with warm water, followed by cool water, and gently pat dry.

Super Sunny Body Scrub

Don't pay big bucks for exfoliating creams and lotions, when you can make this simple formula. In a shatterproof bowl, mix ½ cup of **SUNFLOWER OIL** with enough kosher or sea salt to make a gritty paste. Add a few drops of your favorite essential oil to give it a pleasing scent. Then bring the bowl with you into the shower and rub the mixture over your wet skin—face, hands, elbows, and knees.

Soak in the Sunshine

Here's a relaxing, skin-pleasing bath routine: Add ¼ cup of **SUNFLOWER OIL** and 2 or 3 drops of your favorite essential oil to your bathwater, and settle into the tub. To maximize the softening effect, soak for five minutes first, then add the oils to seal in the moisture. Relax for a half hour, then carefully step out of the tub and pat your skin dry.

Back in the Day...

When your locks have lost their luster, bring back the shine with this old-fashioned **SUNFLOWER OIL** treatment: Shortly before bedtime, mix 2 tablespoons of sunflower oil with two raw egg yolks, and massage the mixture thoroughly into your hair from roots to tips. Cover your head with a shower cap, and leave it on overnight. (Put a towel over your pillowcase to catch any drips.) Come morning, wash the mixture out with your usual shampoo, then follow up by rinsing with a solution of 2 tablespoons of apple cider vinegar in 1 quart of warm water.

Oils & Vinegars

Ditch Dull Skin

Say good-bye to dull, dry skin with this **VEGETABLE OIL** face pack. In a small bowl, combine 2 tablespoons of vegetable oil, 1/2 tablespoon of honey, and 1 teaspoon of lemon juice. Mix until smooth. Apply the mask to your face in small circles from forehead to chin. Remove it with a warm, wet washcloth, then rinse with cool water and gently pat dry.

Beat Back Brittle Nails

In order to fix dried-out nails for good, you have to address the root of the problem, which is too little moisture. So do what dermatologists recommend: At bedtime, massage **VEGETABLE OIL** into your hands and nails, and put on a pair of rubber gloves, which will force the oil to penetrate your skin. Leave the gloves on overnight, and by morning, you should see signs of improvement. Repeat each night until your nails are in good shape. Then perform the procedure once every few weeks, or as needed, to maintain their strength and appearance.

Very Veggie Hair Treat

Want shiny, silky hair? Of course you do! So turn to this treatment for instant results. Heat a cup of **VEGETABLE OIL** in the microwave for 10 seconds, until it's just warm, not hot. Pour the oil over your dry hair, and massage it in from roots to ends. Cover your head with a shower cap or wet towel and leave it on for 30 minutes. Shampoo and condition as usual.

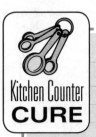

Kitchen Counter CURE

Overnight Heel Repair

Lots of folks suffer from dry, cracked heels, but you don't have to be one of them. This **VEGETABLE OIL** treatment will have your heels soft and smooth in no time at all. The simple fix: Start by washing your feet with warm, soapy water, and use a pumice stone to exfoliate. Dry your feet thoroughly, then rub your heels with a generous amount of vegetable oil, pull on clean cotton socks, and crawl into bed. Come morning, your skin will be noticeably softer. Keep this up until your heels are healed, then continue the treatment several times a week to keep them soft and smooth.

ACV Is OK for Me!

Don't bother with beauty-aisle astringents and toners. **APPLE CIDER VINEGAR** (ACV) has natural alpha hydroxy acids and acetic acid to stimulate circulation and minimize pores, just like those pricey products. In a small bowl, combine 2 cups of cool water with 1 tablespoon of apple cider vinegar. Dip a cotton ball into the bowl, and wipe the mixture over your clean, dry face and allow to air-dry (the scent will vanish quickly).

Balanced Bath

The pH level of **APPLE CIDER VINEGAR** is similar to the pH level of the protective acid mantle layer of our skin, and this soothing soak will help restore balance. Add 1 cup of apple cider vinegar to a bathtub filled with warm water, and soak for 20 minutes or so. No need to rinse afterward; just pat your skin dry.

Razor Bump Remedy

The anti-inflammatory properties of **APPLE CIDER VINEGAR** help soothe irritated skin. Moisten a cotton ball with the vinegar, and gently press it on the rash. For especially aggravated bumps, apply a light layer of honey to the area first, wait five minutes, then rinse, pat dry, and apply the vinegar treatment.

For Whiter, Brighter Teeth...

Try **APPLE CIDER VINEGAR**. Every morning and night, saturate a cotton pad with the vinegar, rub it across your teeth, and rinse thoroughly with clear water.

BEAUTY
Bonus

CURB CELLULITE

If you're trying to get rid of those unsightly "cottage cheese" patches on your skin—that is, cellulite—try **APPLE CIDER VINEGAR** before spending big bucks on spa treatments. Mix 3 tablespoons of apple cider vinegar with 1 tablespoon of olive oil, and massage it into the problem spots for 10 minutes twice a day. This will increase circulation and help reduce the fatty deposits.

Oils & Vinegars

Back in the Day...

For centuries long before Grandma took her very first breath, women have been using **APPLE CIDER VINEGAR** to shine and condition their hair. But with a few herbal additives, you can tailor the treatment to accomplish more than that. All you do is add 1 cup of dried herbs to 1 quart of high-quality vinegar, let the mixture steep for a few weeks, strain out the solids, and pour the liquid into a clean bottle. As for the type of herbs, it really depends on the effect you're looking for. Here's the rundown:

• Calendula is a good, all-around conditioner.

• Chamomile puts highlights in blonde or light brown hair.

• Lavender and lemon verbena add enticing fragrance.

• Nettles control dandruff.

• Parsley and rosemary make dark hair come alive.

• Sage darkens graying hair.

Whichever combo suits your fancy, use the potion as a final rinse after shampooing, at a ratio of roughly 2 tablespoons of herbal vinegar per cup of warm water.

ACV Hair Repair

Over time, hair sprays, gels, and other styling products can build up in your hair, making it dull, drab, and tangle prone. Fortunately, there's a fast, simple way to rout out that residue. Mix equal parts of **APPLE CIDER VINEGAR** and water in a spray bottle. After shampooing, spritz the mixture onto your hair, and massage it into your scalp. Let it sit for three minutes, then rinse with clear water. You'll soon have shiny, silky-smooth hair that's easy to manage.

Time to Shine

Restore your hair's natural luster with **APPLE CIDER VINEGAR**. Mix 1 cup of warm water with 2 tablespoons of vinegar, and pour it over your freshly washed hair. Rinse thoroughly, and follow with a light conditioner.

Down with Dandruff

Bid those flakes "adieu" with the acidic power of **APPLE CIDER VINEGAR**. Simply combine equal parts of vinegar and warm water. Pour the solution over your head and massage it into your scalp. Leave it on for two minutes, then shampoo it out.

Radiant Rice Toner

Oily, acne-prone skin can use all the help it can get, and an assist from **RICE VINEGAR** is one way to stop the breakout cycle and leave your face radiant. In a small bowl, mix 6 tablespoons of lukewarm water with 1 tablespoon of the vinegar. Use a cotton ball to apply it all over your face, then dab more on specific trouble spots and let it air-dry. Use twice a day to clear up your skin and help keep it blemish-free.

Age-Spot Eraser

While you can't stop the aging process, you can slow down its telltale signs, such as dark "liver" or age spots that typically appear on the back of your hands. Mix equal parts of **RICE VINEGAR** and onion juice and use a cotton ball to dab the mixture on each spot. Let it air-dry. Use twice a day until the spots are less noticeable, then once a day to keep them at bay.

Handy Heel Softener

Soften hard, calloused heels with a vigorous **RICE VINEGAR** scrub. In a small bowl, combine 2 tablespoons of the vinegar with 1 tablespoon of honey and 1 tablespoon of kosher or sea salt. Mix well, then apply the paste to your heels, massaging it into the skin for several minutes. Then rinse it off with warm water and thoroughly dry your feet.

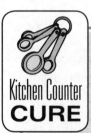

Kitchen Counter CURE

Fungus Fighter

Like other acidic vinegars, **RICE VINEGAR** can change the skin's pH value and soften skin—while fighting the fungi that cause athlete's foot and toenail fungus. Use it as a foot soak by putting equal parts of the vinegar and water in a footbath. Soak your feet for 30 minutes, twice a day. No need to rinse afterward, just thoroughly dry your feet before putting on shoes.

Alternatively, some people have gotten relief from toenail fungus simply by applying undiluted vinegar directly under, over, and around the affected nails.

Cut-the-Oil Cubes

Here's a very cool way to get oily skin under control: Combine equal parts of **WHITE VINEGAR** and water. Pour the solution into a clean ice cube tray and freeze. Every morning, pop out a cube and gently rub it all over your face, from your forehead to your chin, and let your skin air-dry. The vinegar's acidic properties make it an excellent astringent, and the frozen cubes are a great way to tone your skin during those hot and humid summer months.

Anti-Acne Paste

This bedtime treatment combines the healing powers of vinegar and honey and will leave your skin soft and smooth as it fights the bacteria that produce pimples. In a small bowl, combine 2 tablespoons of **WHITE VINEGAR**, 1 tablespoon of flour, and 1 tablespoon of honey. Mix well, adjusting the ingredients until you have a paste-like consistency. Using your fingertips, apply the paste directly onto the acne-prone areas and allow it to air-dry. Then toddle off to bed. In the morning, wash the paste off with lukewarm water, then rinse your face with cool water and dry.

Conserve Your Color

Whether you dye your hair at home, or spend money having it done in the salon, you want that vibrant color to last. Here's one way to prevent hair color from fading. Before washing your hair for the first time after it's been dyed, seal in the color by rinsing your dry hair with a solution of 2 parts cold water and 1 part **WHITE VINEGAR**. And when you do shampoo, use a sulfate-free product, which will also help to prolong color life.

BEAUTY
Bonus

LET NAIL POLISH LINGER LONGER

When you paint your finger-nails and/or toenails, you want the look to last, but before you know it, your polish starts chipping off. Well, you can put a stop to that by adopting this simple prep routine: Soak your nails in **WHITE VINEGAR** for about one minute. Let them air-dry thoroughly, and paint the surfaces as usual. The vinegar will remove the natural oils from the surface of your nails, so instead of chipping off, your polish will hang on tight!

SPOTLIGHT ON
HEAD-TO-TOE BEAUTY

The beauty benefits of using oils and vinegars begin at the very top of your head and end way down at your toes. In fact, they're probably the most versatile ingredients in your pantry. Here's just a handful of the beautifying magic they can perform for you:

◆ **De-stink your feet.** The antiseptic properties of **APPLE CIDER VINEGAR** can help to deodorize and disinfect feet. Plus, its antifungal attributes prevent and combat athlete's foot. Mix 1 cup of vinegar with 4 cups of water in a basin. Soak your feet for 15 minutes, then rinse with warm water and dry them thoroughly before you put on shoes.

◆ **Smooth your body.** This homemade body lotion will last up to two months. Scoop ½ cup of solid **COCONUT OIL** into a microwave-safe bowl. Add 1 tablespoon of grated beeswax. Nuke for short bursts, stirring after each, until the mixture is melted. Add 10 drops of your favorite essential oil and stir well. Let cool for 10 minutes, then add 1 to 2 tablespoons of water and blend with a hand mixer, until it's the consistency of thick pudding. Pour into a clean container with a tight-fitting lid and store away from sunlight.

◆ **Treat your tresses.** For shiny, soft hair, mix one egg yolk with 2 tablespoons of extra virgin **OLIVE OIL** and 1 teaspoon of lemon juice. Pour the mixture over your dry hair, and work it in well from roots to tips. Wait 15 minutes, then shampoo and condition.

◆ **Tame frizz.** Warm ¼ cup of extra virgin **OLIVE OIL** and pour it over your dry hair. Work it in well from roots to tips, then cover your head with a shower cap. Let it sit on your locks for an hour, then shampoo and condition as usual.

◆ **Clean your mitts.** Slicing strawberries, picking blueberries, or dicing beets can stain your hands. And your paws can get mighty grimy from working in the garden, and super stinky from filleting fish. Wash them down with **WHITE VINEGAR** and you'll get them clean faster than if you scrub them with soap and water, and it won't dry out your skin.

Oils & Vinegars

Hydrating Chocolate Mask

Eating dark **CHOCOLATE** does a body good (you can read all about it on page 139). But did you know that putting chocolate on your skin is equally beneficial? Chocolate that is at least 70 percent cacao is loaded with antioxidants, which can help your skin stay younger looking and clear. This mask is one great way to feed your face: Melt one square of dark chocolate in the microwave or in a double boiler. Add one raw egg yolk and 1 tablespoon of extra virgin olive oil, and stir well. Using your fingertips or a clean makeup brush, apply the mask to your face and neck. Leave it on for 15 minutes, then remove it with a warm, wet washcloth, rinse with cool water, and gently dry.

Chocolate Skin Saver

Put the power of **CHOCOLATE** to work on exfoliating dry, rough body parts such as knees, elbows, and heels. Melt five squares of dark chocolate in the microwave or in a double boiler. Add ½ cup of brown sugar and ¼ cup of extra virgin olive oil, and stir until smooth. Using your fingertips, apply the scrub to your rough knees, elbows, and heels, massaging it in for several minutes. Remove it with a warm, wet washcloth, and dry.

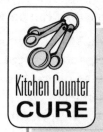

Kitchen Counter **CURE**

A Real Chocolate Smoothie

This tutti-frutti **CHOCOLATE** face mask will remind you of an ice cream topping, but don't eat it! Instead, use it to hydrate and tone your skin.

- **1 square of dark chocolate (at least 70 percent cacao)**
- **3–4 small watermelon cubes, seeds removed**
- **3 fresh strawberries, hulled**
- **2 apple slices, peeled**
- **½ of a ripe banana, peeled**

Melt the chocolate in the microwave. In a blender, combine all of the fruit and blend to a pulp. Pour the pulp into a bowl and stir in the chocolate. Mix well. Apply the paste to your face and neck. Leave it on for 15 minutes, then remove it with a warm, wet washcloth. Rinse with cool water, and pat dry.

Decadent Dessert Mask

Once you've tried this delectable **CHOCOLATE** facial treatment, you'll turn to it again and again for a quick pick-me-up for your face. Melt three dark-chocolate squares in the microwave or in a double boiler, then stir in 1/8 cup of honey, 1 tablespoon of plain Greek-style yogurt, and 2 teaspoons of ground oats (grind uncooked rolled oats in a coffee grinder or food processor). Mix until you have a smooth, creamy paste. Using your fingertips, massage the paste onto your face in small circles from forehead to chin and down your neck. Leave it on for 15 minutes, then remove it with a warm, wet washcloth. Rinse with cool water, and gently pat your skin dry.

Healthy Hair Helper

You probably haven't thought about putting **CHOCOLATE** on your hair, but maybe you should. Here's why: Antioxidant-rich dark chocolate can help boost blood circulation to your scalp, which encourages hair growth. And besides, it makes your hair incredibly shiny and smooth. Just melt three squares of dark chocolate in the microwave or in a double boiler, let it cool slightly, and then vigorously rub it into your wet scalp. Leave it on for three minutes, then shampoo and condition as usual.

HOW'S THAT?

Q *My friend swears by her homemade* CHOCOLATE *pedicures. Is chocolate really good for your feet?*

A It sure is! As long as the chocolate is dark (at least 70 percent cacao). Try this simple treatment and see for yourself: Melt two squares of dark chocolate in the microwave or in a double boiler. Let it cool down a bit, then stir in 1 tablespoon of kosher or sea salt. Put a towel under your just-washed and slightly damp feet to catch any drips, and scoop up the chocolate scrub with your hands. Massage it well into your feet, paying attention to dry heels. Leave it on for 10 minutes, then remove it with a warm, wet washcloth, rinse with lukewarm water, and thoroughly dry your tootsies.

A Honey of a Healer

This **HONEY** mask is ideal for oily, acne-prone skin. It contains sage, which helps clear up blemishes, and the honey soothes congested skin. Start by coring an unpeeled apple and cut it into slices. Put the slices in a food processor or blender, and add 2 tablespoons of warmed honey (warm it in the microwave until it becomes runny, but not hot) and 1/2 teaspoon of fresh sage. Puree until you have a smooth paste. Put the paste in the refrigerator for 20 to 30 minutes. Apply the cooled paste to your face and neck. Lie down and relax for 30 minutes, then remove it with a warm, wet washcloth. Rinse with cool water, and gently pat your skin dry.

Spicy Complexion Clearer

Add a little spice to your life, er, face mask, and wake up to clearer skin! At bedtime, warm up 2 tablespoons of **HONEY** in the microwave until it's runny, but not hot. Stir in 1 teaspoon of fresh-squeezed lemon juice, 1/4 teaspoon of ground cinnamon, and 1/4 teaspoon of ground nutmeg, mixing until you have a smooth paste. Using your fingertips, apply the paste to your face and neck, massaging in small circles. Wait 15 minutes, then remove it with a warm, wet washcloth. Rinse with cool water, and pat your skin dry.

BEAUTY
Bonus

ICE THE BURN

This skin treatment is actually a frozen **HONEY**-sicle. Use it as a cooling facial cleanser in the summer, or as a super soother for sunburned skin anywhere on your body. Start by whipping one egg until it's frothy. Heat 1/2 cup of solid coconut oil in the microwave until it's just melted, but not hot. Slowly pour the liquid coconut oil and 1 tablespoon of honey (warm it up to make it runny) into the whipped egg. Mix gently until you get a creamy consistency. Stand an empty toilet paper roll in a small bowl and spoon the mixture into the cardboard roll. Leaving it in the bowl, put the whole shebang in the freezer overnight. The next day, peel off the cardboard and use the honey stick to clean your face and neck, or gently rub it anywhere you have sunburn. Leave it on for five minutes, then remove it with a cool, wet washcloth and dry. Cover the stick with plastic wrap or put it in a ziplock freezer bag, and store it in the freezer for future use.

Fountain of Youth Mask

Nothing can make you look 25 (or even 40) forever. But this once-a-week mask has been known to keep women's skin looking soft, smooth, and firm well into their senior years. In a small bowl, thoroughly mix 2 tablespoons of heavy cream, 1 tablespoon of **HONEY**, and the contents of one vitamin E capsule. Spread it onto your face and neck, and leave it in place for 20 minutes. Then rinse it off with lukewarm water, and gently pat your skin dry. Before long, your friends will be demanding to know where you found the Fountain of Youth!

Out, Out, Darn Spots!

There are many natural spot-removal remedies floating around (and a few in this book), but this is one of the simplest and gentlest: Once a day, mix 1 teaspoon of **HONEY** with 1 teaspoon of plain yogurt. Apply the mixture to the problem areas, and let it dry. Then wait another 30 minutes, and wash it off with lukewarm water.

Say "Bye-Bye, Blackheads"

Here's a sweet way to banish blackheads: Just heat about 1/8 cup of **HONEY** until it's lukewarm, and dab it onto your blemishes. Let it sit for a couple of minutes, wash it off with warm water, and rinse with cool water. Pat your skin dry, and follow up with your usual moisturizer.

Back in the Day...

The classic milk and honey cleanser has been around since Cleopatra's time for good reason—the milk soothes while the honey attracts moisture and keeps it within your skin. Warm up 1 teaspoon of dark **HONEY** until it becomes runny, but not hot. Stir in 1 tablespoon of whole milk or cream. Mix well, then using your fingertips, apply the cleanser to your face and neck. Leave it on for 20 minutes, then remove it with a warm, wet washcloth. Rinse with cool water, gently pat your skin dry, and apply your usual moisturizer to lock in the goodness.

Blackstrap Beautifier

When you think of **MOLASSES**, you probably conjure up images of delicious cookies. Well, it's time to rethink this pantry staple. Why? Because blackstrap molasses is chock-full of minerals that can do wonders for your skin. So treat your face to this simple mask: Apply about 1 tablespoon of blackstrap molasses to your face, massaging in small circles from forehead to chin. Leave it on for 15 minutes, then remove it with a warm, wet washcloth. Rinse with cool water, and pat dry.

Mighty Fine Molasses Mask

This facial mask will tighten and tone your skin and leave you glowing. In a medium bowl, mix ½ cup of uncooked rolled oats, 2 tablespoons of honey, and 2 tablespoons of blackstrap **MOLASSES**. Pour in enough boiling water and stir to make an oatmeal consistency. Let the mixture cool down until it is just warm, and then scoop up the mask with your fingertips. Apply it to your face and neck, massaging in small circles. Leave it on until it is completely dry, then remove it with a warm, wet washcloth. Rinse with cool water, and pat dry.

Intensive Molasses Hair Conditioner

This treatment works wonders for revitalizing dry, brittle, and heat-damaged hair. Whisk together 3 tablespoons of cold-pressed sweet almond oil (available online), 1 tablespoon of blackstrap **MOLASSES**, and two raw egg yolks. Add 2 teaspoons of aloe vera gel and stir to form a smooth paste. Apply the mixture to your dry hair, and cover your head with a plastic shower cap, topped with a warm towel. Leave it on for 30 minutes, then rinse with warm water and let your hair air-dry.

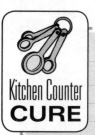

Kitchen Counter CURE

Reverse the Gray

Here's good news: Blackstrap **MOLASSES** may actually reverse the graying process. The recommended dose is 1 to 2 tablespoons each day, first thing in the morning. You can take it straight from the spoon, spread it on toast, or mix it into herbal tea. You could start getting results in as little as two weeks.

Hey, Sugar, How 'Bout a Scrub?

Sure, there are a lot of fancy facial scrubs in the beauty aisles, but don't be tempted. Instead, head into the kitchen and whip up an all-natural scrub, like this one: In a bowl, combine 5 tablespoons of brown **SUGAR**; 1/4 of a medium cucumber, grated; 1 tablespoon of extra virgin olive oil; and 1/2 teaspoon of vitamin E oil. Stir until you have a smooth paste. Massage the paste on your clean face for several minutes. Rinse it off with lukewarm water, then cool water, and gently pat your skin dry.

BEAUTY Bonus

REMOVE A FADING FAKE TAN

Self-tanning products can give you a great faux glow—until it starts to fade, which leaves your skin dry, patchy, and flaky. You could resort to a commercial tan remover, or you could take this more natural approach. In a bowl, mix 1 cup of raw **SUGAR** (available in health-food stores and supermarkets) with 3/4 cup of lemon juice. Rub the mixture over your skin, and leave it on for a few minutes. Rinse it off with warm water, pat your skin dry, and apply your usual moisturizer.

Sweet Cheeks

Granulated **SUGAR** might not be good for the *inside* of your body, but *outside* it can do a couple of big favors for your face. Reach for the sweet stuff when you want to:

- **Clear up pimples.** Just mix a spoonful of sugar with a few drops of water, and dab it onto the spots.

- **Supercharge your cleanser.** Add 1 teaspoon of sugar to the lather when you wash your face.

Sweet-and-Sour Body Scrub

This rub will make your skin feel squeaky clean and satiny soft all over. In a shatterproof bowl, combine 1/2 cup of brown **SUGAR**, 1 teaspoon of honey, and the juice of half a small lemon. Bring the mixture into the shower and gently massage it all over your dry body, then rinse it off with warm water and pat dry. No need to moisturize afterward because your skin will be soft and smooth.

Sugar Water Cleanser

Exfoliate and cleanse your skin with this **SUGAR** and water combo: Add 1 heaping tablespoon of granulated sugar to ½ cup of warm water and stir to completely dissolve. Massage the sugar water onto your face in small circles from forehead to chin. Leave it on for 15 minutes, then remove it with a warm, wet washcloth, rinse with cool water, and pat dry.

Sugar-and-Spice Body Scrub

When you buy a commercial body scrub, there's no telling what chemicals might be in it. But this one's so safe, you could eat it! In a large bowl, combine 1 cup of brown **SUGAR**, 1 cup of granulated sugar, ¾ cup of almond oil or melted coconut oil, and 2 teaspoons each of ground cinnamon, ground ginger, and ground nutmeg. Mix thoroughly, then spoon it into a plastic container with a tight-fitting lid and keep it in the bathroom. At bath time, scoop out a small handful of the blend, and massage it all over your damp body. Then rinse with warm water.

I Gotta Hand It to You . . .

And here it is—my extra-strength hand cleaner for those times when work or play leaves you with grimy paws. In a bowl, mix 2 ½ cups of granulated **SUGAR**, 1 cup of extra virgin olive oil, and 4 tablespoons of lemon juice to make a gritty paste. Pour it into a container with a tight-fitting lid, and stash it somewhere handy in your kitchen, workshop, or garage, and reach for it whenever you need to clean up fast.

Back in the Day...

While commercial hair sprays have been around for ages, the age-old problem of spray buildup that makes hair dull and lifeless hasn't gone away. So give this time-tested, all-natural, gunk-free alternative a try: Dissolve 1 tablespoon of granulated **SUGAR** in 1 cup of hot distilled water, and mix in 1 tablespoon of vodka to act as a preservative. Pour the potion into a plastic spray bottle, and use it as you would any other hair spray.

SPOTLIGHT ON SWEET BEAUTY TREATS

For most of us, eating sweets is a guilty pleasure, and one that we try hard not to indulge in too often. But there's no reason to feel guilty about using sweets on your face and body. In fact, it's just what the dermatologist ordered because sweets such as chocolate, honey, molasses, and sugar are very beneficial to your skin. Here are just a few ways to sweeten the deal:

◆ **Moisturize your face.** Heat two dark-**CHOCOLATE** squares in the microwave until just melted. Stir well, then allow the chocolate to cool slightly. Using a clean makeup brush, apply the chocolate to your face from your forehead to your chin, avoiding the eye area. Wait five minutes, then remove it with a warm, wet washcloth, and gently pat your skin dry.

◆ **Clean and shrink your pores.** Mix 2 tablespoons of **HONEY** with 1 tablespoon of baking soda. Splash your face with warm water, then use your fingertips to gently massage the scrub on your face in small circles from your forehead to your chin. Remove it with a warm, wet washcloth, rinse with cool water, and gently pat dry.

◆ **Get soft, shiny hair.** Wet your hair and work in about ¼ cup of **MOLASSES** from roots to tips. Leave it on for at least 30 minutes, then rinse thoroughly with warm water. Shampoo and condition.

◆ **Smooth your lips.** Put a little water on your finger, then dip it in granulated **SUGAR** and gently apply it in a circular motion to your lips. The sugar will slough off dry, flaky skin.

◆ **Get a closer shave.** Whether it's your face, legs, or underarms, exfoliating dead skin cells helps the razor make a closer cut. Apply slightly wet brown **SUGAR** to your skin, working it in with a circular motion. Then rinse it off with warm water and start shaving.

◆ **Soften your feet.** In a shatterproof bowl, mix ½ cup of raw **SUGAR** with a few drops of peppermint oil, then bring it into the shower. Scrub the mixture onto your wet feet to slough off dead skin cells and soften rough heels.

Sweeteners

Brightening Beet Treatment

Give your face a youthful glow with this invigorating scrub. Finely grate three slices of peeled fresh **BEET** into a bowl. Stir in 2 tablespoons of ground oats (grind uncooked rolled oats in a coffee grinder or food processor) until you have a thick paste. If the beet isn't juicy, add a few drops of warm water to the mixture. Apply the mask to your face, massaging in small circles from forehead to chin. Wait 10 minutes, then remove it with a warm, wet washcloth. Rinse with cool water, and dry.

Best Beet Beautifier

Here's a simple way to freshen your face and get into the pink of health. Cook one **BEET** in boiling water until soft, and use a potato masher to mash the beet into a pulp. Then use a clean makeup brush to apply the pulp evenly to your face and neck. Lie down and relax for 30 minutes before washing it all off with lukewarm water, and gently dry.

Beat Dry Skin

If you've tried everything to combat dry skin, beat it once and for all with **BEETS**. Finely grate three slices of peeled fresh beet into a bowl. Add 2 tablespoons of plain whole-milk yogurt and 2 teaspoons of almond oil. Stir well. Apply the mix to your face with your fingertips. Leave it on for 10 minutes, then remove it with a warm, wet washcloth. Rinse with cool water, and gently dry.

BEAUTY
Bonus

YOU CAN'T BEAT BEET BLUSH

That is, if you're looking for a super-simple and ultra-healthy way to color your cheeks. Just cut a small red **BEET** in half, and rub the cut side over your cheekbones until you get the shade you want. Then, for good measure, run a cotton swab over the beet's surface, and smooth the juice onto your lips to tint them rosy red. If you want a glossier look, finish by dabbing on a bit of solid coconut oil.

Outstanding Onion Mask

Using **ONIONS** on your skin is just as beneficial as including them in your diet (see page 146 for more on onions' health-giving properties). For this facial mask and many of the recipes in this section, you'll need fresh onion juice; see "Easy Onion Juicing" (below) for instructions. This facial mask exfoliates and brightens your skin. In a small bowl, combine 2 tablespoons of flour, 1 1/2 tablespoons of fresh onion juice, 1/2 teaspoon of milk, and a pinch of ground nutmeg. Stir to form a thick paste, adding more flour or milk as needed. Using your fingertips or a clean makeup brush, apply the mask to your clean face and neck. Leave it on for 20 minutes, or until it's completely dry. Then dab some milk on your face and massage in small circles to help dissolve the mask. Finish by removing it with a warm, wet washcloth, then rinse with cool water and gently pat your skin dry.

Brighten Up with Onions

You can lighten and brighten your skin with this treatment: Puree one peeled, chopped pear, 1/4 cup of whole milk, and 2 tablespoons of fresh **ONION** juice (see "Easy Onion Juicing," below) in a blender or food processor. Using your fingertips or a clean makeup brush, apply the mixture to your freshly cleaned face, and leave it on for 20 minutes. Rinse it off with lukewarm water, and follow up with your usual moisturizer. Repeat two or three times a week.

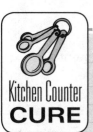

Kitchen Counter CURE

Easy Onion Juicing

Don't waste your money on store-bought bottled **ONION** juice. Instead, make your own so it's fresh when you need it. Just grate one or more raw onions, or chop them finely in a food processor, squeeze the pieces through cheesecloth, and pour the liquid into a jar with a tight-fitting lid. You can store it in the refrigerator for up to two weeks. Just remember, the juice loses its potency quickly, so for best results, make only as much as you'll use within a day or two.

Cure Complexion Woes

Although acne is infamous for targeting teenagers, almost anyone can break out in annoying pimples. One simple cure: Slice a medium-size **ONION** and simmer it in ¹/₂ cup of honey until the onion is soft. Then puree the mixture in a blender or food processor (or mash it by hand) to make a paste. Let it cool to room temperature, and dab it on the blemishes. Leave it on for at least 60 minutes, rinse it off with warm water, and gently pat your skin dry. Repeat the routine every evening until a clear face stares back at you in the mirror.

Another Way to Tackle Acne

To treat large areas of acned skin, give this full-face mask a try: Peel, chop, and heat seven plums until their flesh is soft. (You can do the job in either the microwave or a conventional oven.) Mash the fruit, and mix it with 1 tablespoon of **ONION** juice (see "Easy Onion Juicing" on page 329) and 2 teaspoons of extra virgin olive oil. Using your fingertips or a clean makeup brush, spread the mixture evenly onto your just-washed face, and leave it on for 30 minutes or so. Remove it with lukewarm water, rinse with cool water, and gently pat your skin dry. Follow up with an oil-free moisturizer. This mask is also good for treating acne that is on your back and/or shoulders.

Back in the Day...

Here's a real old-time, farm-fresh facial treatment that women have been using for decades to tone, nourish, and soften their skin: In a small bowl, mix 1 tablespoon each of carrot juice, **ONION** juice, and extra virgin olive oil, and add one raw egg yolk, stirring until well combined. Using your fingertips or a clean makeup brush, apply the mask to your face and neck. Leave it on for 20 minutes, then wash it off with lukewarm water, rinse with cool water, and gently pat your skin dry. Repeat weekly for best results.

Hold On to Your Hair

You'd think that by now, some genius would have come up with a pill to prevent hair loss. Unfortunately, at least so far, there is no foolproof solution. There are, however, plenty of homemade formulas, and some of the most effective ones feature **ONIONS** in the starring role. Here's a pair of choices that just might keep the hair on your head from fading fast:

- Slice a raw onion in two, and massage your scalp with the cut surface. Cover your head with a shower cap, and leave it on overnight. Then shampoo and rinse your hair thoroughly. Repeat three times a week.

- Mix 1/4 cup of onion juice (see "Easy Onion Juicing" on page 329) with 1 tablespoon of raw honey, and massage the mixture into your scalp every day. Then shampoo and condition as usual.

> # BEAUTY
> ## Bonus
> ### A RUMMY GOOD KEEPER
>
> If you're lucky enough to have held on to a full (or almost-full!) head of hair, count your blessings. And help keep those locks in place with this simple routine: Chop a medium-size **ONION** and soak it overnight, peels and all, in 8 ounces of dark rum (don't refrigerate it). Strain out the solids, and massage the liquid into your scalp. Then shampoo, condition, and style your hair as usual. Repeat the procedure every week.

Skins for Soft Tresses

Believe it or not, **ONION** skins can soften your hair and enhance its color. Put 2 1/2 cups of lightly packed onion peels in a pan, and pour 1 quart of boiling water over them. Steep, covered, for 50 minutes. Strain the brew into a fresh container, and let it cool to room temperature. Then wash your hair as usual, and towel-dry it slightly. With your head over a basin to catch the runoff, rinse three or four times with the onion-skin tea. Finish by rinsing with clear water. Use this treatment weekly to keep your hair amazingly silky, and help minimize the gray.

This Spud's for You

Rejuvenate your tired, aging skin with a **POTATO**. Simply peel and finely grate a small spud into a bowl. Add enough warm water (or a scented version like rose water) to make a paste. Then stir in 1 teaspoon of warmed honey and mix well. Using your fingertips, apply the paste to your face and leave it on for 15 minutes. Remove it with a warm, wet washcloth, rinse with cool water, and gently pat your skin dry.

Give Your Face a Lift

This intensive anti-wrinkle mask is especially tailored for dry skin. To make it, boil a peeled, medium-size **POTATO** in 1 cup of whole milk until the spud is soft. Mash it, and mix in 1 tablespoon each of onion juice (see "Easy Onion Juicing" on page 329) and honey. After washing your face as usual, smooth the blend onto your face and neck. Wait 20 minutes, then rinse thoroughly with lukewarm water, gently pat your skin dry, and apply your normal moisturizer.

Erase Dark Circles

POTATOES are natural under-eye brighteners, so applying them directly on the affected area can banish dark eye rings. Here's how to perk up your peepers: Peel and slice one raw potato. Lie down and place one potato slice over each eye. Rest for 20 minutes, then remove the slices, splash your eyes with cool water, and very gently pat them dry.

HOW'S THAT?

Q *I've heard that POTATOES are good for your skin, but are there any hair treatments that use potatoes?*

A Yes, indeed, there are. Here's one way to use spuds to put highlights in brown locks. Boil a large, unpeeled baking potato in a quart of water, then dip a pastry brush in the liquid, and saturate your hair. (Be careful not to get the spud water in your eyes!) Wait for 30 minutes, then rinse with cool water. Repeat every two to three weeks to retain the "spudtacular" highlights.

SPOTLIGHT ON
HEALTHY HAIR

You wash it, condition it, spray it, and probably dye it, too. So you can't really be surprised when a bad-hair day turns into a bad-hair month. Reverse the ill effects of that not-always-good attention you've been paying to your hair, and use some or all of these treatments to coax it back to good health:

◆ **Defeat dandruff.** Good old red **BEETS** can help in healing a flaking, itchy scalp. Finely shred a raw beet over a small bowl. Add 2 tablespoons of apple cider vinegar, and stir to form a pulp. Apply it to your dry hair and leave it on for 15 minutes. Then shampoo it out and condition as usual.

◆ **Keep baldness at bay.** While it may not be possible to cure full-scale baldness, the compounds in **ONIONS** help remove toxins from your body and stimulate blood circulation, both of which strengthen hair follicles and minimize hair loss. Simply add 2 tablespoons of onion juice (see "Easy Onion Juicing" on page 329) to a bottle of your regular shampoo, and use it as you always do. (Just be sure to shake the bottle well before each use.)

◆ **Combat hair loss** with a **POTATO** and honey treatment. Finely grate one peeled raw potato over a bowl. Press the grated potato through a sieve to extract the juice. In a small bowl, mix 2 tablespoons of potato juice with 2 tablespoons of aloe vera gel and 1 tablespoon of warmed honey. Apply this mixture to your dry scalp and massage it in well. Cover your head with a shower cap and leave it on for two hours, then wash and condition your hair as usual. Do this twice a week for best results.

◆ **Bring back the shine.** Finely grate one peeled raw **POTATO** over a bowl. Press the grated potato through a sieve to extract the juice into another small bowl. Beat in one raw egg and 3 drops of lemon juice and stir to mix well. Apply the mixture to your dry hair from roots to tips and leave it on for 20 minutes. Then wash your hair with regular shampoo and condition it as usual. Your hair will look healthy and shiny.

Vegetables

Pretty Pointers from the Pantry

Forever Young Fig Mask

Their claim to fame is delicious Newton cookies, but **FIGS** can also cleanse and exfoliate skin with their active fruit enzymes. So put the power of figs to work for you with this quick and easy face mask: Smash four ripe figs in a bowl, then stir in a heaping tablespoon of plain whole-milk yogurt. Using your fingertips or a clean makeup brush, apply the mask to your face from your forehead to your chin. Wait five minutes, then remove it with a warm, wet washcloth, rinse with cool water, and gently pat dry.

Fantastic Fig Scrub

Revive dull, drab skin with **FIGS**. Cut two ripe figs in half and scoop out the pulp into a small bowl. Add 2 tablespoons of fresh orange juice, 1 tablespoon of granulated sugar, and a few drops of extra virgin olive oil, and stir to make a smooth paste. Using your fingertips, apply the paste to your face, massaging in small circles from your forehead to your chin. Remove with a warm, wet washcloth, rinse with cool water, and pat your skin dry. By the way, you can multiply the ingredients to make enough paste for a whole-body scrub.

BEAUTY
Bonus

FAST FIG FIXES

You don't have to fuss with **FIGS** to extract their beauty-giving potential. Here are a few super-simple ways to use fresh figs, and all you have to do is slice them:

Exfoliate. Cut a fresh fig in half, and scoop out the pulp and set it aside. Take the empty peel and rub the inside of it on your face, from your forehead to your chin. Rinse with lukewarm water, and gently pat your skin dry.

Moisturize. Slice a fresh fig in half, scoop out the pulp, and massage it onto your face. Leave it on for five minutes, then remove it with a warm, wet washcloth. Rinse your face with cool water, and gently pat your skin dry.

Soothe. Moisturize dry, cracked lips by rubbing a dab of fig pulp over them to restore their kissably soft suppleness.

CHAPTER 9

Spice Rack Radiance

Most of us are familiar with the old nursery rhyme saying, "Sugar and spice, and everything nice, that's what little girls are made of." Well, big girls can get good use out of sugar and spice, too! And while there are hundreds of recipes for homemade beauty treatments that contain spices, herbs, and seasonings, we've already done the hard part for you, and winnowed out the best, so you can spice up your beauty routine!

HERBS & SPICES

Straight-Up Scrub

Here's a recipe for a simple face scrub: Mix 1 tablespoon of honey, 1 teaspoon of granulated sugar, and 1 teaspoon of ground **CINNAMON**. Apply it to your face, scrubbing in circular motions from forehead to chin. Rinse with lukewarm water, then cool water, and gently pat your face dry. *Note: Cinnamon can irritate sensitive skin, so before you use this mask or any other cinnamon treatment in this book, apply a dab of the mixture to the inside of your elbow. Wait 10 minutes before proceeding, just to make sure you have no adverse reaction.*

Beautifying Breakfast Mix

Imagine mixing together banana, cinnamon, and yogurt—sounds like a healthy breakfast, right? Well, these ingredients are also the basis of a great beauty treat for your face. This rich mask hydrates your skin and makes it smooth. Start by mashing one ripe banana in a bowl. Add 2 tablespoons of plain whole-milk yogurt, 1/2 teaspoon of ground **CINNAMON**, and 1/2 teaspoon of lemon juice. Stir to make a smooth paste. Apply it to your clean face. Leave it on for 15 minutes, then remove it with a warm, wet washcloth. Rinse with cool water and pat dry.

Bye-Bye, Blemishes

This mask packs a heck of a punch against acne, taking advantage of the antimicrobial properties of **CINNAMON** and honey. Mix 1 1/2 teaspoons of ground cinnamon with 1 tablespoon of honey to make a paste. Apply it to your face, massaging in small circles from forehead to chin. Leave it on for 15 minutes, then rinse it off with lukewarm water, and gently pat your skin dry.

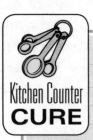

Kitchen Counter
CURE

Super Scented Scrub

Coffee and **CINNAMON** team up to make this super scrub that not only smells great, but will also perk up your skin. So save your morning coffee grounds, let them dry, and use them to make this exfoliating all-over body scrub.

> 1/2 cup of brown sugar
> 1/2 cup of dried coffee grounds
> 1/3 cup of coconut* or sunflower oil
> 1 tsp. of ground cinnamon

Mix all of the ingredients together in a bowl, then spoon the scrub into a clean shatterproof jar with a tight-fitting lid. To use, step into the shower and scoop a generous amount into your hand. Rub your hands together, then apply the scrub all over your dry body, working in small circles. Rinse off with warm water, and pat your skin dry. *If using coconut oil, warm it so it's just soft enough to mix. Don't get it hot; otherwise it'll dissolve the sugar and will be useless as an exfoliant.*

Triple Play for Oily Skin

Balance, moisturize, and stimulate your complexion with this oh-so-fabulous facial mask that curbs oil without overly drying your skin. Warm 2 tablespoons of honey in a small heat-proof bowl by setting it in hot water just until the honey liquefies. Then add 1 teaspoon of fresh-squeezed lemon juice, 1/4 teaspoon of ground **CINNAMON**, and 1/4 teaspoon of nutmeg, and mix to form a smooth paste. Apply it to your clean face and neck, avoiding the eye area. Leave it on for 15 minutes, then remove it with a warm, wet washcloth. Rinse with cool water, and gently dry.

Soothe Stressed Skin

As we all know, emotional stress can take a toll on your body—and, as your body's biggest organ, your skin is no exception. This DIY facial not only calms your complexion, but also reduces swelling and redness and sloughs off dead skin cells. To make the mask, mix 1 teaspoon of ground **CINNAMON** and 1 teaspoon of ground nutmeg in 2 tablespoons of warm honey to form a thick paste. Apply it evenly to your face and leave it on for 30 minutes. Wash it off with a warm, wet washcloth, then rinse with cool water and gently pat your skin dry.

BEAUTY
Bonus

DIY FACE BRONZERS

Commercial bronzers can cost a pretty penny. Plus, you never know what chemicals or other substances you might be putting on your face. So here are two better ideas, straight from your spice rack:

Pretty powder. Put a few teaspoons of cornstarch into a bowl, and mix in pinches of ground **CINNAMON**, cocoa powder, and ground nutmeg until you get the shade you like. Pour the final product into a small tin or empty makeup case and apply it with a makeup brush.

Cute and creamy. Combine small amounts of ground cinnamon, cocoa powder, and cornstarch until you have a color that looks good on your skin. Then add a bit of unscented face or body lotion and stir well. Let the mixture sit for 20 minutes, stir again, and spoon it into a clean jar with a tight-fitting lid. Store the cream in the refrigerator. To use, apply the bronzer with your fingertips.

Color Boost for Brunettes

Give dull brown hair a new lease on life with this easy mixture. It adds shine and highlights to lackluster locks while you sleep: About an hour before you go to bed, pour some of your regular hair conditioner into a bowl, measuring out the same amount you would use after shampooing. Stir in a generous tablespoon of ground **CINNAMON** and mix well. Wash and towel-dry your hair, then apply the spicy conditioner and comb it through your hair. You want to achieve even distribution to avoid streaking. Put on a shower cap, and retire for the evening (cover your pillow with a towel to catch any stray drips). In the morning, thoroughly rinse out your hair, but don't shampoo it. Then dry and style it as usual.

Rise and Shine Hair Treatment

Start your day with this soothing treatment and your hair will reward you by looking its shiny, bouncy best. In a small bowl, combine 1/2 cup of your regular conditioner, 2 teaspoons of ground **CINNAMON**, and 2 teaspoons of honey. Stir well. Wash and towel-dry your hair, then apply the conditioner to the top of your head and work it through your hair from roots to tips. Put on a shower cap and relax for one hour. Rinse your hair well, but don't shampoo. Then dry and style it as usual.

Back in the Day...

When cold weather put the chill right through us, Grandma Putt made sure she had plenty of this bath blend on hand. It not only warms you up, but helps you relax and leaves your skin silky smooth. But don't wait for bad weather to treat yourself to this soothing mixture. In a plastic container with a tight-fitting lid, combine 1 cup of baking soda, 1 cup of dry milk, 3 tablespoons of cornstarch, 2 tablespoons of cream of tartar, and 1 1/2 tablespoons of ground **CINNAMON**. At bath time, shake the container to make sure the contents are blended, and pour about 1/2 cup of the mixture into a tub of water. Then settle in for a good, long soak.

Hello, Cloves...

And good-bye, blemishes! Put the power of **CLOVES** to work on clearing up your breakout-prone skin. This spice helps put a halt to acne thanks to eugenol, a natural antiseptic that can prevent future breakouts. Here's the easy recipe for a skin-clearing mask: Combine 1 teaspoon of ground cloves, 1 teaspoon of honey, and 3 drops of fresh-squeezed lemon juice in a small bowl. Using your fingertips or a clean makeup brush, apply the mixture to your face from forehead to chin. Leave it on for 20 minutes, then remove it with a warm, wet washcloth. Rinse with cool water, and gently pat your skin dry.

Step Right Up to a Steamy Facial

Get your skin deep-down clean and free of airborne toxins with this rejuvenating facial. Start by washing your face and patting it dry. Put 4 cups of water into a saucepan and bring it to a boil. Add ⅓ cup of aniseed, ⅓ cup of whole **CLOVES**, and 3 to 5 drops of peppermint oil to the water. Boil for two more minutes. Remove the pan from the heat, cover, and steep for five minutes. Carefully pour the steamy blend into a large bowl, put your face over it, and cover your head and the bowl with a towel. Keep your eyes closed and let the steam work its magic for three to five minutes, or until the water has cooled. Then gently pat your skin dry.

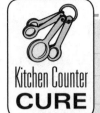

Kitchen Counter CURE

Condition and Color

If you have brown or auburn hair, this recipe is just what you need to rev up your drab locks. Warm ½ cup of olive oil in a saucepan over low heat. Add 2 tablespoons of ground **CLOVES**, and heat until the mixture is hot, but not boiling. Remove the pan from the stove, put the lid on, and let it sit overnight. The next day, strain the liquid into a plastic bottle with a dispenser top (a clean shampoo or conditioner bottle is perfect). To use, squirt a bit of the mixture onto one of your palms, and rub it between your hands to warm it up. Work the potion into your scalp, and comb it through to the ends of your hair. Cover your head with a plastic shower cap, and go about your business for 20 minutes. Then rinse the oil out, and shampoo as usual.

Get Cute with Cumin

This face mask contains **CUMIN** and will give your skin a natural glow. In a small bowl, combine ¼ cup of warmed honey, 3 tablespoons of finely ground organic turmeric, and 1 tablespoon of finely ground organic cumin. Stir to mix well. Apply the mask to your face, massaging in small circles. Leave it on until it's completely dry, then remove it with a warm, wet washcloth. Rinse with cool water, and gently pat your skin dry.

Fantastic Face Pack

Soothe sunburned skin with this cool pack, which also helps calm breakout-prone skin. Put ¼ cup of very cold plain yogurt in a small bowl. Stir in 3 tablespoons of finely ground organic turmeric and 1 tablespoon of finely ground organic **CUMIN**. Mix well, then slather the pack evenly on your face and neck. Leave it on for five minutes, then rinse it off with cool water and pat dry.

BEAUTY
Bonus

HAIR'S TO CUMIN!

Silky, smooth hair is just a shampoo away when you use this **CUMIN** concoction. Bring 1 cup of water to a boil. Stir in 1½ tablespoons of whole cumin seeds, remove from the heat, and let steep for 10 minutes. When the mixture is warm, strain out the seeds. Add one raw egg yolk and mix until creamy. Pour the mixture over your hair, and massage it well into your scalp and down from roots to tips. Put on a shower cap and leave it on for 30 minutes. Wash with a mild shampoo and dry.

Smooth, Tone, and Heal

The antibacterial and hydrating powers of **CUMIN** team up to deliver a terrific toner that heals blemishes and helps prevent wrinkles. To make it, bring 3 cups of water to a boil in a saucepan, toss in a handful of whole cumin seeds, reduce the heat, and steep for three minutes. Strain out the seeds, let the liquid cool to room temperature, and mix in a few drops of tea tree and lavender oils. Pour the potion into a dark-colored glass bottle with a tight-fitting lid, and refrigerate. Apply the toner to your clean face morning and evening.

Clarifying Nutmeg Toner

Here's a simple way to soothe and refresh tired skin. In a small bowl, combine 3 tablespoons of whole milk with ½ tablespoon of ground **NUTMEG** and stir well. Using a cotton ball, apply the toner to your clean face, sweeping from your forehead to your chin. Repeat the application several times, until you've used up the toner. Leave it on until it dries completely, then rinse off the toner with cool water and gently pat your skin dry.

Tame Troubled Skin

When your acne flares up and is painful to the touch, this home remedy will ease the pain while it babies your skin. In a small bowl, mix 2 teaspoons of ground **NUTMEG** with a few drops of water until you have a paste. Using your fingertips, apply it evenly to your face, focusing on the breakouts. Leave it on until it dries completely, then, with wet fingers, massage your skin in small circles before removing the paste with lukewarm water. Rinse with cool water, and gently pat your face dry. Continue this treatment for up to three weeks to clear your skin.

HOW'S THAT?

Q *Jerry, I was cleaning out our pantry and found an unopened box of dry milk that was past its expiration date. I was about to toss it, but my sister told me I could put it to good use in a facial. She and I concocted our own mix, making it up as we went along. It was fun, but we ended up creating more of a mess than a good facial! Do you have a recipe I can follow?*

A I sure do, and not only is it a snap to whip up, but it also includes the skin-rejuvenating powers of **NUTMEG**. Mix 3 tablespoons of dry milk, 1 tablespoon of baking soda, and ½ tablespoon of ground nutmeg in a bowl. Then stir in a few drops of water until you have a paste. Apply it to your clean face and neck, and let it dry completely. Remove it with a warm, wet washcloth, and gently pat your skin dry. I think you'll like the results!

Thyme for Beauty

Reap the anti-inflammatory and antibacterial benefits of **THYME** with this soothing face mask. In a small bowl, smash one ripe banana. Add ¼ cup of plain yogurt, 3 tablespoons of chopped fresh thyme, and 2 tablespoons of honey. Stir well until you have a smooth paste. Using your fingertips or a clean makeup brush, spread the paste evenly over your clean face from forehead to chin. Leave it on for 15 minutes, then remove it with a warm, wet washcloth. Rinse with cool water, and gently pat your skin dry.

Distressed-Skin Toner

Whether you're dealing with breakouts, redness, or age-related skin discolorations, this **THYME** toner will leave your face clean and refreshed. Pour ½ cup of organic apple cider vinegar into a glass jar (a mason jar is perfect). Place the jar inside a larger bowl or a pot of very hot water to warm up the vinegar. Then add 3 tablespoons of dried thyme, and let it steep for about two hours. Strain the liquid into a clean bottle with a tight-fitting cap. Store it in the refrigerator for up to two weeks. To use, pour some onto a cotton pad, and apply to your clean face. Let it air-dry, and follow up with your usual moisturizer.

Back in the Day...

Here's a **THYME** and witch hazel toner that has been handed down through generations of women. This legacy recipe can be made in a flash and used after just a short wait to clear your skin of dirt and oil, leaving you aglow. Start with a small, clean jar that has a tight-fitting lid. Put 1 tablespoon of dried thyme into the jar, and pour 4 tablespoons of witch hazel over the thyme. Put the lid on the jar and shake it well. Within 20 minutes, the mixture should have a light brown color. This means the thyme is steeping, and you can go ahead and use the toner, or let it continue to steep overnight. When it's at the strength you want, strain it into a clean bottle with a tight-fitting cap and store the container in the refrigerator for up to one month. To use, pour some toner onto a cotton pad and apply it to your clean face. Let it air-dry, and follow up with your usual moisturizer.

Clay for Your Complexion

When you combine the cleaning, soothing effect of a **THYME** and witch hazel toner (see Back in the Day, at left) with the drying power of white cosmetic clay (available online), you've got yourself a powerful blemish buster. Simply combine 2 teaspoons of cosmetic clay with 2 teaspoons of the thyme toner in a small bowl and stir to mix well, adjusting the ingredients to make a paste. Dab the paste directly onto each blemish and leave it on for 20 minutes, or until it's dry. Remove it with a warm, wet washcloth, rinse with cool water, and pat dry. Then use a cotton ball to apply more thyme toner to your face and let it air-dry.

It's Thyme to Moisturize

Whether your skin is oily, dry, or somewhere in between, it still needs moisture to look its best. That's where this enriching **THYME** moisturizer comes into the picture. To make it, place 1 tablespoon of dried thyme in a small, clean jar with a tight-fitting lid. Pour in 3 tablespoons of argan, jojoba, or sesame oil, cover the jar, and shake it well. Let the mixture steep for two weeks in a cool, dark, dry place, and shake the jar daily. Then strain out the thyme and pour the oil into another clean jar or bottle with a tight-fitting cap. To use, pour a small amount on your fingertips and gently massage it over your clean face in small circles.

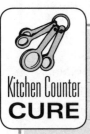

Kitchen Counter CURE

Fresh Thyme Mask

If you're looking for a facial mask to combat blemishes, but one that won't have harsh side effects, this **THYME** mask is just for you.

1 tbsp. of fresh thyme leaves
1 tbsp. of full-fat sour cream
1 tsp. of organic honey
½ tsp. of lemon juice

In a blender, combine all of the ingredients and blend until the thyme is in very small pieces. Apply the mask to your clean face and neck. Leave it on for 15 minutes. Remove it with a warm, wet washcloth, then rinse with cool water and gently pat your skin dry.

SPOTLIGHT ON
SPICING UP YOUR LOOKS

A sprinkle of spices and a handful of herbs are just what you need when you're looking for a better beauty routine. Add volume to your kisser, soothe your skin, and treat yourself to a relaxing bath, all with the help of these hardworking spice rack heroes:

◆ **Plump up your lips.** Simply apply olive oil or petroleum jelly to your lips, then gently pat a pinch of **CINNAMON** across them. You'll feel a tingle, but if the tingle becomes uncomfortable, rinse your lips immediately.

◆ **Clear your complexion.** Combine 2 tablespoons of plain yogurt, 2 tablespoons of uncooked rolled oats, and 1 teaspoon of ground **CLOVES**. Apply to your face and leave it on for 10 minutes. Remove it with a warm, wet washcloth, rinse with cool water, and pat dry.

◆ **Banish breakouts.** Combine 2 tablespoons of ground **NUTMEG**, 2 tablespoons of organic honey, and 2 teaspoons of whole milk. Stir until you have a smooth paste. Apply to your face in small circles, and leave it on for 15 minutes. Remove it with a warm, wet washcloth, rinse with cool water, and gently pat dry.

◆ **Tighten and tone your skin.** Bring 2 cups of water to a boil. Place ½ cup of chopped fresh **THYME** leaves and 1 tablespoon of dried green-tea leaves in a heat-proof bowl. Pour the boiling water over the leaves and let them steep until the water has completely cooled. Strain out the leaves and pour the remaining liquid into a clean jar or bottle with a tight-fitting lid and store it in the refrigerator. To use the toner, apply it to your clean face with a cotton ball and allow it to air-dry on your skin.

◆ **Relax and refresh.** Tie 1 cup of dried **THYME** sprigs in a piece of cheesecloth or old panty hose. Draw a bath, and as the tub fills, drop the thyme pouch into the water. Add 2 cups of whole milk to the water, and swish it around to mix. Leave the pouch in the water and settle in for a good, long, beauty-enhancing soak.

Positively Peppery Scrub

If you've never thought about using **BLACK PEPPER** in a skin treatment, you're in for a surprising treat. This pungent seasoning is loaded with antioxidants and has anti-inflammatory properties, which means it's just the ticket for getting your skin clean, refreshed, and glowing. This mask is a perfect introduction: Grind black peppercorns until you have $1/2$ teaspoon. Put the pepper in a small bowl and stir in 1 teaspoon of plain Greek yogurt. Mix well. Using your fingertips, apply the scrub to your face, massaging in small circles from forehead to chin. Rinse it off with lukewarm water, and gently pat your skin dry.

Tantalizing Toner

Skin that's prone to inflammation and blemishes is begging for a soothing toner like this one. In a small saucepan, boil $3/4$ cup of water. Add 1 tablespoon of whole **BLACK PEPPERCORNS** and 1 sprig of fresh rosemary, and continue boiling until half the water has evaporated. Remove the pan from the heat and let the liquid cool to room temperature. Strain it into a clean glass bottle with a tight-fitting cap, add 2 tablespoons of apple cider vinegar, and gently shake to mix. Store the bottle at room temperature. To use, apply the toner to your clean face with a cotton pad and allow your skin to air-dry.

BEAUTY
Bonus

PEPPER POTION FOR HAIR

Got dandruff? This potent **BLACK PEPPER** treatment will stimulate circulation in your scalp and help slough off all those telltale flakes. In a small bowl, combine $1/2$ cup of plain yogurt and 1 teaspoon of ground black pepper. Apply the mixture to your scalp, massaging it in, and leave it on for 30 minutes. Rinse it off with warm water, but don't shampoo. The best time to use this treatment is in the evening, then shampoo and condition your hair the next morning.

Conquer Cellulite

Besides revving up your circulation, **CAYENNE PEPPER** improves the efficiency of your lymphatic system, thereby allowing your body to eliminate toxins—including the ones that cause cellulite. Each time you consume cayenne pepper, you help the detox process along, but here's a specific remedy that has proven to be effective: Squeeze the juice of one lemon into a glass, and add a pinch of ground cayenne pepper. Fill the balance of the glass with cold water, stir, and drink up. (You'll want to gulp this spicy-sour concoction down quickly.) Perform this routine three times a day, and within 30 days or so, you should begin to notice a difference in your "cottage cheese" areas.

Halt Hair Thinning

Because **CAYENNE PEPPER** increases the blood flow to your scalp, it can help promote hair growth. So if you've got thinning hair, try this treatment: Mix 2 teaspoons of ground cayenne pepper with enough olive oil to make a thick paste. Massage it thoroughly into your dry scalp and hair, cover it with a shower cap, and leave it on for 10 minutes. Then remove the cap, and follow up with your usual shampoo and conditioner.

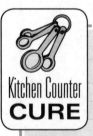

Kitchen Counter CURE

Vodka and Cayenne Hair Stimulant

Put the invigorating power of **CAYENNE PEPPER** to work stimulating blood flow to your balding scalp and encouraging hair growth.

¼ cup of vodka (plain, not the flavored kind)
3 tbsp. of ground cayenne pepper

Pour the vodka into a glass bottle with a tight-fitting cap. Add the cayenne pepper and shake the bottle to mix. Leave the bottle in a cool, dark place for a week. Then pour the liquid into a shatterproof bowl, add ½ cup of warm water, and stir. Bring it into the shower with you, and after shampooing your hair, pour the mixture over your head, massaging it into your scalp. Leave it on for five minutes, then rinse it out with warm water and condition as usual.

Improve Your Skin Tone

It's no surprise that **SALT** is the main ingredient in a lot of skin treatments. One reason is because it's a natural exfoliator—especially coarse sea salt granules, which remove dead skin cells, leaving your complexion soft and supple. Try this simple mixture and see for yourself: In a small bowl, combine 2 tablespoons of extra virgin olive oil and 2 tablespoons of sea salt. Using your fingertips, apply the combo to your face and neck, massaging in small circles. Remove it with a warm, wet washcloth, rinse with cool water, and gently pat your skin dry.

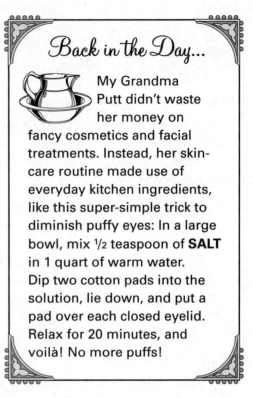

Back in the Day...

My Grandma Putt didn't waste her money on fancy cosmetics and facial treatments. Instead, her skin-care routine made use of everyday kitchen ingredients, like this super-simple trick to diminish puffy eyes: In a large bowl, mix ½ teaspoon of **SALT** in 1 quart of warm water. Dip two cotton pads into the solution, lie down, and put a pad over each closed eyelid. Relax for 20 minutes, and voilà! No more puffs!

Salty Shrinker

Here's a mask that will tighten up enlarged pores and improve the elasticity of your skin. Mix equal parts of buttermilk and sea **SALT** to form a paste. Using your fingertips, apply it to your face, massaging in small circles from forehead to chin. Leave it on for five minutes, then remove it with a warm, wet washcloth. Rinse with cool water, and gently pat your skin dry.

Salt of the Sea Toner

Sea **SALT** naturally absorbs impurities from your skin, which makes it an ideal toner for oily or problem-prone complexions. Mix 1 teaspoon of sea salt per ¼ cup of warm water in a bottle that has a tight-fitting cap. Give it a shake and let it sit overnight so the salt can dissolve completely. Then dampen a cotton pad with the brine, and smooth it over your freshly washed face. Or you can make the mixture in a spray bottle and mist your face with it, then allow your skin to air-dry. Whichever method you use, follow up with your usual moisturizer.

Spice Rack Radiance

SPOTLIGHT ON
BEAUTIFUL HAIR

From dull, limp locks to itchy, flaky dandruff, your hair can suffer from many indignities brought about by heat, humidity, and even air pollution. Here are some easy hair treatments that use spice rack ingredients to bring back the luster, shine, and manageability you've been looking for:

◆ **Hot-oil treatment.** In a clean jar or bottle with a tight-fitting cap, combine ½ cup of extra virgin olive oil, 1 tablespoon of ground **BLACK PEPPER**, and 3 drops of tree tea oil. Shake to mix, and leave the container in a cool, dark place for a week. When you're ready to use the treatment, warm it up by placing the jar or bottle in a pan of very hot water, then pour the oil over your dry hair and comb it through from roots to ends. Cover with a shower cap, and leave it on for 30 minutes. Then shampoo it out and follow up with your usual conditioner.

◆ **Scalp tingler.** Pour one bottle of beer (use the cheapest brand) into a shatterproof bowl. Stir in 2 tablespoons of ground **CAYENNE PEPPER**, cover the bowl tightly with plastic wrap, and let it sit at room temperature away from sunlight for an hour. When you're ready to wash your hair, bring the bowl with you. Pour the mixture over your dry hair, being careful to avoid your eyes, and leave it on for 15 minutes before shampooing it out. Follow up with your usual conditioner.

◆ **Limp-hair lifter.** Fill an 8-ounce spray bottle about a third of the way with sea **SALT**. Add ⅓ teaspoon of lemon juice and 3 drops of lavender oil. Fill the balance of the bottle with warm water, and shake until the salt is dissolved. Spray the mixture lightly onto your wet hair, and then blow-dry and style it as usual, or let your hair air-dry.

◆ **Super scalp scrub.** For dandruff-prone hair and/or an itchy scalp, take a handful of sea **SALT** and massage the granules into your dry scalp for two minutes. Then shampoo and condition as usual.

CHAPTER 10

Bouquets of Beauty

Floating rose petals in a bath is nothing new, but how about mixing fresh herbs for a facial? Or using tomatoes in a skin toner? Or reviving damaged hair with chives? The truth is, you can create dozens of beauty treatments from the herbs on your windowsill and the plants in your kitchen garden. So read on to put your green thumb to good use and grow some beautiful additions to your skin-care repertoire.

ON THE WINDOWSILL

Basic Basil Toner

Put the potent powers of **BASIL** to work for you with this gentle facial toner: Start by boiling 1 cup of water in a saucepan. Add 3 tablespoons of crushed fresh basil leaves (or 3 teaspoons of dried, crushed leaves). Boil for five minutes. Place a lid on the pan and remove it from the heat. Let it steep until it cools to room temperature. Strain out the leaves, setting them aside. Pour the water into a bottle with a tight-fitting cap. Add 1 teaspoon of witch hazel and shake the bottle to mix. Store in the refrigerator, where it will keep for up to one week. To use, pour some toner onto a cotton pad and wipe it across your freshly washed face, allowing it to air-dry on your skin.

Foil Fine Lines

Get ready to look years younger! Place the leftover **BASIL** leaves described in "Basic Basil Toner" (see page 349) in a small bowl. Add 4 tablespoons of plain yogurt and stir to make a paste. Apply it to your face, leave it on for 10 minutes, then remove the paste with a warm, wet washcloth. Rinse your face with cool water, and gently pat dry.

Wake Up Your Face

For a refreshing way to start your day, pour the Basic **BASIL** Toner (see page 349) into an ice cube tray and freeze it. In the morning, pop out a toner cube and rub it all over your face and neck to clean and refresh your skin, plus minimize the look of enlarged pores.

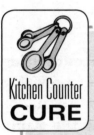

Kitchen Counter CURE

Basil Beauty Bonanza

Your **BASIL** bounty can leave you with a smooth, youthful complexion. Once you whip up the basic basil paste, you have the basis for a face wash, mask, and toner.

> **20–30 fresh basil leaves**
> **Organic plain yogurt**
> **Distilled water**

In a bowl, crush the fresh basil leaves so that the natural oils are released. This basil paste can be used in three wonderful ways:

- **Face wash.** Mix a few drops of the distilled water into the paste, and apply it to your face in small circles from forehead to chin. Leave it on for five minutes, then remove it with a warm, wet washcloth.
- **Mask.** Mix 1 teaspoon of the yogurt into the basil paste and stir. Apply the paste evenly to your face and leave it on for 20 minutes. Rinse it off with lukewarm water, followed by cool water, then gently dry.
- **Toner.** Crush the fresh leaves as described above, then add 2 cups of boiling water to the bowl. Allow the mixture to steep for 15 minutes, then strain it over a bowl to separate the leaves from the liquid. Store the basil water in a bottle or jar with a tight-fitting lid. Use morning and evening by pouring some onto a cotton pad, wiping it across your just-washed face, and allowing your skin to air-dry. Store the toner for up to one week in the refrigerator.

Brighten Your Eyes

When a night on the town (or seasonal allergies) leaves your eyes bleary and puffy, treat your peepers to **CATNIP**. Just bring 3 cups of water to a boil in a saucepan, and add 2 tablespoons of fresh catnip leaves. Reduce the heat to low, and simmer for three minutes (no more!). Remove the pan from the burner, and let the brew steep for another 50 minutes. Then strain out the solids, pour the liquid into a clean glass jar with a tight-fitting lid, and store it in the refrigerator. When the need arises, soak a washcloth in the solution, lie back, and put it over your eyes for half an hour—then face the world bright-eyed and bushy-tailed!

(Cat) Nip and Tuck

Don't go under the knife to rid your face of fine lines and wrinkles. Instead, pluck some **CATNIP** from your windowsill plant and put this herb's antioxidant and anti-aging properties to work on your skin. Here's the easy treatment: Put 2 tablespoons of fresh catnip leaves (or 1 tablespoon of dried leaves) in a small heat-proof bowl. Pour 1 cup of boiling water over the leaves and let steep until the water is completely cool. Strain out the leaves and pour the liquid into a glass bottle or jar with a tight-fitting cap. Store it in the refrigerator for up to one week. To use, pour some of the liquid onto a cotton ball, and apply it to your face and neck, allowing it to air-dry on your skin.

Back in the Day...

Here's an old-time treatment that my Grandma Putt used weekly to condition her hair. It can also serve as a daily rinse to keep your locks looking their best. Put ¼ cup of fresh **CATNIP** leaves (or 2 tablespoons of dried leaves) in a heat-proof bowl, and pour 2 cups of boiling water over them. Let steep overnight. Then strain out the leaves and pour the liquid into a spray bottle or a jar with a tight-fitting cap. Store in the refrigerator for up to one week. Here are two ways to apply this right after washing your hair:

• Pour the solution over your freshly washed hair, work it through from roots to tips, put on a shower cap, and leave it for 30 minutes. When the time is up, no need to rinse. Simply dry and style.

• Spray your hair from roots to tips with the rinse, comb it through, and then dry and style your hair as usual.

On the Windowsill

Beauty

Awesome Oregano Toner

You love it on your pizza and in your tomato sauce, so I know you'll love **OREGANO** on your face, too! To use it in this terrific toner that refreshes and tightens pores, start by putting ¼ cup of fresh oregano leaves (or 2 tablespoons of dried leaves) in a heat-proof bowl. Pour 3 cups of boiling water over them, and let steep until cool. Then strain out the leaves and pour the remaining liquid into a glass jar with a tight-fitting lid. Store the toner in the refrigerator for up to one week. To use, pour some onto a cotton ball and apply all over your clean face.

No-Frills Face Mask

Soothe and smooth your skin and make it glow with this oh-so-gentle **OREGANO** and aloe face mask. In a small saucepan, bring ½ cup of water just to a boil. Remove from the heat and immediately stir in 2 tablespoons of fresh oregano leaves or 2 teaspoons of dried leaves. Let steep for 10 minutes. Meanwhile, split one aloe vera leaf in half and squeeze the gel into a heat-proof bowl. Strain out the oregano leaves from the tea, and pour the remaining liquid into the bowl with the aloe vera gel. Stir to make a sticky paste. Using your fingertips, massage the paste in small circles from your forehead to your chin. Leave the mask on for 15 minutes, then remove it with a warm, wet washcloth. Rinse with cool water, and gently pat your skin dry.

BEAUTY
Bonus

HERBAL HAIR DETANGLER

This leave-in **OREGANO** hair treatment will make your tresses smooth as silk. Put ¼ cup of fresh oregano leaves (or 2 tablespoons of dried leaves) in a heat-proof bowl. Boil 1 cup of water and pour it over the leaves. Let steep until the tea is completely cool. Strain out the leaves, pour the remaining liquid into a spray bottle, and store it in the refrigerator for up to one week. After shampooing and conditioning your hair, towel-dry your tresses, then spray the detangler all over your hair and comb it through. Dry and style your hair as usual.

Perfect Parsley Toner

If you're tired of spending your hard-earned money on expensive cosmetics, but you don't have time for elaborate DIY routines, give this ultra-simple toner a try. Just put $1/2$ cup of chopped fresh **PARSLEY** in a heat-proof bowl, and cover it with 1 cup of boiling water. When it's cooled to room temperature, strain the liquid into a glass jar that has a tight-fitting lid. Store it in the refrigerator, where it will keep for about two weeks. Then every morning and evening, pour some onto a cotton pad and sweep it over your freshly washed face. Let your skin air-dry.

Rejuvenating Facial Mask

Exfoliating skin treatments are designed to slough off dead skin cells—leaving you with a smoother, more radiant complexion. This one does the job like a champ. To make it, puree $2/3$ cup of fresh pineapple chunks (at room temperature) in a blender or food processor. Pour in $1/4$ cup of extra virgin olive oil, and blend until the mixture is almost paste-like. Finally, add $1/4$ cup of chopped fresh **PARSLEY**, and pulse a few seconds at a time, making sure the mask doesn't liquefy. Spread the mixture onto your face and neck, and leave it on for 15 minutes. Rinse it off with lukewarm water, and follow up with your usual moisturizer.

On the Windowsill

HOW'S THAT?

Q *Jerry, my hair is starting to get a little sparse. I can't afford those fancy drugstore hair restorers, so do you know of something more natural (and way cheaper) that I can try?*

A I sure do, and the answer is **PARSLEY**! It stimulates the blood circulation in your scalp, which can lead to the growth of strong, healthy hair. Here's my recipe for a great get-up-and-grow tonic: Puree a big handful of fresh parsley sprigs with 2 tablespoons of water in a blender or food processor. Massage the mixture into your wet scalp, wrap a towel around your head, and go about your business for about an hour. Then shampoo as usual, and follow up with a conditioner. Repeat every week or so until your head is a growth industry again.

BEAUTY
Bonus

ROSEMARY RINSE

ROSEMARY restores the bounce and shine to stressed tresses. In a heat-proof bowl, steep ¼ cup of fresh rosemary sprigs in 3 cups of boiling water for an hour. Strain out the solids and pour the remaining liquid into a spray bottle. After shampooing and conditioning your hair, towel-dry it, then spray it from roots to tips with the rinse. Leave it on your hair for 30 minutes, then rinse it out with lukewarm water.

Savory Steam Treatment

A steam facial opens up your pores, preparing it for any treatment that follows. Pick a handful each of fresh **ROSEMARY**, basil, and mint from your windowsill plants and kitchen garden. Place the herbs in a large pot, and pour in enough water (about 7 cups) to completely cover them. Bring the water to a boil and simmer for 25 minutes. Turn off the heat and let the mixture steep for 15 minutes. Strain out and save the solids. Pour the remaining liquid into a large bowl, bend over it, cover your head and the bowl with a towel, and allow the steam to bathe your face until the water cools.

Perfectly Pretty Paste

Put the leftover herbal solids from "Savory Steam Treatment" (above) in a bowl. Add 3 tablespoons of **ROSEMARY** leaves and a teaspoon of water. Use a handheld blender to make a paste, adding more water as needed to make one of these facial treatments:

- For a refreshing facial, massage the paste onto your face and neck in small circles. Wait five minutes, then remove it with a warm, wet washcloth, rinse with cool water, and gently pat your skin dry.

- For a blemish-blasting mask, mix the paste with one raw egg yolk, 1 teaspoon of honey, and 1 teaspoon of turmeric. Apply the mask evenly to your face. Allow it to dry completely, then remove it with a warm, wet washcloth, rinse with cool water, and gently pat your skin dry.

- For an anti-aging facial scrub, mix the paste with four crushed uncoated aspirin tablets. Massage the scrub onto your damp face, then rinse it off with lukewarm water, and gently pat dry.

Sage Skin Solution

Harvest **SAGE** from your windowsill plant and you'll push back the hands of time. Put ¼ cup of fresh sage leaves in a heat-proof bowl, and pour 3 cups of boiling water over the leaves. Let steep for 30 minutes, then strain out the solids and pour the remaining liquid into a glass bottle with a tight-fitting lid. Store it in the refrigerator for one week. Use a cotton ball to wipe the toner across your clean face and neck, letting it air-dry on your skin.

Go, Gray, Go!

Are you looking for a way to conceal the silver strands in your hair? Then give this all-natural treatment a try: Bring 2 cups of water to a boil, and toss in a handful each of fresh or dried **SAGE** and rosemary. Reduce the heat, and let the mixture simmer for 30 minutes. Remove it from the stove and let it steep overnight. The next day, strain out the herbs, massage the remaining liquid into your dry hair, and let it air-dry. Then shampoo, condition, and style as usual. Repeat the procedure every three to five days, and before long, the gray will be a lot less noticeable.

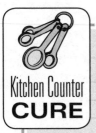

Kitchen Counter CURE

Sage Super Soak

This bath blend will calm nerves, increase mental alertness, and stimulate senses. Plus, it'll soften your skin and relieve any irritation caused by weather, insect bites, or allergies.

¼ cup of dried rosemary, crumbled
¼ cup of dried SAGE, crumbled
2 tbsp. of dried parsley
2 tbsp. of sea salt
2 tbsp. of uncooked rolled oats

Grind all of the ingredients in a blender to make a coarse powder. Put ¼ cup of the blend in a cheesecloth bag, and tie the top securely. Toss the pouch into the tub as you run hot water into it. Then step in, lean back, and relax. Squeeze the bag occasionally to release more of the potent essences into the water. *Note: Store leftover powder, either loose or in individual pouches, in a lidded container away from heat and light.*

FROM THE KITCHEN GARDEN

Calendula Cleanser

Baby your skin with a calming cleanser. Put 1/4 cup of fresh **CALENDULA** flowers in a heat-proof bowl, and add 1 cup of boiling water. Let steep for 15 minutes, then strain out the solids. Allow the remaining liquid to cool, then stir in 1 tablespoon of dry milk. Using a cotton ball, apply the cleanser all over your face, then rinse with lukewarm water. Cover and refrigerate any unused mixture, and discard it after 48 hours.

Scrub for Sensitive Skin

Some facial scrubs can be too harsh and irritating. But not this gentle blend: Grind 1 cup of uncooked rolled oats, 1/3 cup of cornmeal, and 1/3 cup of dried **CALENDULA** into a fine powder. Store the mixture in a tightly sealed container in a cool, dry location for up to one month. To use, scoop out some of the powder and add enough warm water to make a paste. Gently massage the scrub onto your face, then rinse and gently pat dry.

Calendula Conditioning Rinse

This recipe needs to "marinate," but it's worth the wait! Pour 1 quart of high-quality vinegar into a jar with a tight-fitting lid. Add 1 cup of dried **CALENDULA**, put on the lid, and let it sit for two weeks. Then strain out the solids and pour the liquid into a spray bottle. After washing your hair, spray the rinse all over your head and comb it through from roots to tips. Keep it in the fridge and use the rinse within a month.

HOW'S THAT?

Q *My son's feet stink! Do you have any recipes for fighting foot odor with natural ingredients?*

A Yep, and it's as easy as 1, 2, 3. Finely chop **CALENDULA** flowers until you have 1/4 cup, and put them in a small bowl. Stir in 1/4 cup of arrowroot powder (available online). Tell your son to rub the combo onto his feet, especially between his toes.

Look Lively with Chives

Or, I should say, look lovely with **CHIVES**. Here's how: In a medium saucepan, bring 2 cups of water to a boil. Add a handful of fresh chives and simmer for 30 seconds. Using tongs, remove the chives from the boiling water and plunge them into a bowl of ice water. Leave them for two minutes, then remove them to paper towels and gently squeeze out the water. Put the chives in a blender, add 1/2 cup of extra virgin olive oil, and puree for two minutes. Using a clean makeup brush, apply the chive puree evenly to your face. Wait 30 minutes, then remove it with a warm, wet washcloth.

Pamper Your Hair

Follow the recipe for making **CHIVE** puree, above, to make a rich hair mask. Work it into your hair from roots to tips. Cover with a shower cap and leave it on for one hour. Then shampoo and condition your hair as usual.

Fight Foul Flakes

Versatile **CHIVES** contain volatile compounds that spell defeat for dandruff. Put 1 tablespoon of chopped fresh chives in a small bowl, and add 1 cup of just-boiled water. Cover the bowl, and let the mixture steep for 20 minutes or so. Shampoo your hair as usual, and rinse with the chive tea. Repeat this routine daily, and after a few weeks, you'll find that your white flakes have flown the coop.

Back in the Day...

As a boy, one of my jobs was to pick the **CHIVE** blossoms. Once I'd gathered a bowlful, Grandma Putt got to work on this beauty blend: Put 1 cup of fresh chive blossoms in a large heat-proof bowl. Add 3 cups of boiling water and steep for 30 minutes. Strain out the flowers and put them in a jar with a tight-fitting lid. Pour the remaining liquid into a bottle with a tight-fitting cap. Store both in the refrigerator for up to two weeks. To use the flowers, scoop some out and mash them to make a paste. Apply it to your face in small circles, remove it with a warm, wet washcloth, and dry. Use the liquid as a facial toner on your cleansed skin, and as a hair rinse after shampooing.

From the Kitchen Garden

Love Your Looks with Lavender

Besides smelling absolutely divine, **LAVENDER** is a wonderful addition to your beauty repertoire. Use it in this fragrant toner that will firm your skin and give you a nice healthy glow. Put 1/4 cup of fresh lavender buds in a bowl, and pour 1 cup of boiling water over them. Let steep for several hours, then strain out the solids and pour the remaining liquid into a bottle with a tight-fitting cap. Store it in the refrigerator for up to two weeks. To use the toner, pour some onto a cotton ball and wipe it all over your clean face.

Luxuriate in Lavender

Make your own **LAVENDER** oil and use it to soothe dry skin or to have a relaxing bath. Here's the how-to: Place several freshly cut lavender flowers, stems, and leaves on a large, flat surface, and bruise them with a wooden mallet by gently pounding on them. Place the bruised floral pieces in a quart-size mason jar, and pour in enough almond or jojoba oil (available online) to cover them completely. Put the lid on the jar and let it sit away from heat and light for 48 hours. Strain out the lavender, replace with newly bruised fresh pieces, and again let it sit for 48 hours. Strain out the floral pieces and store the remaining oil in a dark glass jar away from heat and light. Then use it to:

- **Soothe dry skin.** Rub lavender oil on dry arms, legs, and hands. This is especially good to do at bedtime because the soothing lavender aroma will ease you into sleep.

- **Have a relaxing bath.** In a large bowl, mix together 1 cup of Epsom salts, 1/2 cup of sea salt, 3 tablespoons of baking soda, and 10 drops of lavender oil. Mix well and store in a sealed jar. To use, pour 1/3 cup under running bathwater and enjoy your fragrant soak.

BEAUTY
Bonus

AROMATIC HAIR HELPER

Infuse your hair with fragrance and shine with this super-simple **LAVENDER** rinse. Put 1/4 cup of dried lavender in a heat-proof bowl, and pour 2 cups of boiling water over it. Let steep for one hour. Strain out the solids, and use the remaining liquid as a final rinse over your shampooed hair. Leave it on for 15 minutes, then dry and style.

Purifying Scrub

Buff away dead skin cells with this **MINT** scrub. Using a coffee grinder, crush dry mint leaves until you have 2 tablespoons. Put it into a bowl, and add 1 tablespoon each of honey and whole milk. Stir to make a paste. Apply the scrub to your face, massaging in small circles from forehead to chin. Remove with a wet washcloth, rinse, and gently pat dry.

Destroy Dark Circles

Dark under-eye circles make you look years older, and who needs that? Regain your youthful appearance with this **MINT** treatment. In a blender, puree a handful of fresh mint leaves and 3 tablespoons of water. Scoop the puree into a small bowl and stir in 4 tablespoons of rose water (available online, or make your own following the recipe on page 360). Refrigerate the mixture for at least one hour. Then dip two cotton balls into it and place them over your closed eyes for 15 minutes a day.

Remarkable Mint Rinse

Is your scalp irritated? Well, this remarkable rinse can stop the itch. Just steep 2 tablespoons each of chopped fresh **MINT** and chopped fresh parsley in 8 ounces of just-boiled water for 10 minutes. Strain out the herbs and pour the liquid into a plastic bottle. After shampooing, rinse your hair with the mixture, and then use your favorite conditioner. Follow this procedure twice a week to keep your scalp healthy.

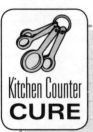

Kitchen Counter CURE

Soothing Foot Soak

Stimulate the circulation in your feet, fight fungus, and deodorize your toes—all at the same time—with this mighty **MINT** footbath. Start by putting ½ cup of fresh mint leaves in a large heat-proof bowl. Pour 3 cups of boiling water over the leaves and let steep for 30 minutes. Then pour the liquid and solids into a foot basin, and add ½ cup of apple cider vinegar. Drop in a handful of marbles and wait for them to settle on the bottom. Then sit down and soak your feet, rolling them back and forth over the marbles to relax your tired, aching dogs.

From the Kitchen Garden

Stop and Smell the Roses

This fragrant facial steam treatment opens clogged pores and stimulates blood circulation. But it also preps your skin for deep cleansing and toning. The simple process: Bring 7 cups of water to a boil in a large pot. Remove it from the heat and stir in 1 cup of dried **ROSE** petals. Let it steep for 15 minutes, then lean over, carefully drape a towel over your head and the pot, and allow the steam to bathe your face until the water cools.

Scented Splash

The keys to maintaining healthy, young-looking skin are to drink plenty of water and to use a mildly astringent splash like this one to help hydrate your skin and keep it supple. Put 1 cup of fresh **ROSE** petals in a clean glass jar, and pour in 4 cups of white-wine vinegar that's been heated to near boiling. Cover the jar with a lid or plastic wrap, and leave it in a dark place at room temperature for 10 days, occasionally shaking the jar. Then strain the liquid into a fresh jar and add 1 cup of rose water (see the recipe in Back in the Day, above). To use, mix 1 tablespoon of the rose potion in ½ cup of lukewarm water, and splash it onto your clean face. You can let it air-dry on your skin, or gently pat dry. Store the potion in the refrigerator for up to two weeks.

Back in the Day...

Back in Grandma Putt's day, rose water was a staple in every woman's beauty-care kit, and for good reason: It can purify and tone any type of skin, heal blemishes, hydrate dry skin, reduce redness and swelling, and much more. Of course, you can buy rose water in health-food stores and online these days, but it's easy as pie to make your own. Just put 1 cup of fresh **ROSE** petals into a heat-proof bowl, and pour in just enough boiling distilled water to cover them (about 2 cups). Cover the bowl, let the petals steep for 30 to 60 minutes, and strain the liquid into a bottle or jar with a tight-fitting lid. Store your rose water in the refrigerator, where it will keep for up to 10 days.

Everything's Just Rosy...

Especially when you use your homemade **ROSE** water (see Back in the Day, at left). Here are a few ideas to get you started:

- Splash it on your face after cleansing.

- Spray it on all over to cool and refresh your whole body.

- Dab it onto your legs and underarms to soothe freshly shaved skin.

- Add 1 cup to your bathwater for a softening, scented soak.

Super-Softening Body Oil

ROSES and almond oil soften skin and reduce irritation. So put them on your beauty team with this easy formula: Place 1 cup of fresh rose petals in a jar with a tight-fitting lid, crush them with a wooden spoon, and pour in 1 cup of almond oil. Cover and let the mixture sit for a week in a cool, dark place, then strain the oil into a clean bottle. Massage it into your damp skin after you shower. You'll feel—and smell—fabulous!

Anti-Acne Duo

What do you get when you combine the skin-healing power of **ROSES** with the circulation-boosting ability of mint? A fast way to dry up pimples, that's what! Grind enough fresh mint leaves with a mortar and pestle to equal about 2 tablespoons, then stir in 1/4 cup of rose water and mix well. Using your fingertips, dab a generous amount of the mixture onto each individual spot and let it air-dry on your skin. Do this twice a day after washing your face, and your pimples will soon be history.

BEAUTY Bonus

THE SCENT OF SUMMER!

Enjoy the heady scent of your summer bloomers all year round by making your own **ROSE** perfume. Simply pack a mason jar with as many fresh rose petals as it will hold. Then fill the jar with glycerin. Put the jar in a cool, dark place and let it sit for three weeks. Then strain the liquid into a clean bottle with a tight-fitting cap. Dab it on, and enjoy your signature scent.

From the Kitchen Garden

A Tomato Tone-Up

Here's an easy way to tone oily skin: Mash a medium-size **TOMATO** and spread the mush onto your face. Wait about 30 minutes, then rinse with lukewarm water, splash with cool water, and gently pat your skin dry. *Note: Tomatoes are mildly acidic, so if your skin is sensitive, use yellow tomatoes, which are lower in acid.*

Let's Get Glowing

This super scrub will leave you radiant. Cut one ripe **TOMATO** into quarters and push the pieces through a sieve over a small bowl to separate the solids from the juice. Discard the solids. Add 1 teaspoon of ground oats (grind uncooked rolled oats in a coffee grinder or food processor), 1 teaspoon of plain yogurt, and ¹/₂ teaspoon of honey to the liquid and stir well to combine. Using your fingertips, apply the scrub to your face, and leave it on for 30 minutes, or until completely dry. Remove it with a warm, wet washcloth, rinse with cool water, and gently pat dry.

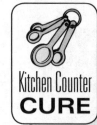

Kitchen Counter CURE

Terrific Tomato Hair Treatment

TOMATOES help balance the pH levels in your hair, making your locks more manageable. To perform this balancing act, just mix 1 teaspoon of cornstarch with 1 cup of tomato juice, and comb the solution through your clean, wet hair. Leave it on for about 10 minutes, and rinse well. Then dry and style your hair as usual.

Tomato Face Mask

Improve the texture of your skin with this purifying mask. Cut one large, ripe **TOMATO** into quarters. Bring 4 cups of water to a boil in a saucepan. Drop the tomato quarters into the boiling water and boil for just one minute, no longer! Remove the tomatoes from the water (with a slotted spoon) onto a plate and let them cool a bit. Carefully peel off the skins and use a teaspoon to scoop out the seeds. Put the remaining pulp into a bowl and smash it with a wooden spoon. Stir in 1 teaspoon of slightly warm honey and mix well. Using a clean makeup brush, apply the mask to your clean face. Leave it on for 30 minutes, then remove it with a warm, wet washcloth. Rinse your face with cool water, and gently pat your skin dry.

Index

Index

Index

Index